Medical Treatment of Glaucoma

Xinghuai Sun • Yi Dai
Editors

Medical Treatment of Glaucoma

Springer

Editors
Xinghuai Sun
Eye & ENT Hospital
Shanghai Medical College of Fudan University
Shanghai
China

Yi Dai
Eye & ENT Hospital
Shanghai Medical College of Fudan University
Shanghai
China

ISBN 978-981-13-2732-2 ISBN 978-981-13-2733-9 (eBook)
https://doi.org/10.1007/978-981-13-2733-9

This Springer imprint is published by the registered company Springer Nature Singapore Pte Ltd.
The registered company address is: 152 Beach Road, #21-01/04 Gateway East, Singapore 189721, Singapore

Preface

The management of glaucoma has been considerably improved in the last three decades. On the basis of deeper understanding about the cellular, molecular, and genetic levels associated ocular changes, a large number of medications have been developed for the treatment of glaucoma. A number of potential new agents and new methods addressing the underlying pathophysiology of the disease are promising and may develop new therapeutic targets for the treatment of glaucoma in the future.

All chapters in this book are contributed by experts in the medical therapy and basic research of glaucoma around the world. With the great appreciation for chapter authors' hard work, it is our sincere hope that this book will provide a comprehensive introduction to various aspects of medications in glaucoma and generate a deep re-understanding on medical treatment of glaucoma in practice. We are looking forward to hearing from the readers, whose critical comments will be much appreciated.

Shanghai, China — Xinghuai Sun
Shanghai, China — Yi Dai

Contents

Glaucoma Related Ocular Structure and Function

1

Dao-Yi Yu, Stephen J. Cringle, and William H. Morgan

Abstract

Glaucoma is an aetiologically complex disorder of optic neuropathies. Stressors related to age and intraocular pressure lead to progressive degeneration of the retinal ganglion cells. Clinically ophthalmic testing has been used to identify and quantify the functional and/or structural defects for diagnosis, assessing progression and therapeutic outcomes of glaucoma.

There are multiple ocular structures, which could involve the causes and consequences of glaucoma at the cellular, molecular and genetic levels associated with functional changes. In this chapter, we would like to describe some ocular structures and functions highly relevant to glaucoma.

No doubt, knowledge and information of retinal ganglion cells are critical for understanding glaucoma. The retinal ganglion cells are specialized projection neurons actively receiving visual signal through their dendrites and transmitting integrated visual information from the retina to the brain. Each subcellular component of the retinal ganglion cell is remarkably different in terms of structure, function and extracellular environment. Simplifying the retinal ganglion cells into a series of compartments, rather than attempting to understand it as a single, homogeneous structure, could be more useful for understanding pathogenic processes involved in optic neuropathies.

To understand the mechanisms of maintaining normal intraocular pressure and pathogenesis of elevated intraocular pressure, the only treatable risk factor, we need to understand aqueous humour formation, aqueous fluid dynamics and outflow pathways. This knowledge and information are fundamentally important for understanding the pathogenesis of glaucoma, particularly primary open angle glaucoma, and therapeutic interventions. The epithelium of the ciliary body, posterior surface of the iris and the lens play a role in aqueous humour production and/or barrier function. Endothelial cells line the inner surface of the cornea, trabecular meshwork, Schlemm's canal, the collector channels and aqueous vein plexus, and the aqueous vein. This chapter provides updated information about the structure and function of the endothelium and epithelium.

D.-Y. Yu (✉) · S. J. Cringle · W. H. Morgan
Centre for Ophthalmology and Visual Science, The University of Western Australia, Nedlands, WA, Australia

Lions Eye Institute, The University of Western Australia, Nedlands, WA, Australia
e-mail: dyyu@lei.org.au

X. Sun, Y. Dai (eds.), *Medical Treatment of Glaucoma*,
https://doi.org/10.1007/978-981-13-2733-9_1

Keywords
Glaucoma · Optic nerve head · Retinal ganglion cells · Trabecular meshwork Aqueous humour

1.1 Introduction

Glaucoma covers a group of complex optic neuropathies characterized by a progressive loss of retinal ganglion cells (RGCs) and their axons, and associated alterations in the retinal nerve fibre layer (RNFL) and optic nerve head (ONH) with a concomitant loss of the visual field [1–3]. Although the exact pathogenesis of glaucoma is not understood, elevation of intraocular pressure (IOP) is the only treatable risk factor [4].

In this chapter, we attempt to describe some major ocular structures and functions, which are highly related with glaucoma. We focus on two major issues relevant to the loss of retinal ganglion cells (RGCs) and elevated intraocular pressure (IOP).

Firstly, we would like to describe the aqueous humour fluid dynamics and key cells involved. Two critical cell types, the epithelium and the endothelium play important roles in aqueous humour circulation. To understand the mechanisms of maintaining normal intraocular pressure (IOP) and pathogenesis of elevated IOP, we need to better understand aqueous humour formation, aqueous fluid dynamics and outflow pathways. Aqueous humour is produced by the ciliary epithelium. There are abundant publications, which provide detailed information about aqueous formation. In this chapter, we would like to describe the endothelium and its role in aqueous humour circulation and the outflow pathway in detail.

Secondly, the RGCs are one of the most critical cells for understanding glaucoma. Each RGC has different subcellular components. They have different structure, function and extracellular environment. Enhanced knowledge of the RGCs will help us to better understand the glaucomatous insults. The pathogenesis of glaucomatous optic neuropathy is enigmatic and has long been debated. We would prefer to describe RGCs as having different subcellular components. The ONH is a unique region where approximately 1.2 million axons from the RGCs converge to exit the globe. This region has a high metabolic demand as reflected by the regional confinement of cytochrome oxidase enzyme and the presence of a dense capillary network. The efficient supply of nutrients and oxygen and the efficient removal of waste from the retina and ONH are therefore crucial for the survival and function of the axons.

We hope that this information and knowledge could be beneficial for understanding the pathogenesis of glaucoma, particularly primary open angle glaucoma and therapeutic interventions. Some of the statements and concepts discussed in this chapter may not be universally accepted, but they do need addressing and some serious consideration.

1.2 Fluid Dynamics of Aqueous Humour

To maintain normal IOP, proper globe shape and optical properties, aqueous humour must keep a dynamic stability in its production and outflow. Aqueous humour circulation supplies nutrients, such as oxygen and glucose to the avascular anterior tissues, cornea and lens.

Figure 1.1 shows a histological section of the primate anterior segment. The aqueous humour is produced by the ciliary epithelium. It enters the posterior chamber and then flows around the lens and through the pupil into the anterior chamber where it drains via trabecular outflow and uveoscleral outflow.

Interestingly, aqueous humour in the posterior chamber is surrounded by the epithelium of the ciliary body, lens and posterior surface of the iris while in the anterior chamber and outflow pathway including the trabecular meshwork, Schlemm's canal, collector channels, and aqueous vein plexus and veins, it is surrounded by endothelium. In addition, unlike the posterior surface of the cornea, which has a continuous endothelium lining, there is no intact

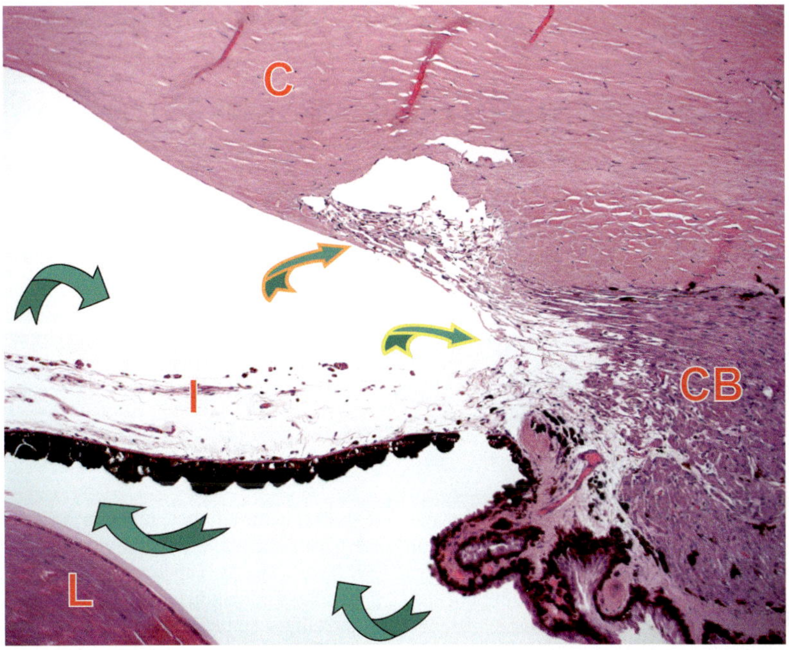

Fig. 1.1 Normal aqueous flow pathways. Histological section of a monkey anterior chamber angle. Arrows illustrate aqueous flow pathways. Aqueous humour is secreted by the ciliary epithelium of the ciliary body (CB) into the posterior chamber between the capsule of the lens (L) and the posterior surface of the iris (I) and circulated through the pupil towards the anterior chamber angle and drains via trabecular outflow (green arrow with orange edge) and uveoscleral outflow (green arrow with yellow edge). Aqueous humour nourishes the avascular lens and cornea (C)

endothelium barrier on the anterior iris surface and ciliary body in the angle (Fig. 1.1).

1.2.1 Aqueous Humour Formation and Flow

Aqueous humour is produced by the ciliary epithelium of the ciliary processes and flows into the anterior chamber through the pupil and into the vitreous cavity and across the retinal pigment epithelium [5, 6].

1.2.1.1 Aqueous Humour Formation

The aqueous fills the anterior chamber, maintains the IOP, and nourishes the avascular cornea and lens and removes the waste from these tissues. Aqueous humour circulates around the anterior chamber and eventually drains into the anterior chamber angle. There is exchange of fluid with the lens and cornea and iris vasculature. In humans, a circadian rhythm of aqueous flow has been reported, with more flow during the day than at night.

The ciliary epithelium consists of two polarized neuroepithelial cell layers, pigmented and non-pigmented. They are opposed each other by their respective apical plasma membranes (Fig. 1.2).

The ciliary epithelium is located between the root of the iris and the beginning of the retina. The pigmented epithelial cell layer of the ciliary body continues with the retinal pigment epithelium, and the non-pigmented epithelium cell layer extends to the neuronal retina.

It is important to understand the cell junctions of the ciliary epithelium. There are multiple isoform-specific gap junctions (connexin proteins) in both cell layers in the ciliary epithelium [7]. These gap junctions establish cell-to-cell communication between the ciliary epithelial cells allowing the intercellular transfer of ions to rapidly respond to stimuli, and in a co-ordinated fashion.

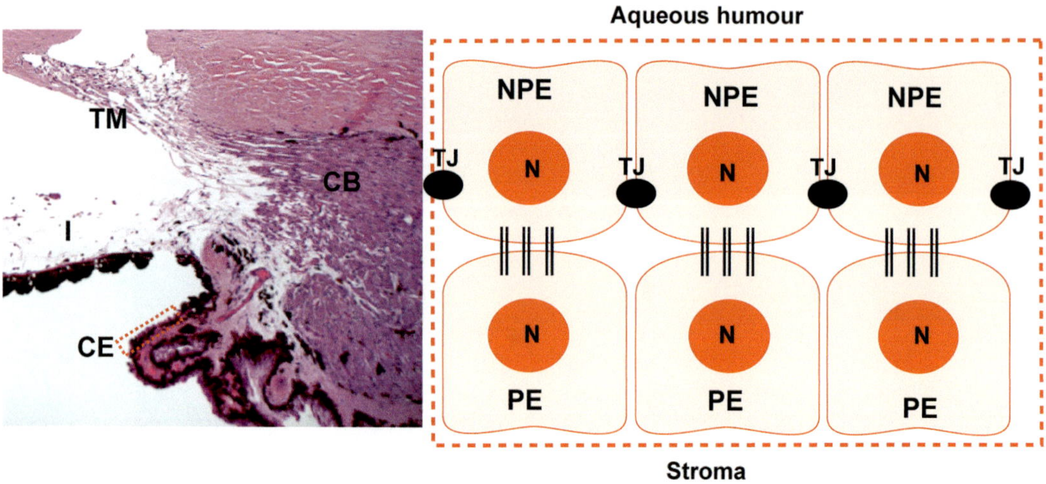

Fig. 1.2 The ciliary epithelium (CE) is located on the surface of the ciliary processes shown in a histological section of anterior chamber angle from a normal monkey. The ciliary body (CB) includes the ciliary epithelium and the underlying tissues, stroma and ciliary muscle. A schematic drawing shows the pigmented epithelial (PE) and non-pigmented (NPE) cell layers opposed to each other by their respective apical plasma membranes. Tight junctions (TJ) in the ciliary epithelium are restricted to the apical plasma membrane of the non-pigmented epithelium cell layer while the gap junctions are present in both non-pigmented epithelium and pigmented epithelial cell layers in the ciliary epithelium. *PE* pigmented ciliary epithelial cell, *NPE* non-pigmented ciliary epithelial cell, *N* nucleus, *TJ* tight junction

Tight junctions in the ciliary epithelium play a role as a functional blood-aqueous barrier between the stroma of the ciliary processes and the anterior chamber, preventing the paracellular passage of proteins through non-pigmented epithelial cells into the aqueous humour.

1.2.1.2 The Source of Proteins in the Aqueous Humour

It is interesting to know the source of proteins in the aqueous humour. Plasma proteins in the aqueous humour are less than 1% of those found in plasma. This could be the result of a process of "ultrafiltration" and paracellular movement from the plasma from the ciliary vasculature through the stroma of the ciliary processes or from the iris to the posterior chamber. However, tight junctions among the non-pigmented epithelial cells (Fig. 1.2) could prevent the diffusion of proteins from plasma through the ciliary epithelium. Later we will describe a potential alternative route through the root of the iris [8].

An additional source of proteins in aqueous humour is the ciliary body itself, after synthesis, processing and secretion [7]. A wide array of molecules have been revealed in the ciliary body including plasma proteins, transthyretin, ceruloplasmin, proteases and protease inhibitors, neuropeptides, anti-angiogenic proteins and chondromodulin, and steroid-converting enzymes. Neuroendocrine and steroidogenic activities have been suggested in the ciliary body.

1.2.2 Aqueous Humour Components

The aqueous volume in the human eye is only ~0.25 ml with low protein content and high ascorbic acid levels. A significant amount of internal fluid exchange (the range from 1.9% to 20% of the aqueous volume per minute has been reported) has been reported [9–12]. Such internal fluid exchange can be altered by many pathological and even some physiological conditions. Therefore, the aqueous humour composition should not be considered constant.

1.2.3 Aqueous Humour Production

1.2.3.1 Ciliary Blood Flow and Aqueous Humour Production

Secretion of aqueous humour requires active transport of ions and water by a complex and energy-dependent transport system comprised of ion-exchangers, cotransporters, the Na+-pump and ion channels. A dynamic relationship between ciliary blood flow and aqueous humour production has been demonstrated [13]. Aqueous production depends on blood flow below a critical level of perfusion, and is independent above that level. It also depends on other factors such as oxygen tension.

1.2.3.2 Age and Aqueous Humour Production

Ageing could also affect the rate of aqueous humour formation [14]. There is an age-related decline in the rate of aqueous production (~15 to 35% decrease) over the 20–80 year age (~2.4% per decade). Interestingly, IOP does not increase with age in normal subjects because the increased resistance to outflow is offset by the reduction in aqueous humour production. The ultrafiltration component of aqueous humour formation is pressure sensitive and decreases with increasing IOP.

1.2.3.3 The Amount of the Fluid Exchange Between Aqueous Humour and Iris

The amount of internal fluid exchange could be significant. It is understandable that avascular tissues in the anterior segment such as the lens and cornea require nutrient support and waste removal by the aqueous circulation. Recent evidence from iris studies by our group and others suggests the fluid exchange between aqueous humour and iris could be much more than previously expected. Recently, our group has studied the iris microvasculature and found that the iris has high density of microvessels and an unusual vascular distribution [15–17]. There are abundant relatively large vessels in the middle of the iris stroma which branch into the superficial microvasculature of the stroma and pupil edge within a short distance. We also found that large diameter of capillary and relatively long spindle-shaped endothelial cells in different orders of iris vasculature. Our results indicate that iris has high blood flow rate and capability for providing sufficient nutrient and waste exchange between the blood stream and the iris stroma.

Some specific features of the iris are highly relevant to fluid exchange with the aqueous humour and iris volume changes. The anterior surface of the iris is unusual. At or soon after birth, the iris surface is not covered with endothelium and only has a modified stroma structure of a relatively dense meshwork of melanocytes and fibroblasts with associated collagen [18–21].

This meshwork of cells does not form a continuous, impermeable blood-aqueous barrier, therefore aqueous humour could freely enter into the iris stroma [21, 22]. The process of fluid and molecules exchange between blood vessels, stroma and aqueous humour is worth further investigation. It has been described that the iris stroma is a sponge-like tissue which has an interwoven, collagenous framework in a matrix of hyaluronidase sensitive substance [23]. There is almost no defined diffusion barrier between the interstitial spaces of the iris and the anterior chamber. A certain concentration gradient of each molecule in the aqueous humour depends on different roles played by aqueous flow, iris vasculature and ciliary body vasculature. It is possible that plasma constituents might diffuse from the ciliary body stroma into the iris stroma and, finally, into the anterior chamber [8, 24]. The iris vascular endothelium may have selective transport functions for some molecules [24]. It is important to further explore the mechanisms of maintaining the concentration gradient for various molecules in normal and diseased conditions, which may be important for understanding the pathogenesis of some common diseases such as glaucoma and cataract and for developing potential interventions.

1.2.3.4 The Blood-Aqueous Barrier Between Aqueous Humour and Ciliary Body

The blood-aqueous barrier between the aqueous humour and ciliary body has been investigated.

Some new concepts have been proposed [25] that suggest that the plasma proteins in the anterior chamber could come from the capillaries of the ciliary body stroma. These proteins diffuse from the capillaries into ciliary body stroma, the iris stroma and finally into the anterior chamber. These proteins could be temporarily stored in the iris stroma, but not derived from the iris vessels. The proteins in the iris stroma are prevented from diffusing posteriorly by tight junctions in the posterior iris epithelium while they can enter the aqueous humour because there is no diffusion barrier in the iris surface. The pupil resting on the anterior lens capsule could act as a one-way valve, which allows the aqueous humour flow from the posterior chamber to the anterior chamber through the pupil, and prevents protein reflux from the anterior chamber into the posterior chamber.

1.2.4 Some Special Roles of Aqueous Humour

1.2.4.1 Oxygen Distribution and Regulation in the Anterior Chamber

Aqueous humour production is a metabolically active process sustained by the delivery of oxygen and nutrients and removal of metabolic waste by the ciliary circulation [13].

In recent years, the importance of oxygen distribution and regulation in the anterior chamber has been increasingly recognized. Clinical and experimental studies suggest that significant oxygen gradients are present in the anterior chamber, and that changes in these oxygen gradients are a major pathogenic factor for cataract and glaucoma.

Oxygen is the only molecule serving as the primary biological oxidant [26]. Since oxygen cannot be stored in tissue, a constant and adequate supply must be guaranteed. However, too much oxygen can be damaging to cells. Thus, both hypoxia and hyperoxia can cause serious consequences for cell survival and function in ocular and systemic diseases [27, 28]. It is well known that mitochondrial oxidative metabolism produces reactive oxygen species (ROS), including superoxide anion and hydrogen peroxide. Increased oxygen tension could potentially produce more ROS by mitochondria [29]. Therefore, oxygen level has to be maintained in a narrow range suitable for each specific cell type.

Extensive studies have been conducted addressing whether different types of contact lenses can reduce corneal and anterior chamber oxygenation [30–36]. In addition to studies on the cornea and contact lenses, the importance of oxygen in the anterior chamber of the eye has been studied [34, 37–41]. Significant oxygen gradients within the anterior chamber have been described in the experimental and clinical studies [34, 37, 40]. It has been shown that the lens normally has a relatively low oxygen environment while the posterior surface of the cornea has a higher oxygen level [34, 40, 41]. There is also evidence that oxygen distribution in the anterior chamber is modulated by local and systemic conditions, and that an altered oxygen environment in the anterior chamber may be a pathogenic factor for nuclear cataract and glaucoma [34, 37–41]. The importance of these findings is also supported by the following observations. The aqueous humour is the only source of oxygen supply for the anterior lens and trabecular meshwork, and some believe that the aqueous may even play a role in supporting the posterior surface of the cornea [36]. Some published data has described the lens as having high oxygen consumption, particularly the lens epithelium which is rich in mitochondria [34, 42, 43]. Oxygen consumption of the cornea has been studied in explanted tissue preparations [32, 44]. The corneal epithelium and endothelium have higher oxygen consumption rates in comparison with the stroma. There is currently no data available on oxygen consumption in the trabecular meshwork. However, we predict that oxygen also plays an important role in the trabecular meshwork. The endothelium in this region is functionally active and plays a critical role in the regulation of aqueous outflow [23]. Mitochondrial damage in the trabecular meshwork has been considered as a pathogenic factor for glaucoma [45]. It is critical to have sufficient but not excessive oxygen supply to maintain the function and survival of the lens, cornea and trabecular meshwork. Oxidative stress has been increasingly considered as a pathogenic factor for cataract and glaucoma. Oxygen reacts with ascorbate in the ocular fluids to produce hydrogen peroxide, which is then converted to water by the action of catalase. The reaction of increased oxygen level with ascorbate may overwhelm the ability of catalase to remove peroxide, thereby exposing the outflow tissues to this toxic metabolite. It seems very likely that there are multiple regulatory mechanisms controlling the oxygenation of different regions of the anterior chamber. Disruption of such mechanisms may be critical to the normal functioning of ocular tissues such as the lens, trabecular meshwork, and the cornea. Mounting clinical evidence implies that oxygen levels in the different tissues within the anterior chamber need to be maintained within narrow limits, suitable to their individual requirements. Unfortunately, accurate measurements of oxygen distribution in key elements within the anterior chamber such as the lens, cornea and trabecular meshwork are yet to be made under normal conditions or in relevant disease models.

1.2.4.2 The Neuropeptides in the Aqueous Humour

The ciliary epithelium is not only an integral component of a secretory neuroendocrine gland, the ciliary body, but also a source of important endocrine signals potentially linking the inflow and outflow of aqueous humour [7]. The neuropeptides in the aqueous humour can serve as messengers to communicate with the trabecular outflow pathway and the uveoscleral pathway. They play a role in the regulation of water and electrolyte homeostasis and in metabolism. Interestingly, some glaucoma-associated genes are highly expressed in the ciliary body. The interlinkage between gene expression, neuropeptides and pathogenesis of the glaucoma could be an important research topic.

1.2.4.3 Immune Privilege

Arguably, the intraocular space is an immune privilege environment. The anti-inflammatory and immunosuppressive molecules in aqueous humour play an important role in keeping the stability of aqueous flow within the eye [46].

For over a century it has been recognized that the foreign tissue grafts can survive long term in the eye. Intraocular lymphatic drainage is conspicuously absent. This ocular immune privilege was originally attributed to a putative sequestration of antigens in the eye [47].

Multiple anatomical, physiological and immune-regulatory processes help keep the stability of the intraocular environment, including aqueous flow resulting in ocular immune privilege. Five important features are present in the eye to maintain ocular immune privilege including blood/ocular barriers, the absence of lymphatic drainage pathways, soluble immunomodulatory factors in aqueous humour, immunomodulatory ligands on the surface of ocular parenchymal cells and indigenous tolerance promoting antigen-presenting cells. There are barriers between the blood and intraocular environment similar to that between the brain and blood. These barriers act to maintain the stability of these important organs and avoid disturbance from blood-borne substances [48]. Three manifestations of ocular immune privilege have been extensively studied, including the intraocular selective anti-inflammatory and immunosuppressive microenvironment; the prolonged acceptance of solid tissue and tumour allografts in the anterior chamber, and the induction of systemic tolerance to eye-derived antigens [49, 50]. Ocular tissues and fluids contain many anti-inflammatory and immunosuppressive molecules, including CD95L (FasL), transforming growth factor-β, macrophage migration inhibitory factor, α-melanocyte-stimulating hormone, calcitonin gene-related peptide, somatostatin and complement regulatory proteins [47]. Furthermore antigens entering the anterior chamber of the eye may evoke a unique form of immune deviation that culminates in the antigen-specific suppression of TH1 immune responses. Cell membranes and some soluble factors in the intraocular environment inhibit both the adaptive and innate immune systems.

1.2.5 Importance of Homeostasis of Aqueous Humour

Aqueous humour is a unique fluid, which plays roles in not only maintaining normal IOP, proper globe shape and optical properties, it also must keep a dynamic stability in its production and outflow. The dynamic nature of aqueous humour is critically important. It means that: (1) Aqueous humour has to be continuously produced and drained, (2) aqueous humour closely communicates with surrounding tissues, supplying nourishment to avascular anterior tissues, such as the cornea and lens, and removing waste, (3) the components of aqueous humour are subject to change, (4) the neuropeptides are involved in a signal pathway between the inflow and outflow and (5) the molecules in the aqueous humour play a role in the intraocular immune privilege. Therefore, homeostasis of aqueous humour is critical for ocular physiology and pathology.

1.3 Aqueous Outflow Pathways in Normal Eyes

Aqueous humour leaves the eye by direct and indirect routes, or called conventional and unconventional pathways at the anterior chamber angle (Fig. 1.1). The conventional pathway is also called the trabecular or direct route. It is through the trabecular meshwork (TM), across the inner wall of Schlemm's canal and into its lumen, and then into collector channels, aqueous veins, and the intrascleral and episcleral venous plexuses. The unconventional pathway or called uveoscleral or indirect route is across the iris root, uveal meshwork and anterior face of the ciliary muscle, through the connective tissue between the muscle bundles, and the suprachoroidal space, and then out through the sclera [51].

In the normal human eye, the importance of the uveoscleral pathway has not been well recognized. The uveoscleral pathway drains ~10% of total aqueous humour drainage in older eyes but could be more in young subjects (>30%). There is no significant net fluid movement across the cornea, iris vasculature or vitreoretinal interface, although fluid exchange and ion fluxes exist. It is generally accepted that aqueous humour outflow through the direct route is pressure dependent, while the indirect outflow route is IOP independent.

1.3.1 Direct Route

1.3.1.1 Trabecular Meshwork

A balance between aqueous production and outflow maintains steady-state IOP. Elevated IOP is mainly due to increase of aqueous humour outflow resistance in open angle glaucoma. Most of the aqueous humour outflow pathway is through the trabecular meshwork, where the dominant outflow resistance is in the cribriform region adjacent to the inner wall of Schlemm's canal in normal and glaucomatous eyes [52].

The trabecular meshwork is a layered structure with few layers at the anterior portion and more than ten layers at the posterior portion. Endothelial cells of the trabecular sheets have some specific features. They have rich cytoplasmic organelles. Cytoplasmic vesicles or vacuoles can be found at many of the endothelial cells located in the internal wall of Schlemm's canal. These vesicles or vacuoles usually have extraordinary dimensions and specific distribution. The functions of the vacuoles are active. There could be a direct pathway for aqueous humour moving from the innermost trabecular space into inside of Schlemm's canal. In addition to be a pathway, they are also capable to be as an active transport for large molecules such as proteins. These proteins could cross the endothelium in order to circumvent the barrier presented to these molecules by closure of the intercellular space by the zonulae occludentes [18]. Furthermore, these vacuoles are also responsible for protein synthesis and secretion. There are some key functions of the trabecular meshwork such as regulation of outflow resistance, phagocytosis and active fluid transport. The involvement of the cytoplasmic vesicles or vacuoles needs to be further investigated.

The trabecular meshwork includes uveal and corneoscleral regions. Aqueous humour first encounters the uveal meshwork, an irregular net-like structure of lamellae, then the corneoscleral meshwork, a number of porous sheets. Uveal and corneoscleral networks of extracellular matrix (ECM) are covered by trabecular meshwork endothelial cells. It is generally accepted that uveal and corneoscleral networks do not generate any significant resistance to aqueous outflow, although the openings in the uveal meshwork, and in the sheets of the corneoscleral meshwork, can vary significantly [53].

There is a pressure gradient between the anterior chamber and Schlemm's canal. The juxtacanalicular tissue (JCT) plays a critical role responding to create the pressure gradient. The JCT is the final portion of the trabecular meshwork through which aqueous humour outflow reaches Schlemm's canal. The JCT is bordered on the one side by the innermost corneoscleral trabecular meshwork sheet and on the other by the basement membrane of the inner wall of Schlemm's canal. Alterations of IOP and episcleral venous pressures, and the distance across the trabecular meshwork and inner wall of Schlemm's canal, can modulate the pressure gradient. Together with associated ECM and the inner wall of Schlemm's canal, the JCT–trabecular meshwork is likely to be a major portion of the resistance to outflow.

The role of the trabecular meshwork cells in maintaining normal aqueous flow has to be recognized. A highly phagocytic function of trabecular meshwork cells has been described. This function allows the continuous removal of particles, cellular debris or protein molecules from the aqueous humour pathway [54, 55]. Cleaning the aqueous humour and preventing obstruction of the inter-trabecular and cribriform pathways are carried out by the trabecular meshwork. Red blood cells and pigment granules, as well as bacteria can be removed by the meshwork cells [56–63]. Phagocytosed materials enclosed in membrane-limited vacuoles fuse with lysosomes forming phagolysosomes. Finally they are stored within the cells. Macrophages can also be found within the trabecular meshwork in the normal condition [57, 64]. It is possible that both macrophages and trabecula cells can lose contact with the trabecular beams and pass the endothelium of Schlemm's canal to enter the aqueous vein system [55, 58].

1.3.1.2 Schlemm's Canal

The inner wall of Schlemm's canal and the JCT are the sites which create normal resistance in the conventional drainage pathway. The JCT consists of trabecular meshwork cells and the endothelium of Schlemm's canal. The JCT region has also been found to be the pathological tissue in glaucoma. It has been implicated that it induces the increased outflow resistance which is responding to elevated IOP in most forms of glaucoma [53]. Understanding the Schlemm's canal endothelium and its contribution to the generation and regulation of outflow resistance is paramount to developing rational therapeutic strategies for glaucoma.

After passing by the JCT–trabecular meshwork cells, aqueous humour passes through the inner wall of Schlemm's canal. This is lined with the only continuous cell monolayer in the trabecular outflow pathway. The inner wall of Schlemm's canal is characterized by elongated endothelial cells aligned parallel to the longitudinal axis of the canal. These endothelial cells are mostly spindle shaped (100–150 μm in length and 8–10 μm in width) with significant variations. When compared with vascular endothelial cells in the eye, the phenotype of these cells is more similar to that in the arterioles rather than veins [65]. These endothelial cells have tight junctions and a discontinuous basement membrane. While the endothelial cells of the outer wall of Schlemm's canal have a continuous basement membrane.

Various size giant vacuoles (1–10 μm in width, 1–7 μm in height) exist in the inner wall of Schlemm's canal, and the size and density of giant vacuoles positively correlates with IOP. The inner wall of giant vacuoles is very thin with various sizes of pores (estimated ~2000 pores per mm^2) and mostly transcellular.

Aqueous humour enters the Schlemm's canal lumen through the inner wall endothelium. Schlemm's canal is a highly elongated ellipse and only 350–500 μm in meridional width [18]. It is expected that the fluid dynamics in Schlemm's canal could be complicated. The inner wall endothelial cells are exposed to shear forces as aqueous humour travels circumferentially on its way to exit the canal lumen and enter a collector channel. A funnelling theory has been proposed, which predicts non-uniform flow patterns across the endothelium of Schlemm's canal. Modelling found that funnelling increases the JCT flow resistance 30-fold.

Whether the endothelial cells are lymphatic or blood vasculature has also been studied. It has been found that the inner wall of Schlemm's canal is unique, sharing extraordinary characteristics with both types of specialized endothelia in addition to having distinctive features of its own [66]. Certainly, Schlemm's canal, and in particular its inner wall, has evolved unique features that enable it to function [53]. However, there are many mysteries to be investigated including the molecular, functional and anatomic features [67] and biomechanics [68].

1.3.1.3 Outer Wall of the Schlemm's Canal and Collector Channels

There are ~25 to 35 collector channels emerging from the external wall of Schlemm's canal. They either join the deep scleral plexus directly or pass to the surface of the eye as aqueous veins. The size of collector channels varies between 20 and 90 μm. They are the principal route for the aqueous humour flow from Schlemm's canal. The distribution of the channels is uneven around the circumference of Schlemm's canal. In terms of the quadrant distribution, the nasal side has more channels than the temporal side. These channels are often connected in groups with each other and with the deep scleral plexus of veins [69, 70]. The collector channels are lined by endothelial cells. The connective tissue of the wall of Schlemm's canal continues outward along the collector channels as a very simple layer, which may show an occasional smooth muscle cell. The adventitia disappears from the walls of those vessels, which join the deep scleral plexus.

The aqueous veins are the major pathway for the aqueous humour flow from Schlemm's canal into the episcleral veins. The aqueous flow pathway is fully lined with endothelial cells which are covered from the trabecular meshwork and Schlemm's canal to the drainage veins. Aqueous outflow pathways are not connected with conjunctival lymphatics. There are marked differences in histochemical labelling between conjunctival lymphatics and normal human aqueous drainage channels [71].

Aqueous humour enters into Schlemm's canal circumferentially. The collector channel ostia (tens of microns in diameter) open from the outer wall of Schlemm's canal. Aqueous humour is transported to collector channels and followed by two parallel pathways, intrascleral plexus and the aqueous veins. There are significant anatomical variations of human collector channel orifices [72]. We recently studied collector channel ostia and found that their orientations are significantly different along with endothelial phenotype differences in different regions of the collector channels in human donor eyes (unpublished data).

1.3.1.4 Aqueous Veins and the Deep Scleral Plexus

Detailed studies of the conjunctival vasculature have been described, but there are many interesting questions regarding the aqueous humour flow pathway. The branches of the anterior ciliary artery supply the bulbar conjunctiva and the anterior episcleral, and form the superficial marginal plexus at the limbus. The episcleral venous plexuses drain the bulbar conjunctival veins and the intrascleral plexuses. The exterior collector channels connect with each other and with the deep scleral venous plexus [69, 73, 74]. The collector channels are fully covered by endothelium. Aqueous veins are aqueous-filled channels at the limbus and can be seen with the slit lamp microscope [75]. The aqueous in aqueous vein can be seen as a clear lamination bordered by blood, but eventual mixing with blood is evident further downstream. Schlemm's canal could be considered as the internal collector channels with increased total surface of the inner wall of the canal [18]. The conjunctival capillaries belong to the non-fenestrated continuous type. Aqueous humour is drained by well-constructed and fully endothelial lined blood vessels [46]. These endothelial cells are relatively uniform in thickness with a well-defined basement membrane. The cell junctions show extensive interdigitations, and a zonula occludens.

It is difficult to study the colourless aqueous outflow and its pathways. Fluorescein dye has been used as a tracer to study the dynamics of aqueous humour outflow experimentally. In order to avoid disturbing the anterior chamber and minimizing IOP changes during the dye injection, a two-syringe system has been used. A 30-gauge needle was inserted into the anterior chamber and a custom-made three-way valve with minimum volume was connected between the needle and two syringes. To keep the volume in the anterior chamber relatively constant, one syringe was used for withdrawal of aqueous and the other for injection of an equal volume of 1% sodium fluorescein. The normal aqueous humour drainage pathways in the conjunctiva were recorded from normal monkeys and rabbits. Figure 1.3 shows selected frames of video clip from a monkey. The fluorescein could be seen gradually filling the aqueous vein and conjunctival vessels after injection into the anterior chamber. We have obtained valuable dynamic information of aqueous outflow pathway. The aqueous drainage pathways increasingly filled with fluorescein over time, and eventually the entire drainage system was visible. Figure 1.3j shows a frame from the late phase. It is clearly evidenced that some vessels are running perpendicular to the limbus but deeper vessels with more random orientations are visible. These vessels running perpendicular

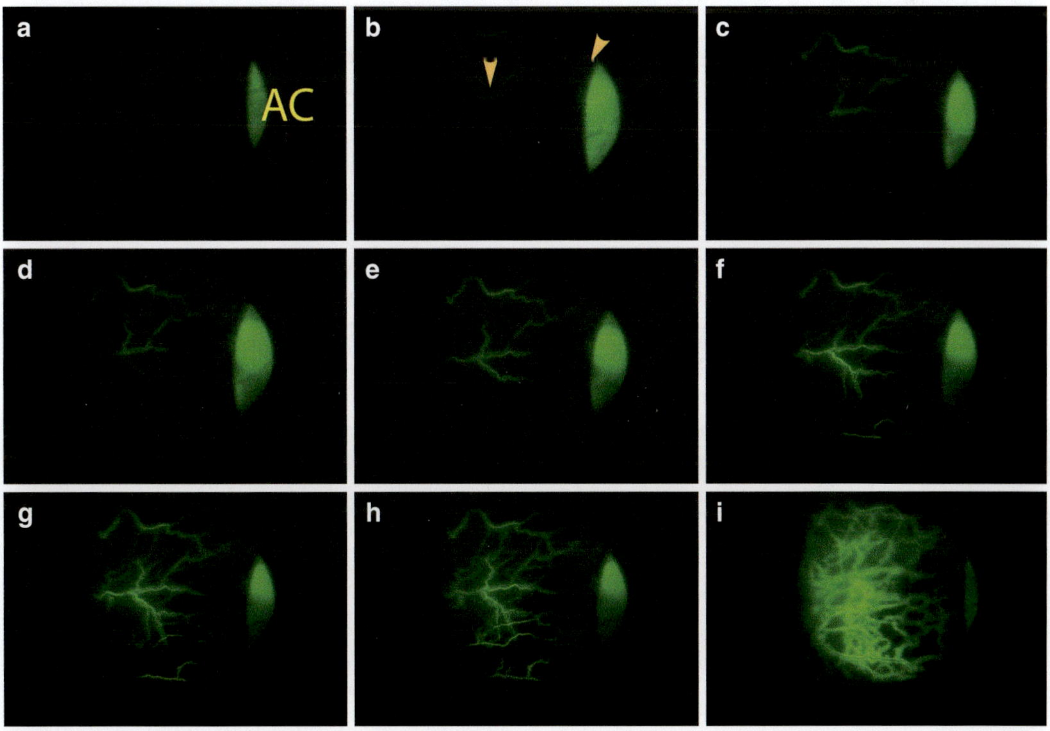

Fig. 1.3 Experimental results of normal aqueous outflow pathways in monkey conjunctiva. Video frames (Panels **a**–**i**) show the sequence of aqueous humour drained from the anterior chamber into conjunctival aqueous humour drainage pathways after fluorescein injection into the anterior chamber. (Panel **a**) is immediately after injection and the fluorescein is confined to the anterior chamber (AC). A few seconds later fluorescein is visible in some superficial vessels (Panels **b** and **c**) and the extent of fluorescein filling increases (**d**–**h**). In the late phase (**i**) there are some vessels with diffused edges in the deeper location. Panel **j** is a magnified image from the late stage (Panel **i**). Reproduced with permission from [46]

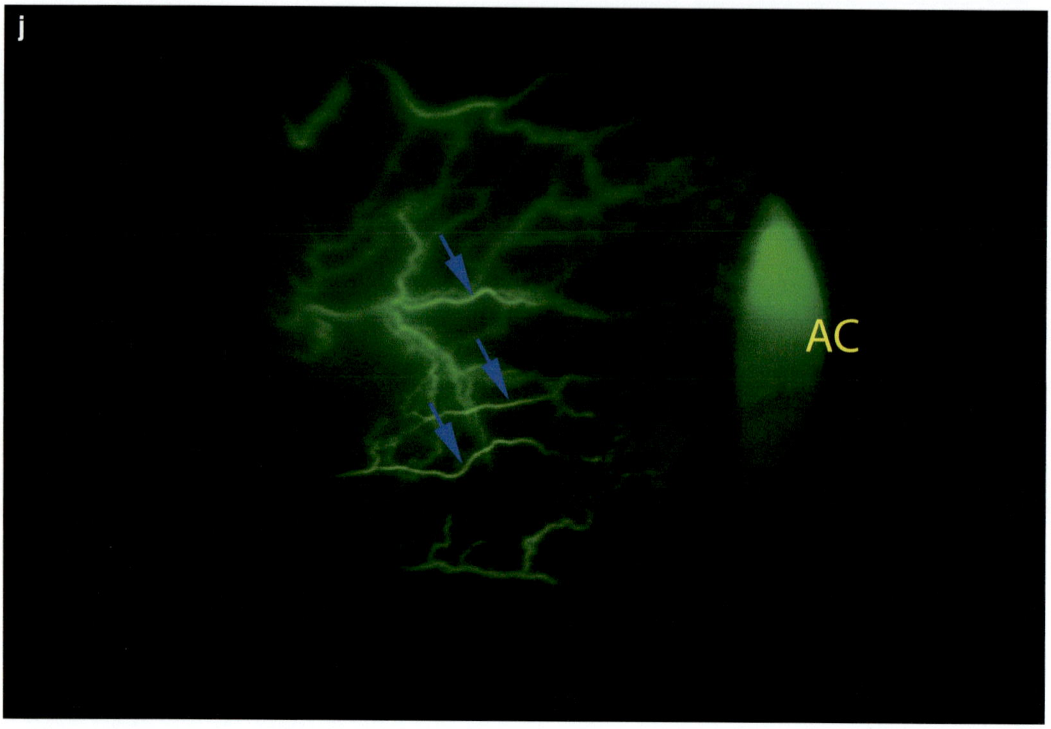

Fig. 1.3 (continued)

to the limbus occurred early (see Fig. 1.3c) and were mostly located superficially. However, the deeper vessels occurred later and seem to be larger in calibre with more interconnections like a vascular plexus. It is very important to find the interrelationship between histological findings and in vivo dynamic information. It is likely these vessels which are running perpendicular to the limbus and are located superficially could be aqueous veins while the deeper plexus could be the intrascleral vein plexus.

Interestingly, the spectral-domain optical coherence tomography technique may help us to visualize the aqueous humour outflow structures including the deep and intrascleral venous plexus in situ in humans [76].

1.3.1.5 Some Concepts of Outflow Resistance and Regulation of Aqueous Outflow

Aqueous fluid traverses the trabecular outflow pathway through the trabecular meshwork, juxtacanalicular connective tissue, endothelial lining of Schlemm's canal, collector channels, aqueous veins and episcleral veins. It is important to study outflow resistance and possible modulation mechanisms. We still do not understand the mechanisms for generating and regulating the outflow resistance, or the cause of resistance increase in glaucoma.

The generally accepted view is that the region providing the main resistance to fluid drainage is the inner wall of Schlemm's canal and the juxtacanalicular connective tissue [5, 6, 77, 78]. Cells in the trabecular meshwork regulate hydraulic conductivity of the inner wall region possibly by modulating extracellular matrix turnover and by actively distorting the meshwork and changing cell shape. This route provides a hydrostatic pressure resistance that is overcome by a hydrostatic pressure gradient between the inside of the eye, the IOP, and the outside of the eye, episcleral venous pressure. The hydrodynamic effect is termed outflow resistance.

Pulsatile flow into the aqueous vein has been carefully studied and is believed to provide important information in normal and glaucomatous eyes [79]. It is unique that the aqueous outflow system can be observed by examining the boundary point of blood and transparent fluid in the conjunctival aqueous veins. In addition, the pulsatile properties of this boundary can be monitored, which may help to determine how an extravascular fluid returns to the vascular system. The patterns of pulsatile flow are synchronous with IOP transients induced by the cardiac pulse, blinking and eye movement. Use of high-resolution spectral-domain optical coherence tomography could be valuable to study pressure-dependent trabecular tissue motion and tissues distal to Schlemm's canal in regulation of aqueous outflow [4].

Hopefully, we can combine both functional and structural studies to investigate the aqueous outflow in the physiological and pathological conditions from experimental models to clinical applications.

1.3.2 Uveoscleral Outflow

Although the bulk of aqueous humour (70–90%) passes through the trabecular outflow pathway, the uveoscleral flow could also play a critical role in aqueous outflow and the understanding of the pathogenesis and therapeutic interventions in glaucoma.

The uveoscleral outflow route has not been sufficiently studied. We have limited knowledge in this field and most information are from relatively few groups [80–86]. Some of the aqueous leaves the eye through the iris root and the ciliary body in the anterior chamber angle [86, 87]. Interestingly, the fraction (40–50%) of aqueous humour flow through the uveoscleral pathway in non-human primates is higher than that in human (in the 5–25% range). Age-dependent reduction of uveoscleral flow has been found in human eyes. Therefore, the fraction of aqueous outflow through the uveoscleral route could be different between the species and with age.

The changes in IOP within the normal range have little effect on uveoscleral outflow. It is possible that changes in IOP do not alter the pressure gradient through the ciliary muscle. The ciliary muscle may play a role in the uveoscleral outflow pathway. Modulation of ciliary muscle may change the uveoscleral outflow and IOP. The uveoscleral outflow could be increased and IOP reduced when the ciliary muscle is relaxed. This could have some potential for developing therapeutic interventions. Epinephrine, for example, has been found to increase uveoscleral outflow, possibly mediated by endogenously synthesized prostaglandins (PGs). In monkeys, observed increases in uveoscleral outflow following administration of very small PG doses equal or exceed the increase that can be achieved with much higher doses of epinephrine. These observations support the concept that the PGs may represent an important new approach to the medical management or glaucoma. Increasing uveoscleral flow can be one of the mechanisms by which prostaglandin $F_{2\alpha}$ and prostaglandin $F_{2\alpha}$-analogues effectively reduce IOP. Whether uveoscleral flow plays a significant role in any other eye disease is not clear. Although we are able to successfully increase aqueous flow through the uveoscleral route, we still have only a limited understanding on its physiological role.

In summary, we have performed extensive studies and accumulated extensive information of aqueous humour outflow pathways. But many fundamental questions still wait for clear answers. We do believe that the aqueous outflow pathway is complex, not only structurally but also functionally. We need to precisely investigate each key component of aqueous humour outflow pathway such as trabecular meshwork, Schlemm's canal, collector channels and the aqueous vein system including aqueous vein, episcleral and deep scleral veins. More importantly, we should understand how these key components work together to keep functional drainage throughout our life. In addition to trabecular meshwork and uveoscleral pathways, it has been described that the aqueous humour enters the ciliary muscle and exits the eye by multiple routes. These routes include the supraciliary space and across the anterior sclera or into the suprachoroidal space and across the posterior sclera, flows through the emissarial canals around the vortex veins or traverses uveal vessels and into the vortex veins or enters the ciliary processes from the ciliary muscle and is secreted back into the posterior chamber [5, 6, 80, 81]. The endothelium plays critical roles for each key component. It may provide important clues for us to understand the aqueous outflow pathways.

1.4 Retinal Ganglion Cell and Its Compartmentation

Retinal ganglion cell (RGC) is the most critical cell involving the pathogenesis of glaucomatous insults. To understand glaucoma induced neurodegeneration on the optic nerve, we have to investigate the interactions of the RGC and the surrounding tissues including glial cells and blood supply because the optic nerve is a part of the white matter of the brain. Glaucoma is believed to be an aetiologically complex disorder of optic nerve neuropathies. It is important to combine knowledge of neuroscience and glaucoma if we would like to have better understanding of the pathogenesis and further improvements in the management of glaucoma.

1.4.1 RGCs Anatomy and Structure

The retina could be seen as a window to the brain because there are close links between the retina and the brain in normal and diseased conditions [88]. All RGC bodies are located in retinal RGC layer. It has different thickness in the inner retina. The thickness in the nasal retina is about 10–20 μm, while it is 60–80 μm thick in the macular region. RGCs are arranged as a single row in the peripheral retina and up to ten rows in the fovea. The size of RGC bodies varies from 10 μm to 30 μm in diameter. Their cell bodies are large compared with other neurons in the retina. Interestingly, the smaller size RGCs are located in the macular region. It is possible to allow more dense RGCs per unit volume. We do not really know the functional difference between different sizes of cell bodies. Unbranched axons of RGCs have significant variation with respect to size. RGC axons travel internally and run parallel to the inner surface of the retina to form the nerve fibre layer of the retina before entering the optic nerve. The axons from different retinal regions entering the optic nerve are well arranged. Axons located in the peripheral portion of the optic nerve come from the peripheral retina while those located in the central portion of the optic nerve come from the posterior retina.

The RGC bodies in the parafoveal region are smaller than in the peripheral retina (Fig. 1.4). The RGC cell body has a rich cytoplasm and RGCs are polarized into dendritic and axonal compartments. The structural polarization is also responsible for some degree of functional polarization and associated with molecular differences within a neuron. The RGC signal inputs are collected by the dendrites and a pulse-coded signal is transmitted from the cell body to the axon. RGCs receive inputs from bipolar cells, which convey signals from photoreceptors to the IPL, and from amacrine cells that branch in the inner plexiform layer (IPL). RGC dendrites extend into the IPL (Fig. 1.4). Abundant synaptic contacts are located in the IPL. Amacrine cells have approximately 20–30 subtypes that are structurally diverse with respect to the distribution of their processes.

There are ~1.2 million axons in the optic nerve. Axons travel through the optic nerve, the chiasm and the optic tracts to synapse with the medial and lateral geniculate bodies, superior colliculi and pretectal nuclei [90]. The lateral geniculate body constrains vast majority of optic nerve axons synapse. The diameter of the axons in the optic nerve varies, with an average diameter of 1 μm in a range from 0.7 to 10 μm. The size of axons corresponds to the size of the cell bodies. The central part of the retina has the smaller RGC bodies and smaller axons while the peripheral retina has the larger axons coming from larger RGC bodies [18]. The axons are organized into ~800 to 1200 inter-anastomosed fascicles, each surrounded by an incompletely segregated pial sheath in the orbital portion of the optic nerve.

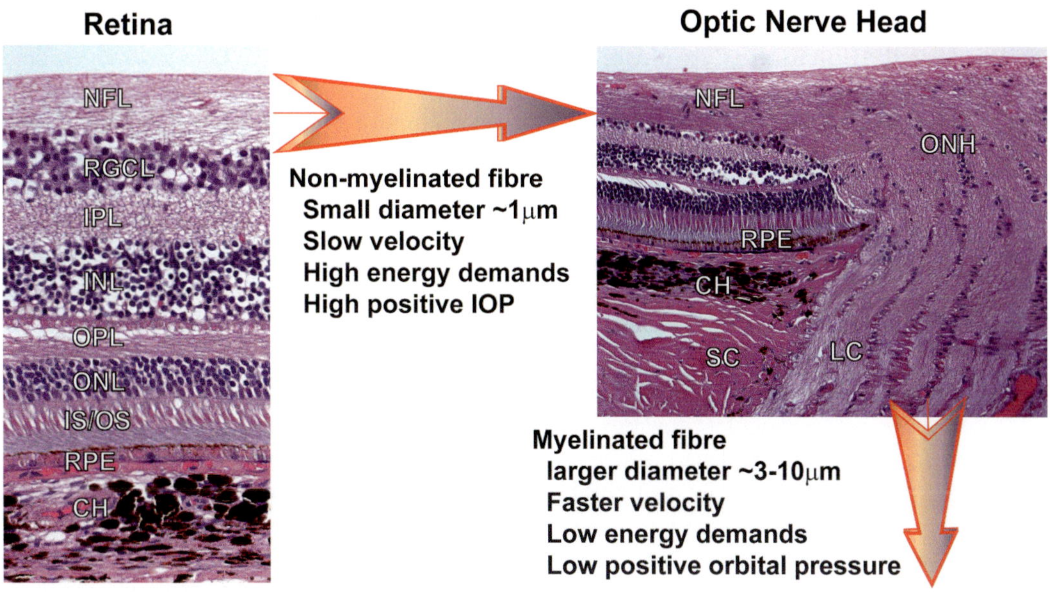

Fig. 1.4 Histological section of the retina from parafoveal region and optic nerve head from a normal monkey [89]. There is a complicated geometric distribution of RGC dendrites, cell bodies and axons located in the inner plexiform layer (IPL), RGC layer (RGCL) and nerve fibre layer (NFL), respectively. RGC bodies are larger than other retinal neuronal cell bodies in the outer and inner nuclear layer (ONL and INL). There are significant differences between non-myelinated fibres in the retina and optic nerve head (ONH), and myelinated axons within the optic nerve, both structurally and functionally. Axons become myelinated after the lamina cribrosa (LC). *IS/OS* the inner/outer segments of the photoreceptors, *CH* choroid, *RPE* retinal pigment epithelium. Reproduced with permission from [89]

1.4.2 Functional Active RGCs

RGCs functional activities are amazing. Visual signals are encompassing the spatial and temporal properties of the light stimulus. There is a tremendous amount of processing within retinal layers prior to transmission by RGC axons to the brain [18]. Most nerve axons are ~1 μm or more in diameter and ~50 mm in length. Although RGC body is larger than other retinal neurons, but axons are on average ~20,000 times larger than the cell body with respect to length and total surface area [91]. Signal conduit via the optic nerve contains 38% of all the afferent fibres contained in cranial nerves [18].

Retinal cells have unusually high-energy requirements. They are exquisitely sensitive to disturbances in the supply of their energy sources (oxygen and other substrates). Importantly, the density of the vascular network in the retina is constrained by the requirement for relative optical transparency. Retinal cells have high metabolic demands, but are only be served by a limited blood supply. Such unusual constraint predisposes the retina to a range of vascular diseases. Retinal blood supply has to have precise regulatory mechanisms that serve to match local blood flow with local tissue demands in order to achieve the delicate balance between oxygen availability and consumption.

1.4.3 Compartmentation of Neuronal Cells

The concept of the micro compartments of neuronal cells has been described in the neurons. We would like to briefly introduce current knowledge of compartmentation before describing the RGCs.

1.4.3.1 Non-uniform of Energy Distribution in the Cytoplasm

The principle of non-homogeneous, intracellular energy distribution and consumption in the cytoplasm of a living cell has been widely accepted. In fact, ATP molecules have only a limited capacity to diffuse within the cytoplasm because they exist mostly in a structure-associated form [92, 93]. There are significant regional variations in ATP concentration within neuronal components resulting in significant energy gradients.

Mitochondria are mobile intracellularly. They can move and accumulate towards sites of high-energy demand and depart when ATP demand decreases [94, 95]. The non-uniform distribution of mitochondria within neurons suggests that intracellular energy consumption is also non-uniform. Non-uniform of energy distribution in the cytoplasm is also supported by the existence of intracellular gradients of oxygen and pH [96, 97].

1.4.3.2 The Concept of Compartmentation of Neuronal Cells

The concept of "micro compartmentation" was introduced decades ago [92] and supported by a large body of accumulated evidence since then [93–95, 98–102].

The concept of the metabolic unit is important for knowing energy homeostasis of the neuronal cell [103]. Micro compartment or simply called compartment is believed to be closely linked with metabolic unit and localized energy generation.

Dynamic modulation of energy generation is critical for maintaining neuronal homeostasis in order to adapt to various conditions including long-term evolving processes such as development and ageing and short-term processes, physiological or pathological such as light adaptation, ischaemia and hypoxia.

A metabolic unit includes three distinct cell populations, neurons, glia and blood vessels. They work in unison to respond to regional changes in metabolic demand. Neurons are the predominant determinants of local metabolic activity based on the momentary demands of electrical processing. Glia (astrocytes and Muller cells) act to couple with blood vessels and neurons to regulate the energy needs of neurons and to buffer the extracellular environment. Blood vessels primarily serve to deliver glucose and oxygen to neurons and remove toxic byproducts from the neuronal environment. These three types of cell populations interact during all aspects of metabolic function, a process referred to as neurovascular coupling, to form a functional energy unit.

The role of glial cells in neurodevelopment, neurophysiology and neuropathology has been particularly emphasized. Knowledge of astrocytes has extensively been derived from CNS studies in recent years. However, such knowledge is largely transferrable from CNS to the retina and optic nerve as they are also embryologically derived from the forebrain [88]. RGCs are intimately dependent upon glial cells for normal function. Glial cells have multiple functions such as the formation of synapses during development and adult life, the formation of synapses and maintaining synaptic structure and arrangement and ensure that neurons receive the correct pattern of innervation [104].

There are two potential mechanisms which may be involved in neurovascular coupling, negative feedback and active control. The local response to the metabolic signals such as oxygen/glucose and carbon dioxide concentrations could alter blood flow. It has been reported that pericytes can attenuate the effects of local metabolic signals by altering capillary diameter. Damage to pericytes can impair a long-lasting supply/demand mismatch [105].

The role of neurotransmitter-mediated signalling, particularly glutamate, in the regulation of regional blood flow has been reported [105]. This is an interesting concept in neurovascular coupling which suggests the roles of astrocytes and neurons in controlling regional blood flow by the release of messenger molecules such as nitric oxide (released from neurons) and arachidonic acid derivatives (released from astrocytes and neurons).

1.4.4 Energy Distribution and Consumption in Different Subcellular Components of RGCs

RGCs have unique geometrical characteristics with a polarized structure, an enormous trajectory and traverse a range of extracellular environments (intraocular, intraorbital and intracranial). RGC is one of the most appropriate neuronal types to fit with the concept of compartmentation. The function of RGCs appears complex when considered as a whole, but it can be easier if breaking down the cell into individual micro compartments because the structural and functional adaptations of each micro compartment are clearly different. Of course, the interconnection of each micro compartment of RGC certainly needs to be considered.

Intracellular energy distribution and consumption is more in-homogeneous in this structure compared to other living cells because the RGC axon has a tremendously long trajectory. The mechanisms to dynamical redistribution of the energy are sophisticated. It requires supporting functional activity within different components of the RGC. These mechanisms are fundamentally important to allow us to understand how RGCs adapt the physiological variations and tolerate the pathological challenges.

Investigations of the pattern of energy distribution and consumption within different subcellular components of RGCs are technically difficult. These techniques include measurements of oxygen distribution and oxygen consumption, mitochondrial distribution and enzyme expression and the presence of neuroglobin. Each technique not only provides valuable information concerning energy distribution and consumption within different subcellular components, but also has certain limitations. Updated information is summarized here which may help identify current understanding and gaps in our knowledge. Hopefully it will stimulate further investigation in this exciting and important field.

RGC cannot attempt to treat as a single, homogeneous structure particularly for understanding pathogenic processes involved in glaucoma and other optic neuropathies. Investigating the RGC as a series of compartments is particularly favoured by understanding RGC degeneration in glaucoma [95].

The pathological responses of RGCs to insults can be interpreted as a set of compartmentalized and inter-related subcellular processes. Assuming that pathologic triggers that initiate a pathogenic chain in one compartment, it can be different to another. Signalling processes allow injury to one compartment to adversely or favourably affect another compartment.

1.4.5 RGC Compartmentation

We propose that it is advantageous to divide RGCs into four different subcellular compartments when considering retinal and optic nerve disease mechanisms: the dendrites of the RGC and their synapses located in the IPL; RGC cell bodies located in the RGC layer; non-myelinated axons in the retina and the optic nerve head, and myelinated axons in the orbit and the cranial region.

The reasons for dividing RGCs into these compartments are based on their differences in structure and function of the RGC, extracellular environment, energetics and the response to pathogenic challenge. The vulnerability of each compartment to insults such as elevated IOP is different. Each compartment does not respond independently to insults but instead is modulated by signals and messengers from other compartments.

1.4.5.1 The Dendrites of RGCs and Their Synapses in the IPL

RGC dendrites integrate with the synapses of bipolar and amacrine cells and summate the total input gathered from the synaptic network. The action potential is initiated at the axon hillock which has greatest concentration of voltage-sensitive sodium channels with high-energy consumption [106].

We have studied capillary morphometry and density measurements in the human IPL at a retinal eccentricity located 3 mm superior to the optic disc [107]. The network supplying the IPL is a complex 3D configuration with smaller capillary diameter and lower capillary density. These structural adaptations serve an important purpose in maximizing nutrient delivery to energy-dependent synapses while at the same time preserving the optical clarity of the retina.

The IPL has relatively low oxygen tension which is close to a "critical" oxygen tension even under normal physiological conditions [108]. But the IPL has a high oxygen consumption during normoxia and oxygen consumption increases during hyperoxia when more oxygen is made available to the IPL [109, 110]. To date we are still unable to explain why oxygen consumption remains almost constant in the inner segments of photoreceptors, while the IPL has the capacity to consume almost all the available oxygen during increased oxygen availability.

The significance of the unique energy demands of RGC dendrites and synapses has not been adequately related back to understanding the susceptibility and tolerance of RGC dendrites to various diseases, such as glaucoma. An interesting question that remains unanswered is whether or not RGC dendrites are the first compartment to be perturbed by various challenges [111, 112]. Conflicting evidence has been found in the literature. It has been suggested that RGCs are relatively tolerant to early ischaemic insults. It could be due to the availability of glucose in the vitreous and the capacity of RGCs to extract ATP from glycolysis [113, 114]. However, an extended period of IOP-induced ischaemia can cause dendritic shrinkage [115].

1.4.5.2 RGC Bodies in the RGC Layer

RGC bodies are located in the RGC layer and significantly larger than other retinal neurons. Each retina has ~130 million photoreceptors and the optic nerve contains ~1 million axons. One RGC transmits through its axon the integrated information from many photoreceptors to the cerebral cortex.

All organelles including mitochondria, endoplasmic reticulum, Golgi apparatus and cytoplasm are synthesized within the RGC cell body. Synthesized organelles are transported to targeted sites. The axon totally lacks any synthetic function, while dendrites have some capacity to synthesize proteins. Almost all RGC compartments are critically dependent on the cell body for the biogenesis of organelles. Damage to the cell body will have a devastating impact on the functioning of the entire cell [116].

The RGC layer has a richer blood supply than the IPL in the human retina [107, 117]. Oxygen tension in the RGC layer is also higher than that in the IPL. The energy demands of RGC bodies appear to be higher than that of other nuclear layers such as the INL and the ONL. The oxygen diffusion model cannot be applied to the RGC layer in a vascularized retina. Using a retinal artery occlusion model we have found that oxygen cannot be delivered to the RGC layer from the choroidal circulation due to the presence of intervening high oxygen consuming layers, particularly the IPL [109]. Currently there is no conclusive evidence from intraretinal oxygen measurements and oxygen consumption analysis regarding oxygen consumption in the RGC layer. However, we have found several forms of experimental evidence from histochemical evidence of COX activity, immunolabelling of cytochrome oxidase subunit Vic, the presence of neuroglobin and the presence of mitochondria around the RGC nuclei suggests that oxygen consumption by RGC bodies is likely to be high.

Nuclear counting using in vivo techniques and post-mortem tissue is a useful means of determining the response of the RGC layer to insults. However, it still cannot define the chronology of cell body death respective to alteration of other RGC compartments. There remains a great deficiency in our knowledge regarding cause–consequence relationships in RGC related diseases.

1.4.5.3 Non-myelinated Axons in the Retina and Optic Nerve Head

RGCs are constantly active and use significant amounts of energy to generate signals. Neurons consume high proportion (50–80%) of total energy for the purposes of signalling. It has been reported that the maintaining resting potentials, counteracting leakage from organelles and the turnover of macromolecules account for less than 20% of total energy consumption. Mitochondrial proton leak and axoplasmic transport could be significant energy consumers but are not accounted for in this analysis [118].

Densely packed RGC axons are a conduit for the transfer of visual information in the form of spike trains. In axons, energy usage is tightly coupled to neural performance [119]. Energy usage links together two fundamental measures of signal quality: signal-to-noise ratio and bandwidth (a measure of speed of response) [120]. Energy demand increases with the spike rate when single axons transmit information in spike trains [121]. Therefore, precise conduit of complex and massive visual information unavoidably requires very high energy. In addition, unlike myelinated axons, non-myelinated axons do not have saltatory properties of action potential conduction which reduce the energy uptake.

Non-myelinated Axons in the Retina

Non-myelinated axons in the retina are located in the nerve fibre layer and optic nerve head. Figure 1.5 illustrates the morphology of these axons (a), their mitochondria location (b) and relationship with blood vessels and astrocytes (c and d). High densely packed mitochondria are concentrated within regularly spaced bulb-shaped varicosities along the course of the axon [122, 123]. The presence of these mitochondria-rich varicosities suggests that the energy demands of non-myelinated axons are high [123]. Mitochondria efficiently produce ATPs

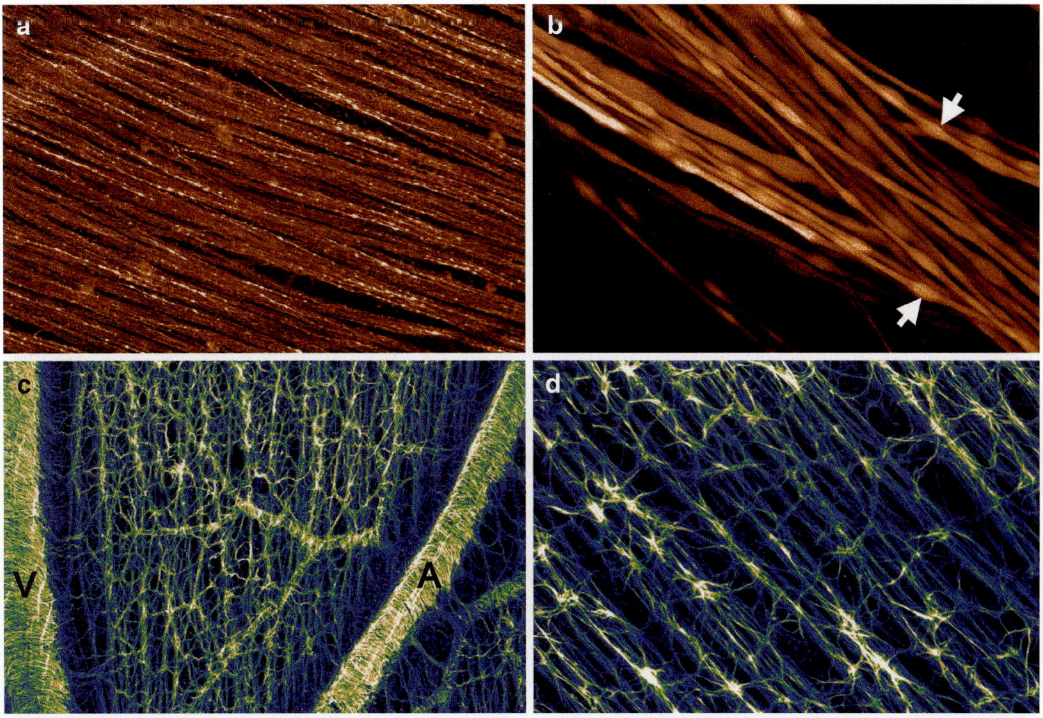

Fig. 1.5 Histology of retinal non-myelinated fibres. (**a**) Low magnification of flat mount staining of normal porcine retina with neurofilament medium illustrates the linear trajectory of non-myelinated axons. High magnification image shows numerous bulb-shaped varicosities (**b**), along the course of the axons (arrows). (**c**) Low and (**d**) high magnification images show the axons, astrocytes and blood vessels. Astrocyte processes were most prominent around vascular structures and run parallel to the direction of axons. Artery (A) and vein (V) are also marked. Reproduced with permission from [89]

through oxidative metabolism to provide high-energy support for non-myelinated axons. They also play a critical role in regulating intracellular calcium, pH and the production of reactive oxygen species, the control of neuronal excitability and synaptic transmission [124].

It has not been possible to determine oxygen consumption in non-myelinated axons in the NFL using intraretinal oxygen measurements and a diffusion model for the same reasons as that described for the RGC layer. However, in addition to the presence of high concentrations of mitochondria in the NFL, there are several other lines of evidence including histochemical evidence of COX activity, immunolabelling of cytochrome oxidase subunit Vic, presence of neuroglobin, presence of a relatively dense capillary network with additional radial peripapillary capillaries [107, 117] and presence of a dense network of astrocytic processes to suggest that the energy demands of non-myelinated RGC axons are likely to be high. There are complex relationships between non-myelinated axons, astrocytes and blood vessels [125]. Again, the delicate metabolic balance between energy demands and energy delivery places non-myelinated axons in a vulnerable position, particularly in the face of ischaemic insults.

Non-myelinated Axons in the Optic Nerve Head

A vast quantity of information about this compartment, non-myelinated axons in the ONH, has been acquired from clinical and animal studies. However, the complex structure of the ONH has posed some limitations in their interpretation. Many fundamental questions are yet to be completely answered.

The intricate embryological processes have been involved in optic nerve development resulting in the complex cellular relationships within the ONH. There are three sources for optic nerve development: RGC axons, which form the nerve proper; the neuroectodermal layers of the optic stalk, which form the glial system of the optic nerve and the associated mesoderm, which is composed of two components. One produces a condensation on the outer surface of the nerve that becomes the meninges; the other is an ingrowth of vascular connective tissue that forms the nerve septa [18]. Interestingly, the optic nerve continues to increase in size until 6–8 years of age.

There is a significant pressure gradient in the ONH. Normal IOP is ~15 mmHg and normal orbital pressure is usually much lower than IOP. Therefore, RGC axons in the ONH are exposed to two different pressure compartments. These compartments have their own unique pressure properties, namely IOP and cerebrospinal fluid pressure (CSFp), respectively, resulting in a pressure gradient that acts upon ONH. Our team has precisely measured the pressure gradient acting across the ONH using a servo-nulling device under a range of intraocular and CSF pressures [126–128]. We demonstrated that the pressure gradient largely falls across the lamina cribrosa.

In Fig. 1.6c, prelaminar (PL) pressure in the ONH is equivalent to IOP and postlaminar pressure (PoL) is equivalent to CSFp in the subarachnoid space. Trans-lamina cribrosa pressure gradient could therefore be determined by calculating the difference between IOP and CSFp. The lamina cribrosa region, characterized by dense laminar plates, is shaded in grey. The absolute pressure is high in the PL region while the pressure gradient falls across the lamina cribrosa. Anterior lamina cribrosa (ALc), posterior lamina cribrosa (PLc) and subarachnoid space (SAS) have also been identified. Figure 1.6c, d illustrates the likely tissue pressures and pressure gradients in the human ONH and pia mater. The pressure gradient in the human lamina cribrosa at an IOP of 15 mmHg is approximately 3.5 mmHg per 100 μm.

Knowledge about tissue pressures in the human ONH is of critical importance for understanding the effects of the tissue pressure on axonal function. It has been evidenced that axonal function is largely tolerant to absolute increases in tissue pressure but exquisitely sensitive to changes in pressure gradient. For example, an absolute pressure increase of 3800 mmHg does not affect nerve conduction or axonal transport [130]. But a pressure gradient of only 4.5 mmHg per 100 μm applied to the vagus nerve signifi-

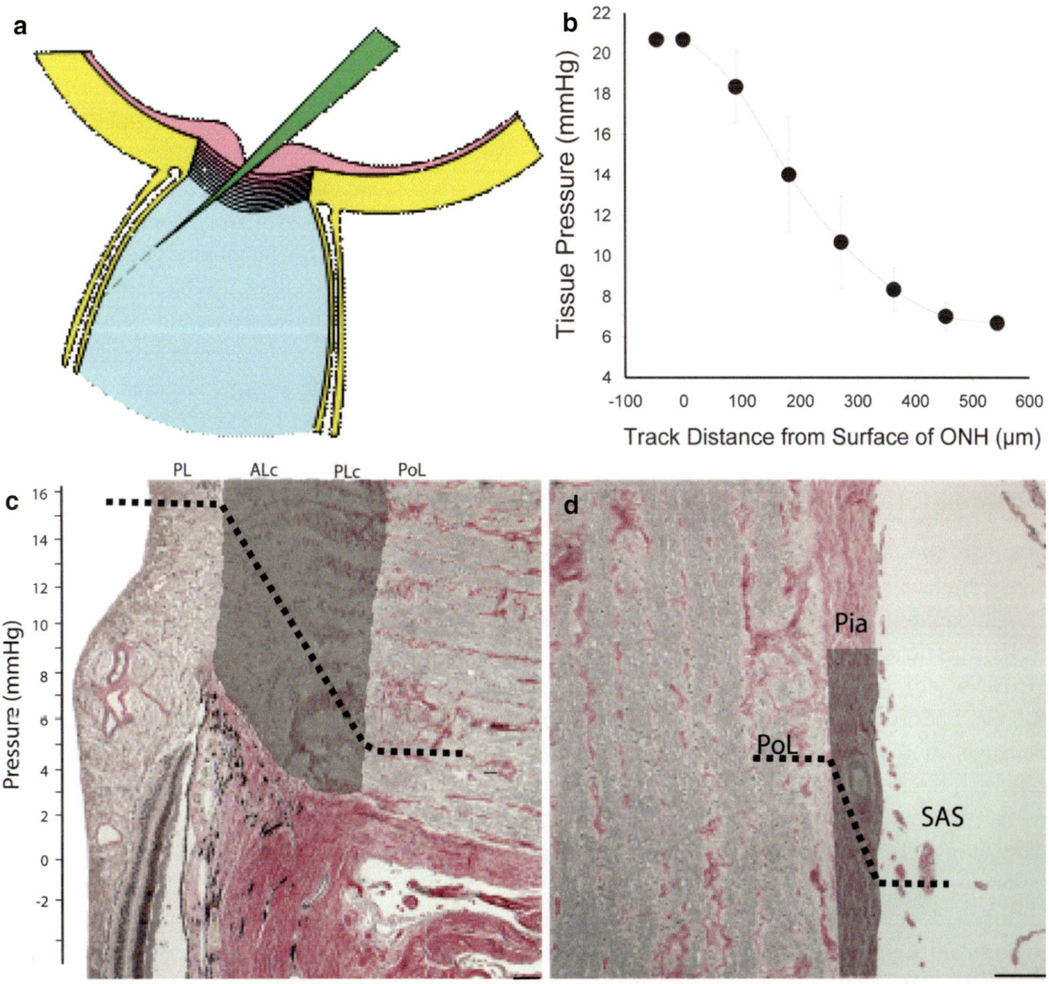

Fig. 1.6 Pressure gradients across the lamina cribrosa and pia mater. (**a**) A schematic drawing illustrating the experimental design used for measuring pressure gradients acting across the lamina cribrosa and pia mater using a servo-null pressure measurement system. (**b**) A typical result of tissue pressure measurements at various depths in the lamina cribrosa. (**c**) Predicted tissue pressure distributions in human laminar compartments [129]. (**d**) Schematic diagram illustrating the predicted distribution of tissue pressure across the pia mater (shaded in grey) of a normal human eye. Reproduced with permission from [89]

cantly retards orthograde axonal transport [131]. One explanation is a pressure-gradient induced reduction in neural perfusion [132] and epineural venular blood flow [133]. The other is a pressure-gradient induced deprivation of neurotrophic factors to the cell body due to axonal transport changes [134, 135].

The ONH has very densely packed axons occupying most of the space in the ONH, leaving limited space for the astrocytes, lamina cribrosa tissue and blood vessels. It is therefore understandable that sufficient blood supply could be a major challenge in this compartment. In addition to mechanical damage, ischaemic insults to the ONH remain a major cause of visual morbidity and for this reason the vascular supply to different laminar compartments of the optic nerve has been a subject of great interest [136, 137].

The central retinal artery (CRA) enters the optic nerve ~10 mm behind the eyeball. Each main posterior ciliary artery (PCA) divides into ~10–20 short PCAs. The ONH is predominantly supplied by the CRA and short PCAs. The ONH can be divided into four regions: the superficial nerve fibre layer, the prelaminar, laminar and retrolaminar regions with different blood supplies. The superficial nerve fibre layer is supplied by the CRA's branches. Short PCAs and branches from the arterial circle of Zinn-Haller supply the prelaminar portion. The laminar region's blood supply is similar to that of the prelaminar region. Small arterioles perforate the lamina cribrosa. These arterioles to the laminar region may also from peripapillary choroid. The retrolaminar region is supplied by pial arteries and the short PCA's branches. Pial arteries that supply the ONH may branch from the CRA, the ophthalmic artery and the PCAs [138]. With regard to venous drainage, the central retinal vein almost exclusively drains all structures in the ONH.

Although there is constrained space in the ONH, the density of capillary networks in the ONH is still greater than most structures in the CNS. This may reflect the high metabolic demands of the ONH. It is also apparent that different laminar regions have significant differences in capillary density and morphometric parameters. The capillaries of the superficial and prelaminar regions are complex and randomly arranged, whereas the capillaries of the laminar region conform to the pattern of the connective tissue septa of the lamina cribrosa. Our knowledge is still limited regarding many aspects of ONH vascular supply, neurovascular coupling and regulatory mechanisms. For instance, why the capillaries within the laminar beams are separated from the astrocytic processes by a large amount of connective tissue remains to be explained [138].

1.4.5.4 Myelinated Axons in the Orbit and the Cranial Region

There are several important distinctions between myelinated and non-myelinated axons. Non-myelinated axons have a significantly smaller diameter and larger surface area per volume when compared with myelinated fibres. In non-myelinated axons, the satellite cell makes just a single wrap around the axon, while in myelinated axons the oligodendrocyte membrane is arranged in a multi-lamellar spiral fashion around the axon. These morphological differences lead to two distinct types of action potential propagation and action current flow in local circuits. In myelinated axons, the sheath is interrupted regularly along the axonal length by nodes of Ranvier, while in non-myelinated axons, action currents flowing in local circuits progressively depolarize neighbouring regions of the membrane and the impulse travels continuously along the axon. In the central nervous system, the predominant cell type that ensheathes axons are oligodendrocytes [139].

Interestingly, the energy required to sustain axonal processes is dependent upon membrane area [139]. The majority of small calibre fibres in the optic nerve are derived from the papillomacular bundle and represent central vision. They have a relatively thin myelin sheath, a rapid rate of firing [140] and a relatively low volume (energy source) to surface area (energy demand) ratio. Energy demands of these fibres are significantly greater than that in other fibres in the optic nerve [140].

The optic nerve from the disc to the chiasm can be divided into four parts: the intraocular nerve (~1 mm long and ~1.5 mm in diameter); the intraorbital nerve (~25 mm in length and ~3 to 4 mm in diameter); the intracanalicular nerve (~4 to 10 mm in length) and the intracranial nerve (~10 mm and ~4 to 7 mm in diameter) [18]. The optic nerve acquires a myelin sheath posterior the lamina cribrosa and is the major determinant of optic nerve diameter. Myelination patterns also vary significantly between the intraocular, intraorbital and intracranial portions.

The velocity of action potential conduction is increased with RGC axon myelination. It is estimated that conduction velocity in myelinated axons is ~3.3 to 10 m/s while that in non-myelinated axons ~0.45 to 1.2 m/s [144]. Energy consumption by myelinated axons is significantly less than in non-myelinated axons.

Myelinated Axons in the Orbit

In the orbit the optic nerve acquires a meningeal sheath which is comprised of dura, pia and arachnoid mater. The arachnoid layer is more closely related to the dura than to the pia mater. The dura mater merges with the outer two thirds of the sclera. The pia and arachnoid mater terminates just before the globe at the lamina cribrosa. CSF is found in the subarachnoid space between pia and arachnoid mater [90]. It may play an important role in nourishing the myelinated optic nerve as well as minimizing stress/strain forces in the optic nerve caused by extraocular muscle movement.

In the orbit, a number of different structures including the rectus muscles and the nasociliary nerve are in contact with the optic nerve and its sheaths. RGC axons are surrounded by glial processes, and organized into segregated bundles at the ONH. Further reinforcement of these bundles begins at the lamina cribrosa where connective tissue septa surround axons.

A pressure gradient exists across the pia mater of the optic nerve. However, it is unlikely that myelinated RGC axons are influenced by the trans-laminar pressure gradient because optic nerve myelination occurs posterior to the lamina cribrosa. Consequently, the susceptibility and response of myelinated and non-myelinated RGC axons could be different. It is possible that IOP is a major modulator of energetics in non-myelinated RGC axons while CSFp may have a greater influence in the functioning of myelinated axons.

Myelinated Axons in the Cranial Region

The environment and structures that surround the orbital and cranial portions of the optic nerve are vastly different. The dura mater is in direct contact with surrounding bone and firmly anchors the nerve to the canal wall in the optic nerve canal. However, the dural sheath at the orbital end of the optic canal separates into two layers: one layer fuses with the orbital periosteum and the other continues as the dural sheath of the nerve. The arachnoid is attenuated in the intracanalicular portion, whereas the dura leaves the nerve to become continuous with the cranial dura in the intracranial portion.

Metabolic activities and energy demands of the lateral geniculate neurons may differ between the species and functional pathways [141]. Regional differences in cytochrome c oxidase staining in the lateral geniculate nucleus have been described. The visual cortex is one of the high-energy demand regions in the brain with richly blood supply. Both capillary diameter and capillary density are higher in layer IV, which has the intense level of cytochrome c oxidase activity [141].

1.5 Other Key Structures of Relevance to Glaucoma

Figure 1.7 schematically illustrates some of these critical anatomic and physiological parameters which are highly relevant to understanding the pathogenesis of primary angle closure glaucoma (PACG).

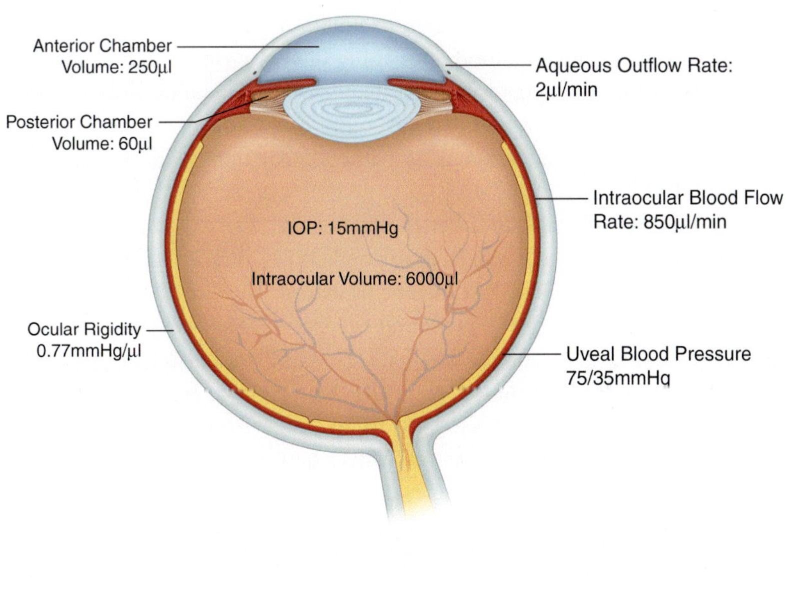

Fig. 1.7 Important parameters relevant to PACG. A schematic drawing to show some critical parameters including ocular rigidity, volume distributions and aqueous and blood flow in the normal eye. Adapted from [142]

These parameters including ocular rigidity, volume distributions and aqueous and blood flow could be useful for predicting the risk of glaucoma, particularly PACG and guide therapeutic strategies. Both the cornea and sclera are dense connective tissues. In fact, most of the intraocular contents such as aqueous humour, vitreous and tissues are almost incompressible and covered by a relatively rigid cornea and sclera. The cornea covers the anterior 1/6th of the total surface area of the globe, while the sclera covers the remaining 5/6ths [143]. The ocular rigidity is ~0.77 mmHg/μl meaning tiny intraocular volume changes could induce significant increase of IOP [144]. The volume of the anterior chamber (250 μl) and posterior chamber (60 μl) is a small fraction of the intraocular volume (6000 μl) [144]. However, the iris is a delicate and movable diaphragm between the anterior and posterior chambers [18] and the lens is suspended in the anterior of the eye by a band of inelastic microfibrils, the zonules. The iris and lens could be moved anteriorly if the volume and pressure increase in the vitreous. The ocular circulation has high intraocular blood flow rate (850 μl/min) in order to support the high demands of the neural retina and avascular tissues in the anterior segments such as lens and cornea. Aqueous outflow rate is about 2 μl/min. Uvea including iris, ciliary body and choroid has rich blood vasculature and uveal blood pressure (systolic 75 mmHg and diastolic 35 mmHg) is higher than normal IOP (15 mmHg). Therefore, input and output fluid including aqueous production and outflow drainage and blood circulation have to be dynamical. Some pathological changes in the iris and choroidal flow and volume could disturb such a delicate balance and be pathogenic factors in PACG.

Arguably, we are now in a better position to investigate the effects of changes in iris and choroid in the pathogenesis of PACG. The structure changes of anterior segment including the geometrics of angle, iris, cornea and lens as well as choroid can be determined clinically using current imaging techniques allowing us to further understand the pathogenesis of PACG and develop new and targeted strategies to manage different stages of the disease.

1.5.1 The Choroid

Choroidal thickness changes, particularly in the macular region, have been studied in different types of PACG. Figure 1.8 illustrates a proposed mechanism of choroidal volume changes inducing PACG. The area of choroid is about 1000 mm^2, which is at least seven times larger than the area of the iris. Increased choroidal volume could induce significant changes in the anterior segment. The area of the iris in Asians is smaller than in Caucasians. Therefore, a small amount of choroidal volume change may cause significant movement of iris diaphragm and lens anteriorly. The iris diaphragm and lens could move forward and also change iris shape (Fig. 1.8b2, b3) from the initial position (Fig. 1.8b1) resulting in pupil block and angle closure. Increased choroidal thickness/volume could very likely be a critical pathogenic factor.

The choroid has a circulation rate 10–20 times that of cerebral cortex and has one of the greatest blood supply rates per tissue volume in the human body [145]. Multiple mechanisms of choroidal volume increase have been proposed including changes in synthesis of osmotically active molecules, increased vascular permeability, fluid flux from the anterior chamber to choroid, movement of fluid across the RPE and changes in the tonus of non-vascular smooth muscle from experimental models [146]. Recently, we have proposed a new mechanism involving changes of the vortex vein system, a major control site in drainage pathway of choroidal circulation [147]. The choroid plays a vital role in sustaining the outer retina's high metabolic demands [110, 148, 149]. There are only 4–6 vortex veins and a large volume of choroidal blood flow must drain into each individual vortex vein.

1.5.2 The Vortex Vein System

The vortex veins drain blood from the choroid and also from some of the anterior portion of the eye. Numerous choroidal veins and some veins from the anterior portion converge into a larger ampulla, then through the scleral channel, finally connecting to the vortex veins which are located outside of the eyeball. The vortex vein system

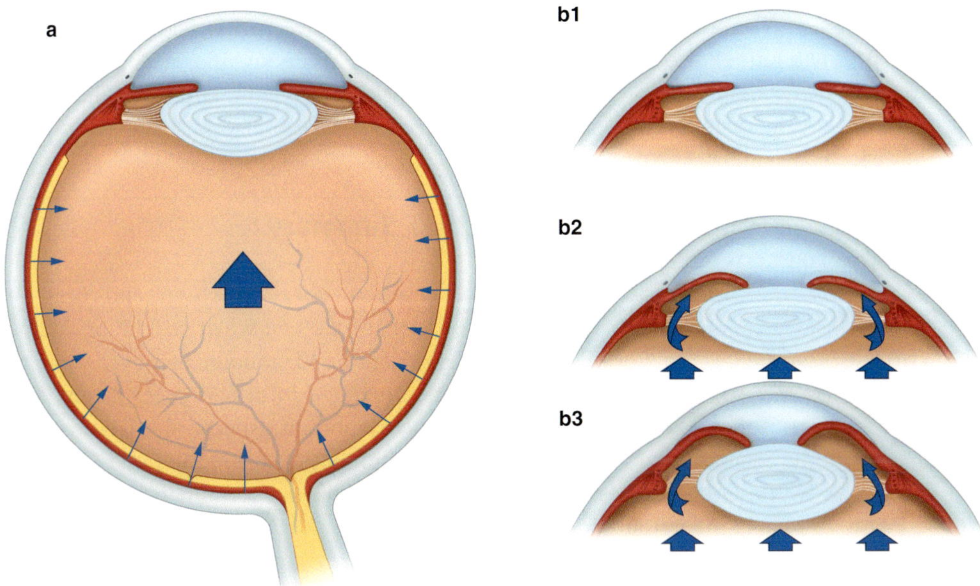

Fig. 1.8 Possible explanation of mechanism of choroidal volume change induced PACG. (**a**) The small arrows indicate choroidal volume expansion, creating a larger forward movement of the lens and iris. Thus, a small change in choroidal thickness can create a significant forward displacement of the lens and iris. (**b1**) Normal situation. (**b2**) Forward displacement. (**b3**) Angle closure. Adapted from [142]

includes all the intraocular, intrascleral and extraocular portions of the drainage pathway [18, 143, 150]. The vortex vein system is a geometrically complex system which includes different regions.

Functionally, the vortex vein system has a major role in maintaining an optimal choroidal blood volume. It must also cope with passing through intraocular, scleral and orbital tissues of different rigidity and significant pressure gradients as it transverses from the intraocular to the extraocular compartments. It is expected that the flow patterns and haemodynamic forces could be significantly non-uniform in the different regions of the geometrically complex vortex vein system.

It is important to investigate how the vortex vein system works under such complex situations in both physiological and pathological condition. The best approach to explore the vortex vein system is to study the regional phenotype heterogeneity in the different regions of vascular endothelial cells. The vortex vein system endothelium had not previously been studied in detail. Nor were the site-specific endothelial phenotypes within the vortex vein system [65, 151–153]. The endothelial intracellular cytoskeleton proteins, cell shape and nuclei position, along with smooth muscle cell distribution have been studied in different regions of the vortex vein system in human donor eyes [151]. The different regions include the choroidal veins, pre-ampulla, ampulla, post-ampulla, scleral entrance, intrascleral channel, scleral exit and extrascleral vortex vein. We found remarkable regional differences of endothelial phenotype and smooth muscle cells distribution in the vortex vein system [151, 152]. These results suggest that distinct haemodynamic changes occur and are very likely to be a control site for the choroidal circulation.

Vascular endothelial cells are vital for normal physiological function. Given the incidence of venous pathology is about 10 times higher than arterial disease, it is important to study the very significant but undervalued vortex vein system. We believe such significant regional differences of endothelial phenotype indicate that haemodynamic conditions are dramatically different. Such sites could be vulnerable site for developing site-specific endothelial dysfunction and induce choroidal volume changes. Certainly, the vortex vein system is an interesting research field for glaucoma and retinal diseases.

We also need to develop clinical assess to evaluate the vortex vein system and determine the role in choroidal thickness changes and PACG. Recent non-invasive imaging techniques have provided some insights suggesting a possible role in the pathogenesis of PACG.

1.5.3 The Iris

Some specific features of the iris are relevant to fluid exchange with the aqueous humour and iris volume changes as we described. It is interesting to know how to maintain a certain concentration gradient of each molecule in aqueous humour if there is no apparent diffusion barrier between the interstitial spaces of the iris and the anterior chamber. Some studies have supported the pathway that plasma constituents diffuse from the ciliary body stroma into the iris stroma and, finally, into the anterior chamber [8, 24]. Some molecules can selectively be transported through iris endothelium [24]. The iris microvasculature, particularly its endothelium, may play a role in selective transport, but this needs to be further explored. Recently, we have studied the iris vasculature and found that the iris has high density microvasculature and an unusual vascular distribution [15–17]. Abundant relatively large vessels are located in the middle of the iris stroma supplying the microvasculature in both superficial sides of stroma and pupil edge within a short distance. Large diameter capillaries and relatively long spindle-shaped endothelial cells have been found in different orders of the iris vasculature. All these findings suggest that iris microvasculature has high blood flow rate and high capability for sufficient nutrient and waste exchange between the blood stream and the iris stroma. It also indicates that the iris volume could be changed during the pathological condition and play pathogeneses of PACG.

Significant change in iris volume has been observed using imaging techniques, and has been postulated to be a major pathogenic factor for PACG [22, 154–158]. The dynamic processes leading to changes in iris and choroid volume could have a more significant and mechanistic effect to its surrounding structures than a mere anatomical observation [154, 159].

1.6 Summary

We describe some structural and functional properties of the eye which are highly relevant to glaucoma, and attempt to cover both general and updated information regarding two of the most important aspects, the RGCs and the aqueous humour. The structure and function of the iris and choroid have only briefly described, but we believe that the importance of the uvea in glaucoma research and clinical practice will be recognized following improved knowledge of the role of vascular endothelial cells and more advanced image techniques. Glaucoma is an aetiologically complex disorder of optic neuropathies with multiple ocular structures involved. It is impossible to cover wide and detailed information at the cellular, molecular and genetic levels associated with functional changes in a single chapter. Knowledge of glaucoma related ocular structure and function could be fundamentally important for understanding glaucoma and for improvements of glaucoma management, including diagnostics and therapeutics.

References

1. Quigley HA. Open-Angle Glaucoma. N Engl J Med. 1993;328(15):1097–106.
2. Vidal-Sanz M, Salinas-Navarro M, Nadal-Nicolas FM, Alarcon-Martinez L, Valiente-Soriano FJ, de Imperial JM, et al. Understanding glaucomatous damage: anatomical and functional data from ocular hypertensive rodent retinas. Prog Retin Eye Res. 2012;31(1):1–27.
3. Hood DC. Improving our understanding, and detection, of glaucomatous damage: An approach based upon optical coherence tomography (OCT). Prog Retin Eye Res. 2017;57:46–75.
4. Xin C, Wang RK, Song S, Shen T, Wen J, Martin E, et al. Aqueous outflow regulation: Optical coherence tomography implicates pressure-dependent tissue motion. Exp Eye Res. 2017;158:171–86.

5. Toris CB. Aqueous Humor Dynamics I: Measurement Methods and Animal Studies. Curr Top Membr. 2008;62:193–229.
6. Toris CB, Camras CB. Aqueous Humor Dynamics II Clinical Studies. Curr Top Membr. 2008;62:231–72.
7. Coca-Prados M, Escribano J. New perspectives in aqueous humor secretion and in glaucoma: the ciliary body as a multifunctional neuroendocrine gland. Prog Retin Eye Res. 2007;26(3):239–62.
8. Freddo TF, Bartels SP, Barsotti MF, Kamm RD. The source of proteins in the aqueous humor of the normal rabbit. Invest Ophthalmol Vis Sci. 1990;31(1): 125–37.
9. Collins R, Van der Werff TJ. Lecture notes in biomathematics. New York: Springer; 1980. p. 1–94.
10. Barany E, Kinsey VE. Rate of flow of aqueous humor. 1. The rate of disappearance of para-aminohippuric acid, radioactive Rayopake, and radioactive Diodrast from the aqueous humor of rabbits. Am J Ophthalmol. 1949;32(6):177–88.
11. Kinsey VE, Barany E. The rate of flow of aqueous humor II. Derivation of rate of flow and its physiologic significance. Am J Ophthalmol. 1949;32:189–202.
12. Moses RA. Adler's physiology of the eye. 5th ed. St. Louis: C.V. Mosby; 1970.
13. Kiel JW, Hollingsworth M, Rao R, Chen M, Reitsamer HA. Ciliary blood flow and aqueous humor production. Prog Retin Eye Res. 2011;30(1):1–17.
14. Gabelt BT, Kaufman PL. Changes in aqueous humor dynamics with age and glaucoma. Prog Retin Eye Res. 2005;24(5):612–37.
15. Yang H, Yu PK, Cringle SJ, Sun X, Yu DY. Quantitative study of the microvasculature and its endothelial cells in the porcine iris. Exp Eye Res. 2015;132C:249–58.
16. Yang H, Yu PK, Cringle SJ, Sun X, Yu D-Y. Iridal vasculature and the vital roles of the iris. J Nat Sci. 2015;1(8):e157.
17. Yang H, Yu PK, Cringle SJ, Sun X, Yu DY. Intracellular cytoskeleton and junction proteins of endothelial cells in the porcine iris microvasculature. Exp Eye Res. 2015;140:106–16.
18. Hogan MJ, Alvarado JA, Weddell JE. Histology of the human eye: an atlas and textbook, vol. 1971. Philadelphia: W.B. Saunders Company; 1971.
19. Tousimis AJ, Fine BS. Ultrastructure of the iris: the intercellular stromal components. Arch Ophthalmol. 1959;62:974–6.
20. Vrabec F. The anterior superficial endothelium of the human iris. Ophthalmologica. 1952;123(1):20–30.
21. Freddo TF. Ultrastructure of the iris. Microsc Res Tech. 1996;33(5):369–89.
22. Oyster CW. The human eye, structure and function. Ophthalmic Physiol Opt. 2000;20(4):349–50.
23. Tasman W, Jaeger EA, editors. Duane's clinical ophthalmology on CD-ROM. Philadelphia: Lippincott Williams & Wilkins; 2005.
24. Raviola G, Butler JM. Morphological evidence for the transfer of anionic macromolecules from the interior of the eye to the blood stream. Curr Eye Res. 1985;4(4):503–16.
25. Freddo TF. A contemporary concept of the blood-aqueous barrier. Prog Retin Eye Res. 2013;32:181–95.
26. Vanderkooi JM, Erecinska M, Silver IA. Oxygen in mammalian tissue-methods of measurement and affinities of various reactions. Am J Physiol. 1991;260(6):C1131–C50.
27. Abu-Amero KK, Morales J, Bosley TM. Mitochondrial abnormalities in patients with primary open-angle glaucoma. Invest Ophthalmol Vis Sci. 2006;47(6):2533–41.
28. Andersen JK. Oxidative stress in neurodegeneration: cause or consequence? Nat Med. 2004;10(Suppl):S18–25.
29. Turrens JF. Mitochondrial formation of reactive oxygen species. J Physiol. 2003;552(Pt 2):335–44.
30. Leung BK, Bonanno JA, Radke CJ. Oxygen-deficient metabolism and corneal edema. Prog Retin Eye Res. 2011;30(6):471–92.
31. Chhabra M, Prausnitz JM, Radke CJ. Modeling corneal metabolism and oxygen transport during contact lens wear. Optom Vis Sci. 2009;86(5):454–66.
32. Chhabra M, Prausnitz JM, Radke CJ. Diffusion and Monod kinetics to determine in vivo human corneal oxygen-consumption rate during soft contact-lens wear. J Biomed Mater Res B Appl Biomater. 2009;90(1):202–9.
33. Alvord LA, Hall WJ, Keyes LD, Morgan CF, Winterton LC. Corneal oxygen distribution with contact lens wear. Cornea. 2007;26(6):654–64.
34. Shui YB, Fu JJ, Garcia C, Dattilo LK, Rajagopal R, McMillan S, et al. Oxygen distribution in the rabbit eye and oxygen consumption by the lens. Invest Ophthalmol Vis Sci. 2006;47(4):1571–80.
35. Bonanno JA, Stickel T, Nguyen T, Biehl T, Carter D, Benjamin WJ, et al. Estimation of human corneal oxygen consumption by noninvasive measurement of tear oxygen tension while wearing hydrogel lenses. Invest Ophthalmol Vis Sci. 2002;43(2):371–6.
36. Stefansson E, Foulks GN, Hamilton RC. The effect of corneal contact lenses on the oxygen tension in the anterior chamber of the rabbit eye. Invest Ophthalmol Vis Sci. 1987;28(10):1716–9.
37. Siegfried CJ, Shui YB, Holekamp NM, Bai F, Beebe DC. Oxygen distribution in the human eye: relevance to the etiology of open-angle glaucoma after vitrectomy. Invest Ophthalmol Vis Sci. 2010;51(11): 5731–8.
38. Chang S. LXII Edward Jackson lecture: open angle glaucoma after vitrectomy. Am J Ophthalmol. 2006;141(6):1033–43.
39. Luk FO, Kwok AK, Lai TY, Lam DS. Presence of crystalline lens as a protective factor for the late development of open angle glaucoma after vitrectomy. Retina. 2009;29(2):218–24.
40. Holekamp NM, Shui YB, Beebe DC. Vitrectomy surgery increases oxygen exposure to the lens: a possible mechanism for nuclear cataract formation. Am J Ophthalmol. 2005;139(2):302–10.
41. Barbazetto IA, Liang J, Chang S, Zheng L, Spector A, Dillon JP. Oxygen tension in the rabbit lens and

vitreous before and after vitrectomy. Exp Eye Res. 2004;78(5):917–24.
42. McNulty R, Wang H, Mathie RT, Ortwerth B, Truscott RJW, Bassnett S. regulation of tissue oxygen levels in the mammalian lens. J Physiol. 2004;559(3):883–98.
43. Edelhauser HF. Cornea and lens oxygen consumption in rabbit and trout: a comparative study. Exp Eye Res. 1974;19:317–22.
44. Freeman RD. Oxygen consumption by the component layers of the cornea. J Physiol. 1972;225(1):15–32.
45. Izzotti A, Longobardi M, Cartiglia C, Sacca SC. Mitochondrial damage in the trabecular meshwork occurs only in primary open-angle glaucoma and in pseudoexfoliative glaucoma. PLoS One. 2011;6(1):e14567.
46. Yu DY, Morgan WH, Sun X, Su EN, Cringle SJ, Yu PK, et al. The critical role of the conjunctiva in glaucoma filtration surgery. Prog Retin Eye Res. 2009;28(5):303–28.
47. Niederkorn JY. Mechanisms of immune privilege in the eye and hair follicle. J Investig Dermatol Symp Proc. 2003;8:168–72.
48. Dermietzel R, Spray DC, Nedergaard M. The blood-brain barrier: an integrated concept. In: Dermietzel R, Spray DC, Nedergaard M, editors. Blood-brain interfaces: from ontogeny to artificial barriers. Weinheim: Wiley; 2006.
49. Streilein JW. Immunological non-responsiveness and acquisition of tolerance in relation to immune privilege in the eye. Eye. 1995;9(Pt 2):236–40.
50. Streilein JW. Ocular immune priviledge: therapeutic opportunities from an experiment of nature. Nat Rev Immunol. 2003;3(November):879–89.
51. Fautsch MP, Johnson DH, Group tSAPRIW. Aqueous humor outflow: what do we know? where will it lead us? Biophys J. 2004;87:2828–37.
52. Bill A. The drainage of aqueous humor. Investig Ophthalmol. 1975;14(1):1–3.
53. Stamer WD. The biology of Schlemm's canal. Amsterdam: Elsevier Ltd.; 2010.
54. Rohen JW, Schachtschabel DO, Berghoff K. Histoautoradiographic and biochemical studies on human and monkey trabecular meshwork and ciliary body in short-term explant culture. Graefes Arch Clin Exp Ophthalmol. 1984;221:199–206.
55. Rohen JW, van der Zypen E. The phagocytic activity of the trabecular meshwork endothelium: an elecron microscopic study of the vervet (*Cercopithecus aethiops)*. Graefes Arch Clin Exp Ophthalmol. 1968;175:143.
56. Broadway DC, Grierson I, Hitchings RA. Local effects of previous conjunctival incisional surgery and the subsequent outcome of filtration surgery. Am J Ophthalmol. 1998;125:805–18.
57. Grierson I, Lee WR. Further observations on the process of haemophagocytosis in the human outflow system. Graefes Arch Clin Exp Ophthalmol. 1978;208:49–64.
58. Grierson I, Lee WR. Erythrocyte phagocytosis in the human trabecular meshwork. Br J Ophthalmol. 1973;57:400–15.
59. Lee WR, Grierson I, McMenamin PG. The morphological response of the primate outflow system to changes in pressure and flow. In: Lutjen-Drecoll E, editor. Basic aspects of glaucoma research. Stuttgart: Schattauert Verlag; 1982.
60. Lutjen-Drecoll E, Futa R, Rohen JW. Ultrahistochemical studies on tangential sections of the trabecular meshwork in normal and glaucomatous eyes. Invest Ophthalmol Vis Sci. 1981;21:563–73.
61. Quigley HA, Addicks EM. Chronic experimenal glaucoma in pimates. I. Production of elevated intraocular pressure by anterior chamber injection of autologous ghost red blood cells. Invest Ophthalmol Vis Sci. 1980;19:126–36.
62. Shabo AL, Maxwell DS. Observations on the fate of blood in the anterior chamber: a light and electron microscopic study of the monkey trabecular meshwork. Am J Ophthalmol. 1972;73:25–36.
63. Sherwood M, Richardson TM. Kinetics of the phagocytic process in the trabecular meshwork of cats and monkeys. Invest Ophthalmol Vis Sci. 1981;20(Suppl):65.
64. Vegge T. The fine structure of the trabeculum cribriforme and the inner wall of Schlemm's canal in the normal human eye. Z Zellforsch. 1967;77:267–81.
65. Yu DY, Yu PK, Cringle SJ, Kang MH, Su EN. Functional and morphological characteristics of the retinal and choroidal vasculature. Prog Retin Eye Res. 2014;40:53–93.
66. Ramos RF, Hoying JB, Witte MH, Daniel Stamer W. Schlemm's canal endothelia, lymphatic, or blood vasculature? J Glaucoma. 2007;16(4):391–405.
67. Alvarado JA, Betanzos A, Franse-Carman L, Chen J, Gonzalez-Mariscal L. Endothelia of Schlemm's canal and trabecular meshwork: distinct molecular, functional, and anatomic features. Am J Physiol Cell Physiol. 2004;286(3):C621–34.
68. Ethier CR, Read AT, Chan D. Biomechanics of Schlemm's canal endothelial cells: influence on F-actin architecture. Biophys J. 2004;87(4):2828–37.
69. Ashton N. Anatomical study of Schlemm's canal and aqueous veins by means of neoprene casts. Part I. Aqueous veins. Br J Ophthalmol. 1951;35:291–303.
70. Dvorak-Theobald G. Schlemm's canal: its anastomoses and anatomic relations. Trans Am Ophthalmol Soc. 1934;32:574–95.
71. Krohn J, Rodahl E. Expression of 5′-nucleotidase and alkaline phosphatase in human aqueous drainage channels. Acta Ophthalmol Scand. 2002;80(6):642–51.
72. Bentley MD, Hann CR, Fautsch MP. Anatomical variation of human collector channel orifices. Invest Ophthalmol Vis Sci. 2016;57(3):1153–9.
73. Dvorak-Theobald G, Kirk HQ. Aqueous pathways in some cases of glaucoma. Trans Am Ophthalmol Soc. 1955;53:301–19.
74. Dvorak-Theobald G. Further studies on the canal of Schlemm: its anastomoses and anatomic relations. Am J Ophthalmol. 1955;39:65–89.

75. Ascher KW. Aqueous veins: preliminary note. Am J Ophthalmol. 1942;25:33–8.
76. Kagemann L, Wollstein G, Ishikawa H, Sigal IA, Folio LS, Xu J, et al. 3D visualization of aqueous humor outflow structures in-situ in humans. Exp Eye Res. 2011;93(3):308–15.
77. Ethier CR. The inner wall of Schlemm's canal. Exp Eye Res. 2002;74(2):161–72.
78. Johnson M, Erickson K. Mechanisms and routes of aqueous humor drainage. Aqueous humor and the dynamics of its flow. 2006. p. 2577–95.
79. Johnstone M, Martin E, Jamil A. Pulsatile flow into the aqueous veins: manifestations in normal and glaucomatous eyes. Exp Eye Res. 2011;92(5):318–27.
80. Bill A, Phillips CI. Uveoscleral drainage of aqueous humour in human eyes. Exp Eye Res. 1971;12:275–81.
81. Bill A. Aqueous humor dynamics in monkeys *(Macaca irus* and *Cercopithecus ethiops)*. Exp Eye Res. 1971;11:195–206.
82. Bill A. The routes for bulk drainage of aqueous humour in the vervet monkey *(Cercopithecus ethiops)*. Exp Eye Res. 1966;5:55–7.
83. Bill A. Conventional and Uveo-scleral drainage of aqueoue humour in the Cynomolgus monkey (Macaca irus) at normal and high intraocular pressures. Exp Eye Res. 1966;5:45–54.
84. Bill A, Hellsing K. Production and drainage of aqueous humor in the cynomolgus monkey (Macaca irus). Investig Ophthalmol. 1965;4(5):920–6.
85. Bill A. The aqueous humor drainage mechanism in the cynomolgus monkey (*Macaca irus*) with evidence for unconventional routes. Investig Ophthalmol. 1965;4:911.
86. Alm A, Nilsson SF. Uveoscleral outflow--a review. Exp Eye Res. 2009;88(4):760–8.
87. Bill A. Uveoscleral drainage of aqueous humor: physiology and pharmacology. Prog Clin Biol Res. 1989;312:417–27.
88. London A, Benhar I, Schwartz M. The retina as a window to the brain-from eye research to CNS disorders. Nat Rev Neurol. 2013;9(1):44–53.
89. Yu DY, Cringle SJ, Balaratnasingam C, Morgan WH, Yu PK, Su EN. Retinal ganglion cells: energetics, compartmentation, axonal transport, cytoskeletons and vulnerability. Prog Retin Eye Res. 2013;36:217–46.
90. Hein K, Bäher M. Optic nerve: optic neuritis. In: Dartt DA, editor. Encyclopedia of the eye. Oxford: Academic; 2010. p. 205–9.
91. Friede RL. The relationship of body size, nerve cell size, axon length, and glial density in the cerebellum. Proc Natl Acad Sci U S A. 1963;49(2):187–93.
92. Friedrich P. Dynamic compartmentation in soluble multienzyme systems. In: Welch GR, editor. Organized multienzyme systems: catalytic properties. Biotechnology and applied biochemistry series. Orlando: Academic; 1985. p. 141–76.
93. Kellermayer M, Ludany A, Jobst K, Szucs G, Trombitas K, Hazlewood CF. Cocompartmentation of proteins and K+ within the living cell. Proc Natl Acad Sci U S A. 1986;83(4):1011–5.
94. Bereiter-Hahn J, Vöth M. Dynamics of mitochondria in living cells: shape changes, dislocations, fusion and fission of mitochondria. Microsc Res Tech. 1994;27:198–219.
95. Whitmore AV, Libby RT, John SW. Glaucoma: thinking in new ways-a role for autonomous axonal self-destruction and other compartmentalised processes? Prog Retin Eye Res. 2005;24(6):639–62.
96. Dubbin PN, Cody SH, Williams DA. Intracellular pH mapping with SNARF-1 and confocal microscopy. II: pH gradients within single cultured cells. Micron. 1993;24(6):581–6.
97. Iturriaga R, Rumsey WL, Lahiri S, Spergel D, Wilson DF. Intracellular pH and oxygen chemoreception in the cat carotid body in vitro. J Appl Physiol. 1992;72(6):2259–66.
98. Clegg JS. Intracellular water and the cytomatrix: some methods of study and current views. J Cell Biol. 1984;99(1 Pt 2):167s–71s.
99. Clegg JS. On the internal environment of animal cells. In: Jones DP, editor. Microcompartmentation. Boca Raton: CRC Press; 1988. p. 1–16.
100. Jones DP, Aw TY. Mitochondrial distribution and O_2 gradients in mammalian cells. In: Jones DP, editor. Microcompartmentation. Boca Raton: CRC Press; 1988. p. 37–54.
101. Minaschek G, Groschel-Stewart U, Blum S, Bereiter-Hahn J. Microcompartmentation of glycolytic enzymes in cultured cells. Eur J Cell Biol. 1992;58(2):418–28.
102. Wang JT, Medress ZA, Barres BA. Axon degeneration: molecular mechanisms of a self-destruction pathway. J Cell Biol. 2012;196(1):7–18.
103. Shetty PK, Galeffi F, Turner DA. Cellular links between neuronal activity and energy homeostasis. Front Pharmacol. 2012;3:43.
104. Allen NJ, Barres BA. Glia and synapse formation: an overview. In: Editor-in-Chief:-á-álarry RS, editor. Encyclopedia of neuroscience. Oxford: Academic; 2009. p. 731–6.
105. Attwell D, Buchan AM, Charpak S, Lauritzen M, Macvicar BA, Newman EA. Glial and neuronal control of brain blood flow. Nature. 2010;468(7321):232–43.
106. Wollner DA, Catterall WA. Localization of sodium channels in axon hillocks and initial segments of retinal ganglion cells. Proc Natl Acad Sci U S A. 1986;83(21):8424–8.
107. Tan PE, Yu PK, Balaratnasingam C, Cringle SJ, Morgan WH, McAllister IL, et al. Quantitative confocal imaging of the retinal microvasculature in the human retina. Invest Ophthalmol Vis Sci. 2012;53(9):5728–36.
108. Yu DY, Cringle SJ, Alder VA, Su EN. Intraretinal oxygen distribution in rats as a function of systemic blood pressure. Am J Phys. 1994;267(6 Pt 2).H2498–H507.
109. Yu DY, Cringle SJ, Yu PK, Su EN. Intraretinal oxygen distribution and consumption during retinal artery occlusion and graded hyperoxic ventilation in the rat. Invest Ophthalmol Vis Sci. 2007;48(5):2290–6.

110. Yu DY, Cringle SJ. Oxygen distribution and consumption within the retina in vascularised and avascular retinas and in animal models of retinal disease. Prog Retin Eye Res. 2001;20(2):175–208.
111. Morgan JE. Retina ganglion cell degeneration in glaucoma: an opportunity missed? a review. Clin Exp Ophthalmol. 2012;40(4):364–8.
112. Stevens B, Allen NJ, Vazquez LE, Howell GR, Christopherson KS, Nouri N, et al. The classical complement cascade mediates CNS synapse elimination. Cell. 2007;131(6):1164–78.
113. Osborne NN, Casson RJ, Wood JP, Chidlow G, Graham M, Melena J. Retinal ischemia: mechanisms of damage and potential therapeutic strategies. Prog Retin Eye Res. 2004;23(1):91–147.
114. Kuwabara T, Cogan DG. Retinal glycogen. Arch Ophthalmol. 1961;66:680–8.
115. Li ZW, Liu S, Weinreb RN, Lindsey JD, Yu M, Liu L, et al. Tracking dendritic shrinkage of retinal ganglion cells after acute elevation of intraocular pressure. Invest Ophthalmol Vis Sci. 2011;52(10):7205–12.
116. Munemasa Y, Kitaoka Y. Molecular mechanisms of retinal ganglion cell degeneration in glaucoma and future prospects for cell body and axonal protection. Front Cell Neurosci. 2012;6:60.
117. Chan G, Balaratnasingam C, Yu PK, Morgan WH, McAllister IL, Cringle SJ, et al. Quantitative morphometry of perifoveal capillary networks in the human retina. Invest Ophthalmol Vis Sci. 2012;53(9):5502–14.
118. Rolfe DFS, Brown GC. Cellular energy utilization and molecular origin of standard metabolic rate in mammals. Physiol Rev. 1997;77(3):731–58.
119. Laughlin SB. Energy as a constraint on the coding and processing of sensory information. Curr Opin Neurobiol. 2001;11(4):475–80.
120. Laughlin SB, Weckström M. Fast and slow photoreceptors - a comparative study of the functional diversity of coding and conductances in the Diptera. J Comp Physiol A. 1993;172:593–609.
121. Zador A. Impact of synaptic unreliability on the information transmitted by spiking neurons. J Neurophysiol. 1998;79(3):1219–29.
122. Andrews RM, Griffiths PG, Johnson MA, Turnbull DM. Histochemical localisation of mitochondrial enzyme activity in human optic nerve and retina. Br J Ophthalmol. 1999;83(2):231–5.
123. Wang L, Dong J, Cull G, Fortune B, Cioffi GA. Varicosities of intraretinal ganglion cell axons in human and nonhuman primates. Invest Ophthalmol Vis Sci. 2003;44(1):2–9.
124. Osborne NN. Mitochondria: their role in ganglion cell death and survival in primary open angle glaucoma. Exp Eye Res. 2010;90(6):750–7.
125. Balaratnasingam C, Morgan WH, Bass L, Kang M, Cringle SJ, Yu DY. Time-dependent effects of focal retinal ischemia on axonal cytoskeleton proteins. Invest Ophthalmol Vis Sci. 2010;51(6):3019–28.
126. Morgan WH, Yu D-Y, Cooper RL, Cringle SJ, Alder VA. The influence of cerebrospinal fluid pressure upon the lamina cribrosa tissue pressure gradient - correspondence. Investig Ophthalmol Vis Sci. 1995;36:2163–4.
127. Morgan WH, Yu D-Y, Cooper RL, Alder VA, Cringle SJ, Constable IJ. The influence of cerebrospinal fluid pressure on the lamina cribrosa tissue pressure gradient. Investig Ophthalmol Vis Sci. 1995;36(6):1163–72.
128. Morgan WH, Yu D-Y, Alder VA, Cringle SJ, Cooper RL, House PH, et al. The correlation between cerebrospinal fluid pressure and retrolaminar tissue pressure. Investig Ophthalmol Vis Sci. 1998;39(8):1419–28.
129. Balaratnasingam C, Morgan WH, Johnstone V, Pandav SS, Cringle SJ, Yu DY. Histomorphometric measurements in human and dog optic nerve and an estimation of optic nerve pressure gradients in human. Exp Eye Res. 2009;89(5):618–28.
130. Ochs S. Energy metabolism and supply of -P to the fast axoplasmic transport mechanism in nerve. Fed Proc. 1974;33:1049–58.
131. Hahnenberger RW. Effect of a pressure barrier on retrograde axoplasmic transport in vitro. A study in the motor neurons of the rabbit vagus. Acta Physiol Scand. 1980;108(2):133–7.
132. Hayreh SS, Bill A, Sperber GO. Effects of high intraocular pressure on the glucose metabolism in the retina and optic nerve in old atherosclerotic monkeys. Graefes Arch Clin Exp Ophthalmol. 1994;232(12):745–52.
133. Rydevik B, Lundborg G, Bagge U. Effects of graded compression on intraneural blood blow. An in vivo study on rabbit tibial nerve. J Hand Surg Am. 1981;6(1):3–12.
134. Rodriguez-Tebar A, Jeffrey PL, Thoenen H, Barde YA. The survival of chick retinal ganglion cells in response to brain-derived neurotrophic factor depends on their embryonic age. Dev Biol. 1989;136(2):296–303.
135. Mansour-Robaey S, Clarke DB, Wang YC, Bray GM, Aguayo AJ. Effects of ocular injury and administration of brain-derived neurotrophic factor on survival and regrowth of axotomized retinal ganglion cells. Proc Natl Acad Sci U S A. 1994;91(5):1632–6.
136. Hayreh SS. Ischemic optic neuropathy. In: Dartt DA, editor. Encyclopedia of the eye. Oxford: Academic; 2010. p. 487–99.
137. Erdogmus S, Govsa F. Anatomic characteristics of the ophthalmic and posterior ciliary arteries. J Neuroophthalmol. 2008;28:320–40.
138. Mackenzie PJ, Cioffi GA. Vascular anatomy of the optic nerve head. Can J Ophthalmol. 2008;43(3):308–12.
139. Waxman SG, Kocsis JD, Stys PK. The axon. Structure, function and pathophysiology, vol. 1995. New York: Oxford University Press; 1995.
140. Sadun A. Acquired mitochondrial impairment as a cause of optic nerve disease. Trans Am Ophthalmol Soc. 1998;96:881–923.

141. Wong-Riley MT. Energy metabolism of the visual system. Eye Brain. 2010;2:99–116.
142. Sun X, Dai Y, Chen Y, Yu DY, Cringle SJ, Chen J, et al. Primary angle closure glaucoma: what we know and what we don't know. Prog Retin Eye Res. 2016;57:26–45.
143. Kaufman PL, Alm A, editors. Adler's physiology of the eye: clinical application. St. Louis: Mosby; 2003.
144. Collins R, Van der Werff TJ. Mathematical models of the dynamics of the human eye. In: Levin S, editor. Lecture notes in biomathematics. Berlin: Springer; 1980.
145. Bill A, Sperber GO. Control of retinal and choroidal blood flow. Eye. 1990;4:319–25.
146. Nickla DL, Wallman J. The multifunctional choroid. Prog Retin Eye Res. 2010;29(2):144–68.
147. Alm A, Bill A. Ocular circulation. In: Hart WM, Moses RA, editors. Adler's physiology of the eye: clinical application. 8th ed. St Louis: Mosby; 1987. p. 183–99.
148. Smith EL, Hill RA, Lehman IR, Lefkowitz RJ, Handler P, White A. Principles of biochemistry: mammalian biochemistry, vol. 1985. 7th ed. Singapore: McGraw-Hill Book Company; 1985.
149. Yu D-Y, Cringle SJ. Outer retinal anoxia during dark adaptation is not a general property of mammalian retinas. Comp Biochem Physiol. 2002;132:47–52.
150. Potter JW, Vandervort RS, Thallemer JM. The clinical significance of the vortex veins. J Am Optom Assoc. 1984;55(11):822–4.
151. Yu PK, Tan PE, Cringle SJ, McAllister IL, Yu DY. Phenotypic heterogeneity in the endothelium of the human vortex vein system. Exp Eye Res. 2013;115C:144–52.
152. Tan PE, Yu PK, Cringle SJ, Morgan WH, Yu DY. Regional heterogeneity of endothelial cells in the porcine vortex vein system. Microvasc Res. 2013;89:70–9.
153. Yu PK, Cringle SJ, Yu DY. Quantitative study of age-related endothelial phenotype change in the human vortex vein system. Microvasc Res. 2014;94:64–72.
154. Quigley HA. Angle-closure glaucoma-simpler answers to complex mechanisms: LXVI Edward Jackson memorial lecture. Am J Ophthalmol. 2009;148(5):657–69.
155. Mak H, Xu G, Leung CK. Imaging the iris with swept-source optical coherence tomography: relationship between iris volume and primary angle closure. Ophthalmology. 2013;120(12):2517–24.
156. Seager FE, Jefferys JL, Quigley HA. Comparison of dynamic changes in anterior ocular structures examined with anterior segment optical coherence tomography in a cohort of various origins. Invest Ophthalmol Vis Sci. 2014;55(3):1672–83.
157. Aptel F, Chiquet C, Beccat S, Denis P. Biometric evaluation of anterior chamber changes after physiologic pupil dilation using Pentacam and anterior segment optical coherence tomography. Invest Ophthalmol Vis Sci. 2012;53(7):4005–10.
158. Baskaran M, Ho SW, Tun TA, How AC, Perera SA, Friedman DS, et al. Assessment of circumferential angle-closure by the iris-trabecular contact index with swept-source optical coherence tomography. Ophthalmology. 2013;120(11):2226–31.
159. Quigley HA, Silver DM, Friedman DS, He M, Plyler RJ, Eberhart CG, et al. Iris cross-sectional area decreases with pupil dilation and its dynamic behavior is a risk factor in angle closure. J Glaucoma. 2009;18(3):173–9.

Mechanism Theories of Glaucoma

2

William H. Morgan and Dao-Yi Yu

Abstract

Glaucoma is a disease of the optic nerve, wherein the anterior part of the nerve, the optic disk, undergoes posterior distortion (cupping and excavation) along with loss of the nerve fibres. This leads to peripheral and finally total visual field loss. The major risk factor is elevated IOP, which along with cerebrospinal fluid pressure (CSFP) largely determines the pressure gradient and forces acting upon the connective tissue, nerve fibres and vessels in that region. Constitutive vulnerability factors like myopic connective tissue thinning play a role in determining the effect of these forces and together broadly form the theoretical planks of the "mechanical" theory of causation. Vascular factors are known to be involved given the common occurrence of disk rim haemorrhages and retinal venous occlusions in the disease. Considerations of these and possible arterial changes have led to a "vascular" theory, although more recent work suggests that features of these two theories are inter-linked. The classification and treatment of glaucoma is currently determined largely by the mechanism of IOP elevation. Given that aqueous production is relatively constant, IOP is largely determined by the rate of aqueous egress from the eye. The passage of aqueous humour within the eye is critical for altering the configuration and function of the drainage angle. The rate of aqueous outflow from the eye via the trabecular meshwork and ciliary body through small channels vitally affects IOP stability and control and is a key factor in glaucoma causation.

Keywords

Glaucoma · Intraocular pressure · Optic disk
Trabecular meshwork · Lamina cribrosa
Aetiology

2.1 Alterations in the Optic Disk in Glaucoma

Glaucoma is an umbrella term to describe a disease in which the optic disk undergoes typical distortion accompanied by matching visual field loss, often but not always associated with elevated IOP above the standard normal range. It is really an umbrella term covering a multitude of causes from congenital through to various acquired and genetic types, most of which have a final common pathway of elevating IOP and causing subsequent optic nerve damage. Glaucomatous optic neuropathy is a term which

W. H. Morgan (✉) · D.-Y. Yu
Lions Eye Institute, Centre for Ophthalmology and Visual Science, The University of Western Australia, Nedlands, WA, Australia
e-mail: BillMorgan@lei.org.au

X. Sun, Y. Dai (eds.), *Medical Treatment of Glaucoma*,
https://doi.org/10.1007/978-981-13-2733-9_2

describes the typical appearance of the optic disk in this disease and its consequences, i.e. the typical visual field loss.

2.1.1 Disk Cupping and Excavation

The optic disk in glaucoma undergoes a typical distortion with thinning of the neuroretinal rim containing the nerve fibres as well as a backwards bowing of the supporting connective tissue, especially the lamina cribrosa (Fig. 2.1). This leads to the appearance of an enlarging empty space in the disk centre, known as the cup with underlying bare lamina cribrosa connective tissue. This process is known as "cupping". The contour of the optic disk changes from a smooth gentle depression into a sharper "cliff edge" to an undercut appearance

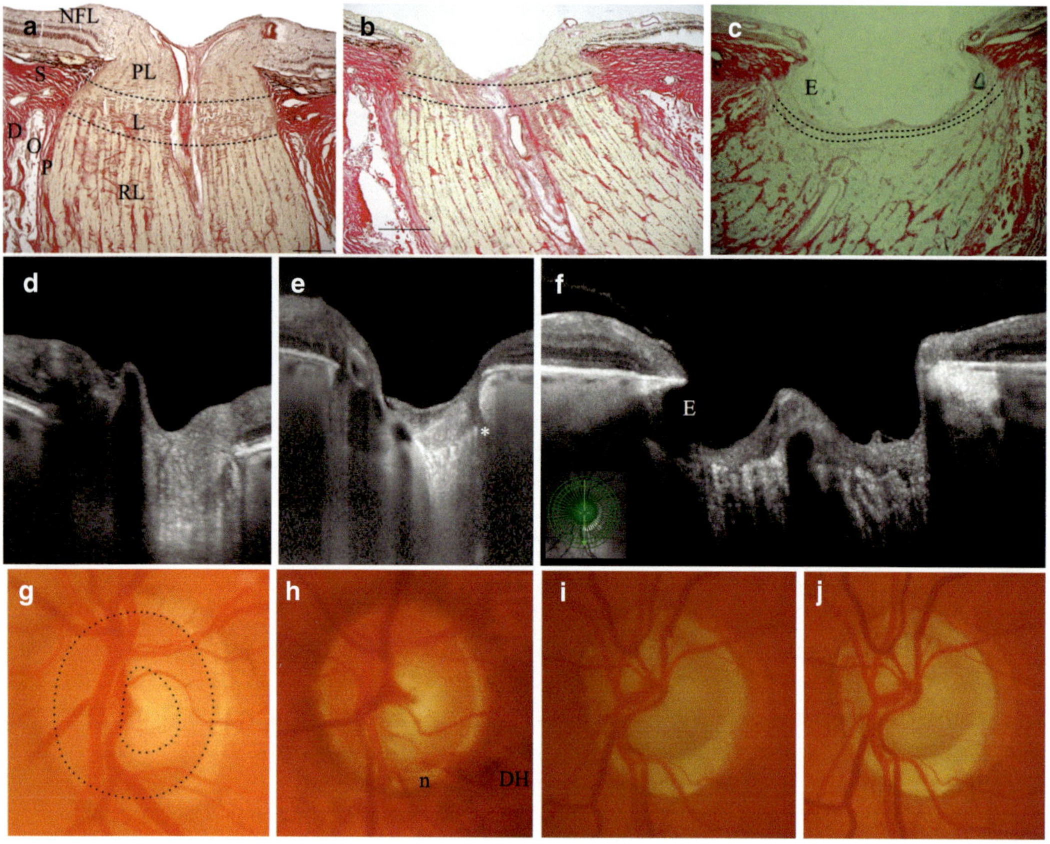

Fig. 2.1 Changes in the optic nerve in glaucoma. From normal (**a**), mild (**b**) to severe (**c**) glaucoma, on histological sections (van Gieson staining), one can see progressive thinning and bowing of the lamina cribrosa (L—between dashed lines) with posterior displacement of its insertion into sclera (S). Excavation is seen (E) with compressed lamina cribrosa is pushed towards the optic nerve subarachnoid space (O). Pia mater (P) and dura mater (D) are seen. The nerve fibre layer (NFL) becomes thinner with disease. These changes are seen in optical coherence tomography scans from patients with mild (**d**), moderate (**e**) and severe (**f**) glaucoma. In (**e**), a lamina defect is seen "asterisk". The inset in (**f**) demonstrates the vertical orientation for all scans. A normal optic disk is seen (**g**) with dotted lines demonstrating the inner and outer neuroretinal rim boundaries. The region inside the inner line is known as the optic cup. In mild disease (**h**) disk excavation with a notch (n) and focal neural loss is often seen (here inferiorly). Disk rim haemorrhages are often seen (DH). A stereo photograph (**i** and **j**) of severe glaucoma can be fused by relaxing your eyes. You will see marked excavation superiorly and also inferiorly with almost total loss of neuroretinal rim. This corresponds to scan (**f**). The visual field worsens from normal (**k**, matching **g** and **d**), mild (**l**) (matching **h** and **e**), moderate (**m**) and severe (**n**, matching **i**, **j** and **f**). Schematic visual field loss and site of optic disk damage with corresponding nerve fibre layer loss is seen in normal (**o**), mild (**p**) and severe (**q**) disease. Only lower half of nerve fibre trajectory pattern is shown for space considerations. Scale bar 400 μm. Histology from Balaratnasingam. Reproduced with permission from Balaratnasingam et al. [2]

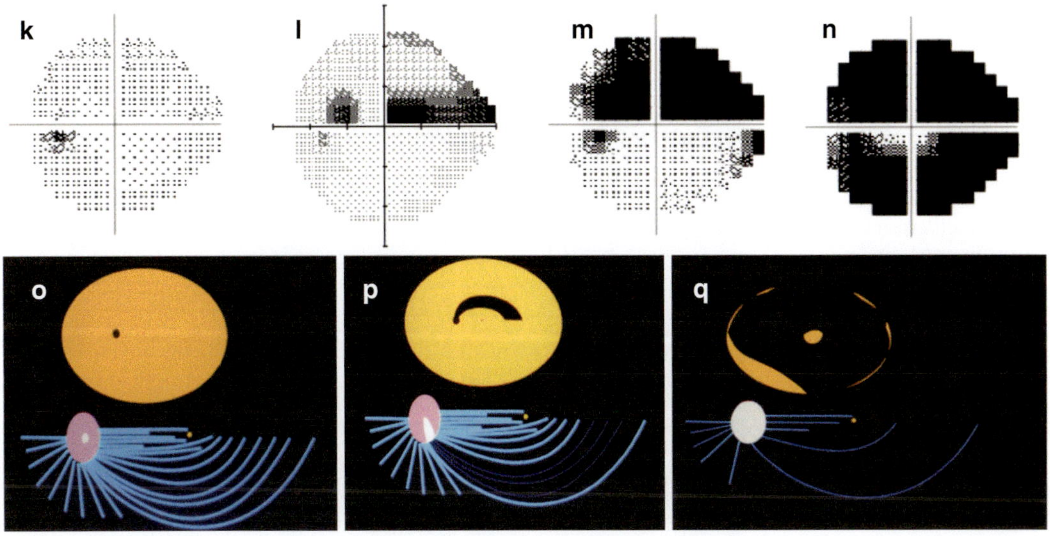

Fig. 2.1 (continued)

known as "excavation" (Fig. 2.1). The degree of excavation can vary and appears to be affected by the tissue differences between surrounding sclera and the lamina cribrosa in the individual. Generally, cupping and excavation should be seen in all cases of glaucoma. If not, other diagnoses should be considered. Cupping and excavation are due to a change in shape of the underlying lamina cribrosa connective tissue (Fig. 2.1) and hence is produced by a force that exceeds the load capacity of the individual's tissue.

In more detail, the optic disk undergoes a process by which the central section devoid of axons, termed "the cup" expands coincidentally with a posterior deformation of the optic disk connective tissue, the bulk of which lies within the lamina cribrosa. The optic cup is not a structure in itself but simply an appearance within the tire-shaped optic disk, of a central hole due to the relative absence of neural tissue (axons and glia). The average optic disk diameter lies somewhere between 1.5 and 2.0 mm vertically, is roughly elliptical with a longer vertical than horizontal diameter in most subjects. This size is more than enough to enclose the one million ganglion cell axons traversing this region from the retina to the optic nerve proper. The axons tend to be displaced towards the peripheral part of the optic disk surface, hence leaving a central absence zone termed "the cup". The junction between the neural (axonal) tissue and the cup is termed "the optic disk margin" and this appears to expand in the disease as nerves are lost and die off leaving the remainder to be pushed peripherally. Additionally, the lamina cribrosa connective tissue just beneath the surface of the central optic disk, distorts posteriorly and also peripherally towards the optic nerve subarachnoid space, creating a bowed, excavated appearance [1].

Surrounding the optic nerve is the optic nerve subarachnoid space which lies approximately 1.0 mm posterior to the disk surface [2]. In glaucoma the peripheral lamina cribrosa deforms towards the optic nerve subarachnoid space. In addition to this posterior deformation in glaucoma the lamina cribrosa undergoes compression [3, 4]. The central cup therefore changes from a gentle circular valley appearance to one where there is a deep cup and often excavation with undermining of the neural rim. The most vulnerable parts of the optic disk tend to be the infero-temporal and supero-temporal regions where such focal changes frequently occur and because of the focal nature are termed "notches". The disk appearance therefore includes increased cupping with excavation and often focal notching. The absence of focal regions of nerve fibres just adjacent to the optic disk can often also be seen macroscopically at the slit lamp using the red free light. Small haemorrhages and absent

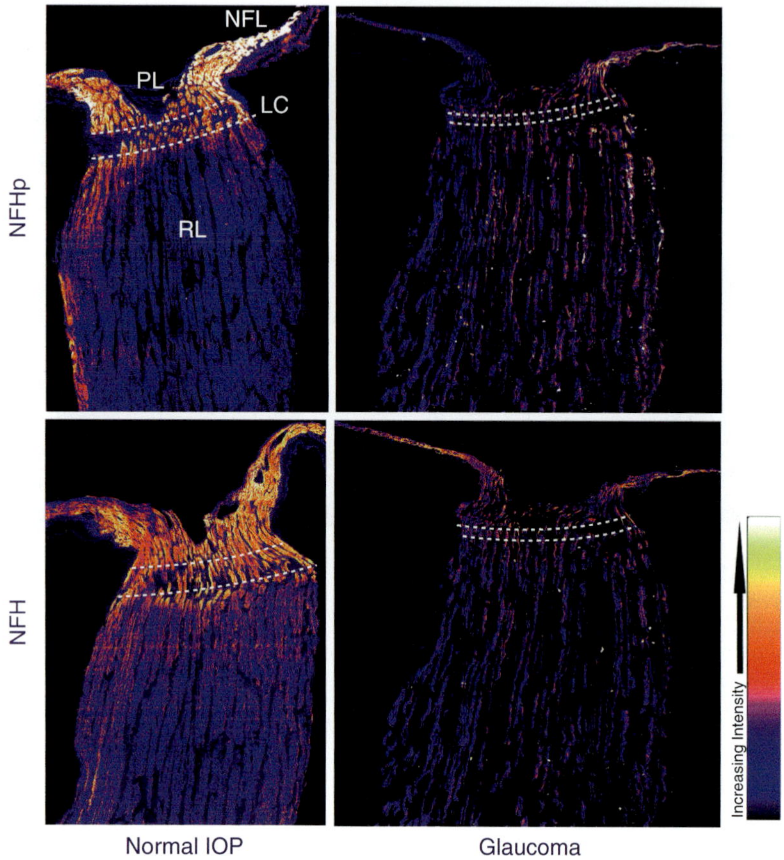

Fig. 2.2 Neurofilaments heavy (NFH) and heavy phosphorylated (NFHp) have been stained with antibodies in sections from normal and glaucomatous human optic nerves. The stain area corresponds to ganglion cell axon distribution and the intensity to the antibody binding levels. The anterior and posterior limits of the lamina cribrosa (LC) are shown by the white dashed lines. Prelaminar (PL) and retrolaminar (RL) optic nerve as well as the nerve fibre layer (NFL) are shown. Unpublished data from Balaratnasingam. Reproduced with permission from Balaratnasingam et al. [2]

venous pulsation are also often seen and will be discussed further [5].

The hallmark pathological feature is the gradual loss of the retinal ganglion cell axons. Figure 2.2 shows the relative loss with sparse distribution of axons in the glaucomatous optic nerve. Thinning of the nerve fibre layer is seen along with reduced neurofilament subtype staining intensity in the laminar and prelaminar regions. There are several theories to explain why nerve axon and cell death occurs in glaucoma. The nerve fibres are the ganglion cell axons, with the ganglion cell bodies residing across the retina. These axons become interrupted at the level of the lamina cribrosa with the formation of retraction bulbs and frustrated growth cones, as described by Vrabec in the 1970s [6]. The mechanism appears to be a form of secondary axotomy induced by forces acting upon the axons leading to local perturbations [7]. Other models of neural stretch injury demonstrate intracellular calcium increase along with neurofilament and microtubule changes leading to axonal transport inhibition, secondary axotomy with retraction bulbs and frustrated growth cone formation [8–10]. The cell body eventually dies through apoptosis. This is a form of Wallerian degeneration, which includes death of the distal axon remnant including loss of synaptic connection in the lateral geniculate body (Fig. 2.3).

An older theory was that bending or movement of the axons in the prelaminar and lamina regions lead to their damage. However, the axons are quite flexible and capable of turning sharp corners without signs of damage [6]. Also, most movement of the lamina occurs when IOP ranges from 5 to 15 mmHg and yet in this pressure range glaucoma is relatively rare [11]. As IOP increases the pressure differential and gradient across the lamina cribrosa this leads to a cascade of various changes to be discussed further. Briefly, they include inhibition of axonal transport at the level

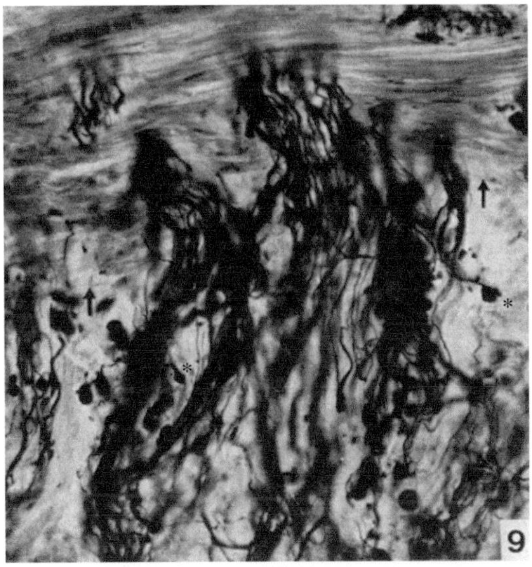

Fig. 2.3 Axons passing through the compressed posterior lamina cribrosa (arrows indicate posterior limit) in a patient with glaucoma. Interrupted axons (axotomy) can be seen with frustrated growth cones "asterisk". Jabonero's method from Vrabec × 270. Reproduced with permission from Vrabec [6]

of the lamina cribrosa, both in the orthograde and retrograde directions such that larger vesicles like mitochondria cannot be transported well across the lamina cribrosa and may not reach regions where energy demand is high [12, 13]. Elevated IOP affects the blood perfusion pressure to the anterior region of the lamina cribrosa. It appears that the lamina cribrosa is the region of prime vulnerability in glaucoma.

2.2 Visual Loss in Glaucoma

2.2.1 Visual Field Loss

Glaucoma is the second commonest cause of blindness worldwide with some ten million people expected to be blind from glaucoma by 2020 [14]. The most vulnerable regions of the optic disk are the supero-temporal and infero-temporal regions, where ganglion cell axon interruption and death tends to preferentially occur [15]. This leads to retrograde loss of the ganglion cell bodies located in an arcuate pattern across the temporal retinal. This leads to loss of retinal function in the retinal regions served by the retinal ganglion cells. The visual loss is spread across the visual field which matches the region of retina affected, allowing for the inverted nature of the eye's optics. Allowing for some individual variation, ganglion cell axons just above the horizontal midline project their axons to the superior optic disk in an upper arcuate pattern. Disease in this region leads to a lower arcuate type or inferior nasal step field defect [16]. Conversely, ganglion cell axons just below the horizontal midline project their axons to the superior optic disk in a lower arcuate pattern. Here, disease leads to an upper arcuate type or superior nasal step field defect. These are the hallmark visual field defects seen in glaucoma.

Visual sensitivity loss is generally measured by the ability of a subject to respond to a spot of added brightness above background illumination (liminal brightness increment). Under a certain range of background illumination, this liminal brightness increment will tend to be a constant ratio (compared to background), allowing for spot size and is known as the Weber–Fechner law. This principle underlies visual field measurements within all modern perimeters. Due to this ratio effect and the characteristics of the measurement error, the sensitivity and deviation from normality are reported using a logarithmic ratio unit (decibel—dB). A key part of glaucoma management is to measure these sensitivities across the visual field and create a visual field map. These are commonly called visual field tests and are frequently repeated for comparison to judge whether the disease is stable or not.

Measurements of structure involving the optic disk neuroretinal rim, surface contour or adjacent nerve fibre layer are often made in order to aid glaucoma diagnosis or to compare with prior measurements to detect change in the disease. These measurements are typically made using a linear scale. Figure 2.4 shows the typical relationship between visual field sensitivity loss vs. the optic disk neuroretinal rim area. The latter is a structural measure of the optic disk axonal and associated tissue content and is normally between 1.8 and 3.5mm^2. One can see that there is a large variability in normal measures. Also, as neural tissue is lost relatively little change in visual field

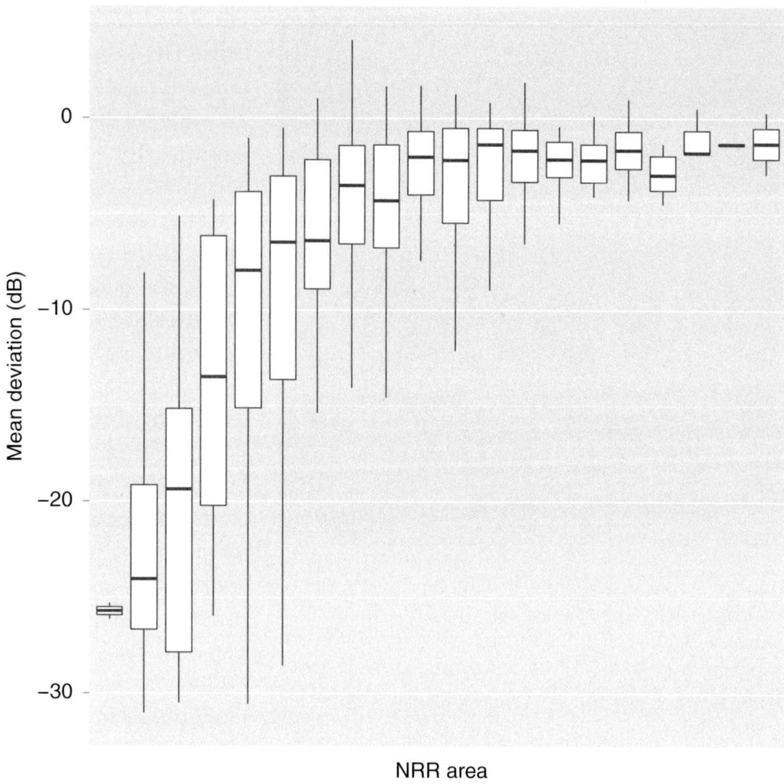

Fig. 2.4 Box plots of average visual field sensitivity loss (mean deviation dB) at different optic disk neuroretinal rim (NRR) areas (mm^2) measured by confocal scanning laser tomography in 460 glaucoma and glaucoma suspect eyes from our clinic

occurs in the early stages, but later in the disease small changes in neural tissue result in large visual field changes. A similar relationship exists between field loss and other neural measures like nerve fibre layer thickness [17]. Visual field loss is not confidently detectable in most cases until it reaches −4 dB. In this and other work it is found that subjects need to lose 30–50% of the optic nerve or nerve fibre layer axons before detectable visual field loss occurs [15].

Typical visual field loss is seen in Fig. 2.1 with a very dense superior arcuate loss in the right eye matching inferior disk excavation in particular. In the left eye the visual field is reduced to a tunnel of vision by dense superior and inferior arcuate scotomas with matching very excavated and cupped optic disk.

Larger diameter axons (magnocellular) appear to be preferentially affected in glaucoma and tend to transmit information from yellow/blue receptive fields as well as certain features of motion detection [18]. Attempts have been made to preferentially test these aspects of visual function in glaucoma [19].

2.2.2 Other Visual Loss

In addition to visual field loss, less easily measured aspects of visual function are impaired in glaucoma. An early change is a subject's ability to adapt to rapid alterations in light levels across his or her visual field. An example of this are complaints about increased length of time to visually adapt from going from a bright outdoors to indoor relative darkness [20]. Additionally, in severe glaucoma, as the optic disk damage becomes very severe and the visual field loss worsens to involve the central visual field, the visual acuity will reduce.

2.3 Pressures and the Eye

In glaucoma, the pressure differential across the optic disk leads to visible changes. The optic disk straddles two pressure compartments: IOP anteriorly and retrolaminar pressure posteriorly. The pressure differential creates forces which promotes disk excavation (Fig. 2.1) amongst other changes. The degree of disk excavation can vary and appears to be affected by the tissue differences between the surrounding sclera and lamina cribrosa within any individual. Specifically, the depth of the vertical part of the cup may be quite deep, approaching 1 mm or more or it may be short, being a fraction of 1 mm and this may partly correspond to differences in strength between the surrounding sclera and lamina cribrosa. Where the surrounding sclera is weak, as in myopia, and there is a smaller difference between the two structures' physical properties the degree of excavation may be smaller, that is the depth of the cup and excavation may be smaller than commonly seen clinically. Others report that there is increased depth of a thinner lamina cribrosa in high myopes [21]. The relationship between the scleral physical properties surrounding the lamina and the lamina cribrosa itself is important for determining some of the forces across the lamina region [22, 23]. The surrounding peripapillary sclera is often thin and weak, as is the lamina cribrosa creating a smaller differential between peripapillary sclera and laminar physical properties. This can add to the difficulties for diagnosing glaucoma in highly myopic individuals. Generally, cupping and excavation should be seen in all cases of glaucoma, if not, other diagnoses should be considered. It is also common to see focal notching, although not essential. The posterior and more peripheral distortion of the lamina cribrosa with compression suggests that there is an increase in force acting upon this tissue, acting in a posterior and slightly peripheral direction towards the optic nerve subarachnoid space and that this force is exceeding the load capacity of the particular individual's optic disk connective tissue.

2.3.1 Optic Disk Tissue Subject to Forces

The optic disk is divided into three broad regions: the prelaminar, laminar and retrolaminar regions (Fig. 2.1) [24]. The prelaminar tissue contains the ganglion cell axons and supporting blood vessels with some glial tissue as the axons pass across the retina into the anterior optic disk region and begin to turn into the disk region. In the laminar region these ganglion cell axons pass posteriorly and group into bundles passing through fenestrations in the connective tissue sheets stretched across the hole within the sclera. This fenestrated collection of connective tissue is termed the "lamina cribrosa" and represents 10–15 semi-discrete connective tissue sheets that are fenestrated with the fenestrations not exactly overlapping but nevertheless allowing the passage of axonal bundles through to the retrolaminar region. Surrounding each ganglion cell axon within the laminar region are glial cell processes and bodies which act as functional and physiological insulating tissues partly to separate the axons from supporting blood vessels which tend to reside within the laminar connective tissue. Just anterior to the laminar collagen is the so-called glial laminar tissue which instead of comprising connective tissue comprises mainly glial supporting tissue (astrocytes). This glial tissue is more densely distributed in this region than the prelaminar region and hence the inclusion in the laminar tissue section. The collagenous lamina cribrosa contains the greatest amount (density) of collagen surrounding and supporting the ganglion cell axons. The tissue in this region appears to be most affected biomechanically by glaucoma [23, 25].

Posterior to the lamina region lies the retrolaminar (also known as postlaminar) region. This is a true white matter tract where oligodendrocytes reside and form myelin sheath surrounding the axons. Pia mater, subarachnoid space and dura mater lie just external to this region. Within the optic nerve subarachnoid space lie many trabeculae which impede cerebrospinal fluid flow from the cranial cavity in certain situations. External to the dura mater lies intraconal orbital fat. The optic nerve subarachnoid space (ONSAS) usually is a narrow space terminating in line with the posterior lamina cribrosa and separated from the overlying retina by thickened sclera (Fig. 2.1). The weakest region separating the ONSAS from the eye and optic nerve is the pia mater. In myopia the termination of the ONSAS is frequently wide with the overlying sclera thin so that any pressure difference between the ONSAS and eye can act upon the sclera leading to a posterior staphyloma

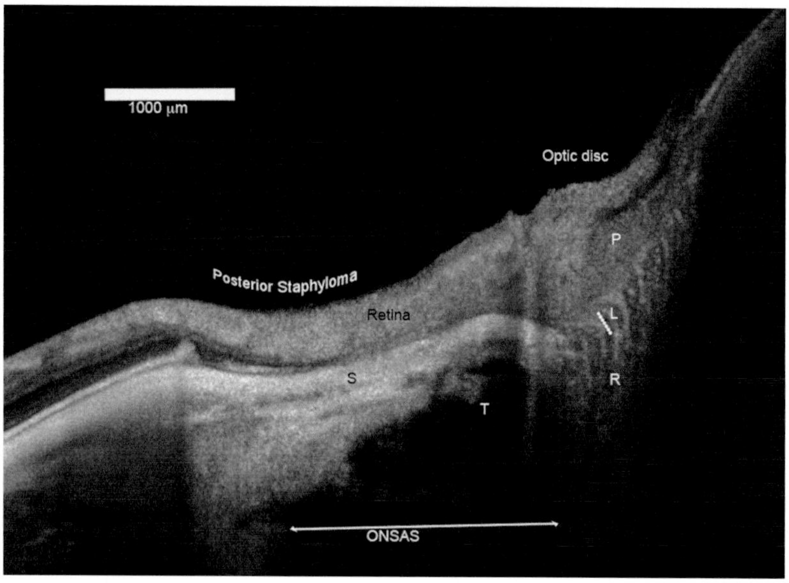

Fig. 2.5 Swept source OCT image of the optic disk and surrounding region in a highly myopic patient. The lamina cribrosa (L) is thin (~200 μm) with prelaminar (P) and retrolaminar (R) tissue on either side. The optic nerve subarachnoid space (ONSAS) is greatly enlarged with overlying thin sclera (S) which is bowing backwards forming a posterior staphyloma containing a posteriorly shifted retina (R). Trabeculae (T) within the ONSAS can be seen

as well as optic disk excavation (Fig. 2.5) [26]. This additional effect upon the overlying sclera can alter the relative degree of excavation and render diagnosis more difficult.

Within the ganglion cell axons reside the machinery for axonal function, namely neurofilaments, microtubules, axons, mitochondria and the biochemical machinery to allow for action potential generation and axonal transport. Microtubules form the tracks along which vesicles are transported both retrogradely (posteriorly) and anterogradely (anteriorly). Small motors, kinesin for anterograde and dynein for retrograde axonal transport move along these microtubule tracks attached to vesicles thereby moving their loads along the axon [27]. Neurofilaments and actin filaments traverse the axonal cytoplasm and have complicated biochemical structures which almost certainly impact upon phosphate moiety delivery and other aspects of energy supply along with local physiological stability in the region. For example, the outer parts of the neurofilaments tend to be phosphorylated in the normal situation but under high pressure situations with a high pressure gradient tend to lose phosphorylation [28] and several consequences occur, including a tendency towards secondary axotomy.

2.3.2 IOP Distribution Across the Eye

2.3.2.1 IOP

The eye is akin to a balloon which is inflated to a certain pressure. This pressure is known as IOP and is mostly applied evenly and equally across all tissue structures within the corneoscleral coat of the eye. There are small exceptions with supraciliary space pressure tending to be 0.8 mmHg lower than IOP with suprachoroidal space pressure reportedly being 4 mmHg lower than IOP at different IOP levels [29]. The reason for this is not clear but is probably due to the elastic Bruch's membrane and ciliary body creating added compression of the more central ocular contents. Additionally, small and variable pressure differences can exist across the lens—ciliary body and lens—iris regions [30]. In the posterior eye the IOP is evenly applied to the prelaminar optic disk region [31].

Fluid pressure within the eye, IOP, can be measured directly with a needle or indirectly with some accuracy using applanation or other techniques [32]. All current clinical techniques for measuring IOP involve various assumptions being made regarding forces applied to the cornea (by the measurement device), corneal physical properties and their relation to IOP [33, 34]. For a more complete understanding of some various techniques and physical principles involved the reader should consult Adler's "Physiology of the eye" amongst other texts [35].

Across various populations the median IOP is 16 mmHg with standard deviation 3 mmHg [36]. Approximately 95% of eyes have IOP between 10 and 21 mmHg. This has tended to become known as the normal distribution of IOP. However, closer inspection of the data reveals a skew distribution to the right (Fig. 2.6) [36]. In this same study, Hollows et al. described the IOP distribution in newly diagnosed glaucoma patients. This demonstrated that a significant proportion of glaucoma patients have IOP within the "normal range".

If subjects without detectable glaucoma are followed for a period of time, a proportion will develop glaucoma. An elevated IOP is known to be the major predictor of future glaucoma within an individual. The relationship between IOP and future glaucoma development risk is exponential, as demonstrated in Fig. 2.7. Similarly, the relationship between reduced glaucoma progression and IOP reduction following treatment follows a similar exponential function [38].

2.3.3 Determinants of IOP

2.3.3.1 Aqueous Production

The aqueous flow within the eye is in a dynamic but equilibrium situation. This means that if IOP is constant then the rate of aqueous production must equal the rate of aqueous outflow from the eye. Aqueous humour is produced by the ciliary processes and enters the vitreal compartment and the posterior chamber. It is produced by an active transport mechanism from the pigmented and non-pigmented ciliary body epithelia joined by gap junctions lining the ciliary processes [39, 40]. Active ionic transporters pump sodium ions as well as bicarbonate ions directly into the vitreous and the posterior chambers. The osmotic load created drags water with it across the epithelium and the ionic imbalance tends to drag chloride and other ions as well. There is selective production and pumping of other substances like glutathione and agents which supply nutrition to the partly avascular structures within the eye (vitreous, lens and cornea). This active transport process requires significant energy delivery and, hence, significant blood flow. So, when blood pressure or perfusion pressure to the eye is significantly compromised then aqueous production will decrease.

In the normal situation, aqueous humour production is relatively constant with some diurnal

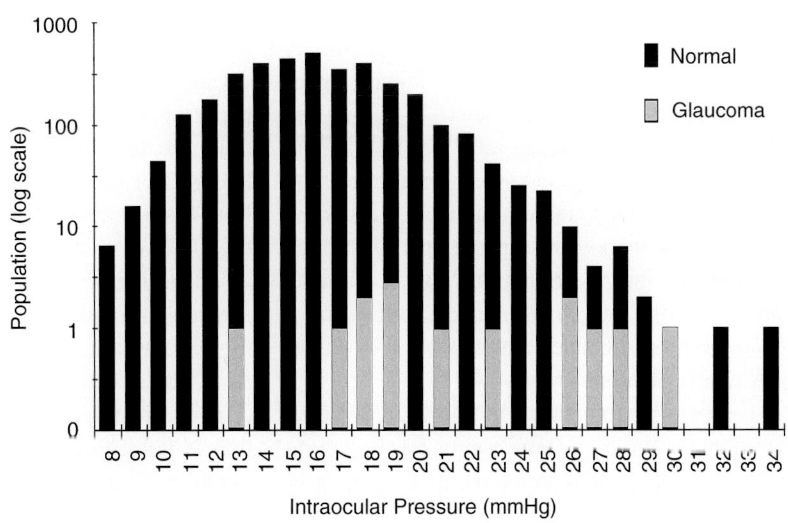

Fig. 2.6 IOP distribution in normal and newly diagnosed glaucoma subjects. Data taken from Hollows et al. [36]

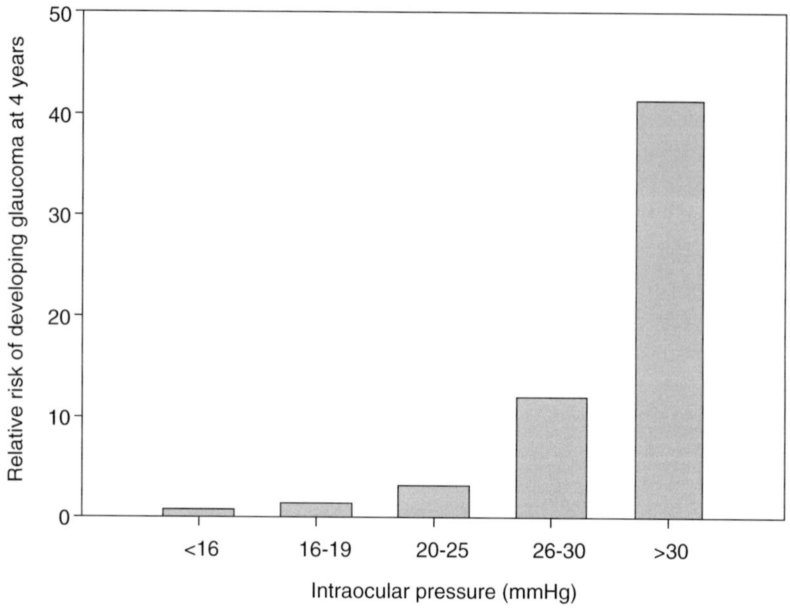

Fig. 2.7 Relative risk of a subject developing glaucoma with visual field loss at 4 years compared to their initial IOP. Relative risk of individuals with initial IOP <16 mmHg is defined as 1. Data derived from Sommer [37]

variation and very little inter-individual variation. We assume that the bulk of aqueous produced flows from the vitreal and posterior chamber compartments between the lens and ciliary processes into the posterior chamber and from there between the lens and iris into the anterior chamber and thence via the trabecular meshwork into canal of Schlemm, collector channels to the aqueous veins (Fig. 2.8) [41]. However, there are other pathways which include the uveoscleral outflow pathway by which aqueous humour passes into the anterior ciliary body between the iris root and trabecular meshwork and enters the ciliary muscle and passes into the supraciliary space adjacent to the sclera [42]. Sclera is porous and allows aqueous to diffuse into the orbit. There are numerous lymphatic vessels within the orbit which can absorb aqueous humour. It is proposed that aqueous humour also passes partly through the vitreous into the retina and can be pumped actively out by the retinal pigment epithelium. It is not known how much aqueous humour passes posteriorly along this route.

It is possible to measure the flow rate of aqueous humour across the pupil using fluorophotometry [43]. This technique relies upon staining of aqueous humour in the anterior chamber with fluorescein and analysing the reduction in fluorescein concentration over time, i.e. a dilution over time effect. This can be mathematically analysed and calculations performed to calculate a rate of aqueous flow across the pupil. For subsequent discussion, it is assumed that all of the aqueous humour produced by the ciliary processes passes anteriorly across the pupil.

The average rate of aqueous humour production is 2.75 μL/min (sd 0.63), with slight reduction with age of approximately 2.4% per decade from ages 20–83. There is a significant diurnal variation with the rate at night (1.6 μL/min) being approximately half the morning production rate (3.1 μl/min). Catecholamines stimulate greater production at night than in the day. Beta-blocker drugs reduce aqueous production by 30–40% in the day time, but not significantly at all at night. Carbonic anhydrase inhibitors and alpha-2-agonists reduce production during the day and at night. These variations may have an effect upon the therapeutic benefit of various drug regimens [39]. The rate of aqueous production is not altered significantly in disease, particularly in glaucoma.

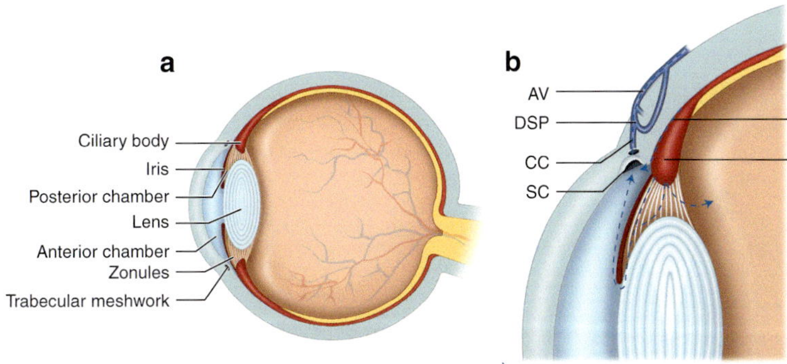

Fig. 2.8 Schematic drawings to illustrate aqueous flow in the normal eye. Major anatomical features are noted in (**a**). Aqueous is produced in the ciliary body and flows across the zonules into the posterior chamber, then anteriorly between the lens and iris to enter the anterior chamber. Most of this aqueous is filtered through the trabecular meshwork and enters Schlemm's canal (SC, in **b** - magnified view). From here it passes into collector channels (CC), deep scleral plexus (DSP) and into aqueous veins (AV) before entering the episcleral veins. Some aqueous in the anterior chamber enters the ciliary body and passes into the supraciliary space (SCS) forming the uveoscleral flow route (USF). Additionally, an unknown proportion of aqueous does not pass through the pupil but passes posteriorly into the vitreous

2.3.3.2 Aqueous Flow within the Eye

As aqueous humour passes between the vitreal compartment into the posterior chamber it traverses a narrow region between the lens equator and ciliary processes. In addition some produced in the posterior ciliary body passes between the zonules of Zinn and across the anterior hyaloid face. The resistance to flow across the anterior hyaloid face can vary and in some patients may be pathologically high [44]. Also in patients with a large lens relative to the size of their eye the lens equator may abut the ciliary processes raising the resistance to flow in this region [45]. Many of these patients may have previously enlarged ciliary processes [46]. Collectively, if aqueous flow resistance across this ciliary region involving ciliary process, lens proximity and anterior hyaloid thickening is increased, then this is termed "ciliary block". The resultant pressure differential between the vitreal compartment and the posterior chamber results in the lens and ciliary processes being pushed forwards like a piston. The ciliary processes rotate anteriorly along with the lens, pushing the iris forwards. The anterior rotation and force upon the iris can cause the iris to block the angle covering the trabecular meshwork, removing the ability of aqueous to enter trabecular meshwork. This is a prime cause of angle closure [47] (Fig. 2.9).

Additionally, from the posterior chamber the aqueous humour must pass between the lens and the iris to enter the anterior chamber. The iris virtually rests upon the lens with a gap of only 3–7 μm forming a significant resistance to flow in this region [30]. Hence, a pressure differential can be produced across the iris. This occurs predominantly in subjects again with a large lens within a small eye, where a greater area of lens/iris contact is induced. The pressure differential acts upon the weakest, thinnest part of the iris, which is the peripheral iris close to the trabecular meshwork. For this reason the peripheral iris may bow forwards and tend to block the trabecular meshwork. This whole process is termed "pupil block". Pupil block and ciliary block remain the two cornerstone hydrodynamic processes causing so-called primary angle closure [48]. The simplest therapy for pupil block is to create a hole in the iris thereby eliminating the pressure differential and this is simply performed using

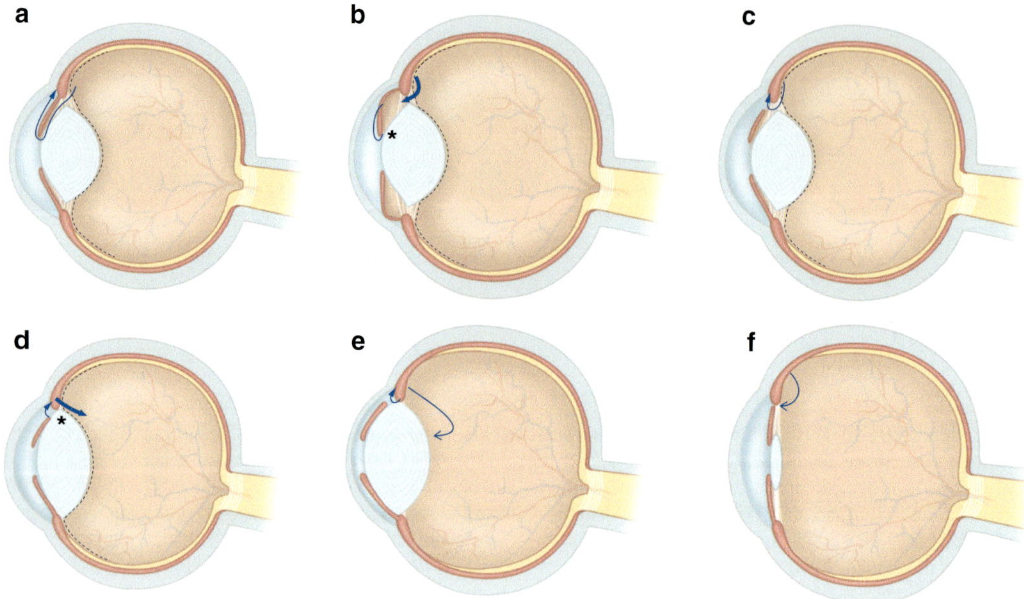

Fig. 2.9 Common sequence of angle closure. Normally, the aqueous flows easily between lens and ciliary body and lens and iris (**a**). Sometimes the angle is crowded and flow resistance between iris and lens is high (pupil block—**b** at "asterisk") cause pressure behind the iris to push it into the angle. This may be relieved by laser iridotomy, creating a hole in the iris (**c**). Over time the lens may enlarge and abut the ciliary processes increasing flow resistance (ciliary block–**d** at "asterisk"). Ciliary block can cause pressure behind the lens to increase pushing it and iris forward to block the angle (**e**). It is usually relieved by lens extraction and insertion of a smaller intraocular lens to allow space between it and the ciliary body for fluid flow (**f**)

a laser iridotomy procedure. The simplest process for eliminating ciliary block is to remove the lens and implant a smaller, thinner plastic lens shifting the lens equator centrally, away from the ciliary processes. This does not eliminate any anterior hyaloid pathology. If anterior hyaloid pathology is present, this will separately require partial removal by creating a hole through the zonules and anterior hyaloid into the vitreal compartment. An alternative is ciliary process shrinkage procedures generally performed with laser to shrink the ciliary process away from the lens equator but, again, this does not address any potential pathology acting within the anterior hyaloid [45].

2.3.3.3 Aqueous Outflow

Aqueous leaves the eye through two major known pathways. One is termed "the conventional pathway" and this comprises passage across the trabecular meshwork. The other, non-conventional pathway is the uveoscleral pathway in which aqueous passes across the ciliary body and into the supraciliary and suprachoroidal space.

In any one individual at any particular time the trabecular meshwork offers a certain resistance to outflow. This has been the standard assumption and is derived from animal experiments in young, healthy monkeys [49]. It is often considered to be the prime explanation for pressure changes in glaucoma. So, if we consider this assumption, then the trabecular meshwork is considered to be the major region for resistance to outflow and comprises the tissue between the anterior chamber and canal of Schlemm. The tissue, in particular, responsible for resistance to outflow is the juxtacanalicular trabecular meshwork tissue just adjacent to the canal of Schlemm. It has been presumed that once aqueous reaches the canal of Schlemm it then directly enters the aqueous veins via the collector channels. This is certainly the pathway but there is some evidence now accumulating that in glaucoma, changes within the canal of Schlemm and collector channels may increase outflow resistance. The collector channels contain functional valves separating them from the canal of Schlemm to reduce back-flow of aqueous [41]. Aqueous humour flow through this system appears to be pulsatile, driven by the cardiac cycle and blinking, which may take advantage of these valvular features [50]. In mathematical models we consider all of this resistance "trabecular resistance" even though we are not specifically assuming that all of the resistance is lying across the trabecular meshwork (Rtrab).

Some investigators believe that the "trabecular resistance" may include some significant resistance distal to the canal of Schlemm within the collector channels and deep scleral plexus as well as the aqueous veins [51]. Experiments removing sclera overlying the canal of Schlemm in ex-vivo eyes have found that most of this distal resistance is close to the canal of Schlemm, within the collector channels and adjacent deep scleral plexus [52]. Removal of the trabecular meshwork in ex-vivo eyes eliminates 14–82% of the flow resistance depending upon various experimental conditions, particularly the IOP [53]. When IOP is elevated and trabecular meshwork is allowed to compress the canal of Schlemm, the fraction of resistance across the trabecular meshwork increases [54].

Uveoscleral outflow (Fuv) was first noted when a fraction of radiolabelled albumin injected into the anterior chamber did not enter the blood circulation [55]. In monkeys approximately half the tracer was found within the ciliary body, supraciliary and suprachoroidal space region and the term "uveoscleral flow" used to describe this route. It is thought that this flow continues through the porous sclera and enters orbital tissue including lymphatics. Some may enter the choroidal vessels [42]. It is not possible to measure this flow rate directly. For various reasons it has been assumed that this flow rate is not significantly altered by pressure differences across the eye: IOP to orbital pressure or IOP to venous pressure. A major reason for this conclusion is that supraciliary space tends to be a constant 0.8 mmHg below IOP across a range of IOP measures [29], providing a constant pressure gradient across the ciliary body. Mathematically, uveoscleral outflow has been treated as the pressure independent outflow pathway, whereas the true situation may not be so clear.

2.3.4 Interaction of Aqueous and the Trabecular Meshwork

The trabecular meshwork is not just a simple filtering tissue which creates a certain outflow resistance. It is vital for the detoxification of the aqueous humour, phagocytosis of cellular debris and pigment and maintaining relative immune privilege within the eye. The detoxification involves removal of reactive oxygen species and other substances. The result is aqueous humour that is less toxic to vascular endothelial cells [41, 56].

Primary open angle glaucoma is the commonest form of glaucoma causing approximately 74% worldwide [14]. It is due to changes in the trabecular meshwork with fibrosis, loss of trabecular cells and thickening of the extracellular matrix [57]. There are likely to be changes in the collector channels and Schlemm's canal also. These changes cannot be seen clinically, but only histologically. Trabecular meshwork cells are post-mitotic and do not divide normally. Autophagy is important for toxin clearance with meshwork cells losing this ability gradually with age. The type of toxins cleared are further discussed in Sect. 2.5.3. Physical stretch of meshwork cells occurs when IOP increases and this leads to cytoskeletal alteration and changes to autophagy [58].

The extracellular matrix is continually being remodelled with some of the remodelling due to endocytosis and autophagy of extracellular matrix components. It seems that changes in meshwork cell autophagy deteriorate with age and cumulative toxin load. This is compounded by any genetic predisposition, e.g. myocilin mutations as discussed in Sect. 2.5.2.

2.3.5 Simplified Aqueous Flow Model of IOP

It is most useful to consider mathematical models of aqueous humour outflow. Most simply, aqueous outflow (Fout) must equal aqueous inflow (production, Fin). Mathematically, Fin = Fout = Ftrab + Fuv, where Ftrab is trabecular outflow and Fuv is uveoscleral outflow: the sum of these two being total outflow. Aqueous production or Fin is measured by fluorophotometry. Trabecular outflow is dependent upon the trabecular region resistance (Rtrab) and pressure differential across the trabecular region. The pressure differential is the difference between IOP and episcleral venous pressure (Pev). Note that Fuv is assumed to be independent of IOP and Pev. So, the mathematical expansion means that Fin = (IOP − Pev)/Rtrab + Fuv. For historical reasons the inverse of resistance is generally considered and called facility of outflow (C), where C = 1/Rtrab. So:

$$\text{Fin} = \text{Fout} = \text{C} \bullet (\text{IOP} - \text{Pev}) + \text{Fuv}$$

Rearranging this to extract IOP reveals the classic Goldmann equation [59, 60].

$$\text{IOP} = \frac{(\text{Fin} - \text{Fuv})}{\text{C}} + \text{Pev}$$

In humans, direct measurement of outflow facility (C) is not possible, but requires calculation. This is classically measured by tonography [35] using Schiotz tonometry techniques [61]. A weight is applied to the cornea and the corneal displacement is measured with a volume shift being inferred. IOP is estimated by the displacement also. The weight can be left on the eye with the change in displacement and hence volume noted over time giving an estimate of outflow (Fout, volume loss per unit time). Measurements of outflow facility range from 0.23 to 0.3 μL/mL/mmHg and don't vary significantly with posture [62]. However, they do reduce by 17–45% at night.

$$\text{C} = \frac{(\text{Fout} - \text{Fuv})}{(\text{IOP} - \text{Pev})}$$

The problem is that Pev and Fuv are required. A solution to this problem is to take measurements at two separate IOP by applying different weights and assume that Pev and Fuv remain constant. Then at different weights (1 and 2):

$$\text{C} = \frac{(\text{Fout}_1 - \text{Fout}_2)}{(\text{IOP}_1 - \text{IOP}_2)}$$

It is impossible to directly measure uveoscleral outflow so it must be derived using the Goldmann equation. So, rearranging to extract uveoscleral outflow reveals:

$$\text{Fuv} = \text{Fin} - \text{C} \bullet \text{IOP} + \text{C} \bullet \text{Pev}$$

One can see that it's heavily dependent upon episcleral venous pressure. Episcleral venous pressure is very difficult to measure [63]. It is generally assumed to be 10 mmHg, but most recent evidence suggests that it's closer to 6–7 mmHg. In most measurements of drug effect upon aqueous flow, Pev has been assumed, generally at values close to 10 mmHg. Assuming a Pev of 8 mmHg, uveoscleral outflow is calculated at being approximately 0.8 μL/min [39]. These assumptions underlie claims that the prostaglandin drugs mainly increase uveoscleral outflow. However, more modern considerations of episcleral venous pressure reveal that these drugs probably have a greater effect upon conventional outflow affecting the so-called trabecular resistance [64].

Episcleral venous pressure was classically measured using a pressure bulb technique applying a small air compressed balloon to the episcleral veins increasing the compression until venous collapse was introduced. More recent work looking at episcleral venous diameter changes with compression demonstrate an inflection point in the pulsation amplitude versus pressure curve at a significantly lower pressure levels at around 7–8 mmHg in normal subjects [63].

It is evident from the above discussion that understanding and measurement of aqueous humour outflow from the eye is heavily dependent upon accurate measurements. These are difficult and in particular fluorophotometry, which measures aqueous total flow, and episcleral venous pressure are both difficult techniques. Classical tonography measuring IOP at different force settings upon the eye makes several assumptions and can roughly estimate conductance or facility of outflow. However, even tomography has problems and contains several key assumptions. It is important to consider these various measurement problems when interpreting the literature regarding drug and other effects upon IOP.

Using this mathematical type understanding helps explain the effect of therapy at various stages of glaucoma. The following graph illustrates the effect of treating facility of outflow at different facilities (Fig. 2.10). It is conventionally considered that facility of outflow reduces and leads to a rise in IOP and that this is the primary reason for IOP elevation in glaucoma [39]. It is generally not considered to be due to a reduction in uveoscleral outflow because uveoscleral outflow accounts for a smaller proportion of normal aqueous outflow. Additionally, aqueous production (Fin) does not alter significantly in glaucoma, whereas facility reduces by more than 50%.

So, trabecular resistance or facility of outflow has a major bearing upon IOP. Figure 2.10 demonstrates the effect of facility of outflow upon IOP at two values of aqueous inflow. Aqueous inflow can be altered by drug therapy by any of the so-called aqueous suppressants like acetazolamide or timolol. One can see that when aqueous

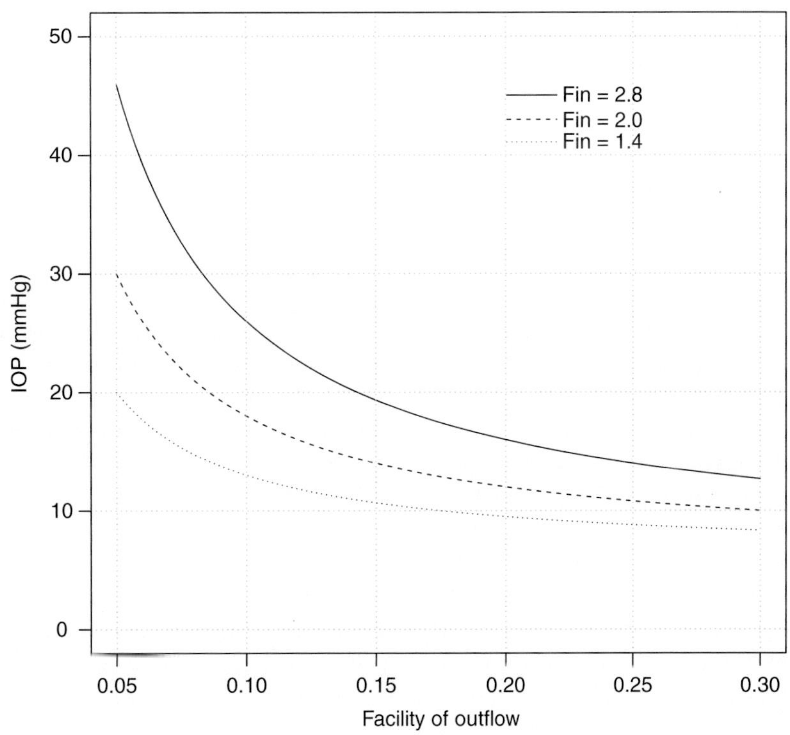

Fig. 2.10 Three curves plotted at various aqueous production rates (Fin, μL/min) using the Goldmann equation plotting IOP (mmHg) vs facility of outflow (C, μL/mL/mmHg). An Fin of 2.8 μL/min is typically normal and can be reduced pharmacologically by 40% to 2 μL/min or lower. However, variations in aqueous production can be seen to cause greater IOP fluctuation with lower facility

outflow facility is low these drugs have a much greater effect upon pressure. An example is with the pressure of approximately 45 mmHg being brought down to approximately 20 mmHg by a 50% reduction in aqueous flow when facility of outflow approximates 0.05. However, when facility of outflow is in the normal range, above 0.25, a 50% reduction in aqueous inflow results in a smaller 7 mmHg reduction, which may still be therapeutically significant. The corollary is the much greater fluctuation in IOP seen due to diurnal and other causes of aqueous production variation when outflow facility is low. IOP fluctuation is significantly greater in glaucoma and is an additional risk factor associated with the disease [65].

Therapeutic maneouvres which increase facility of outflow generally result in a more stable IOP. These tend to include surgical drainage procedures [66].

2.3.6 Cerebrospinal Fluid Pressure

The retrolaminar tissue behind the lamina cribrosa is greatly influenced by cerebrospinal fluid pressure (CSFP) and not subject to IOP. Surrounding the retrolaminar tissue is the pia mater beyond which lies the optic nerve subarachnoid space (ONSAS). Optic nerve subarachnoid space connects hydraulically to the intracranial subarachnoid space and therefore is subject to the influence of intracranial pressure which similarly to the eye pressurizes the cranial contents evenly and equally throughout. This includes the subarachnoid space which extends through the orbital apex surrounding the optic nerve to form the optic nerve subarachnoid space right up to the termination of the optic nerve at the posterior part of the globe. There are numerous trabeculae between the pia mater and dura which possibly limit hydraulic continuity along the subarachnoid space [67]. Animal experiments using dogs, however, do show that above an intracranial pressure of 0 mmHg, the optic nerve subarachnoid space pressure is equivalent to intracranial pressure [68]. Theoretically, it is hypothesized that the orbital tissue pressure creates this breakpoint by compressing the dura when intracranial pressure falls below 0 mmHg [69]. Normal intracranial pressure is at or below 0 mmHg when a person is sitting or standing [70]. This threshold pressure may vary in individuals given that orbital tissue tends to atrophy during life with a likely decrease in pressure. Technically it is extremely difficult to measure orbital tissue pressure with reliability. Presumed extraconal orbital pressure has been measured with needles and found to be close to 2.6 mmHg, although this technique may tend to over-estimate pressure [71].

Cerebrospinal fluid pressure (CSFP) can only be measured directly through a burr hole or via lumbar puncture into the lower spine. Posture and gravitational effects need to be considered when estimating intracranial CSFP [70]. Orbital tissue pressure sets a floor below which ONSAS pressure cannot fall, i.e. a buffer. Another buffering factor which alters the relationship between retrolaminar tissue pressure and CSFP is the physical property of the pia mater. The pia mater has some elasticity similar to a sausage skin and there exists a small but definite pressure gradient across the pia mater, particularly when ONSAS pressure is low [68]. Figure ONSAS illustrates these relationships in the dog, and one can see that below an intracranial pressure of 4 mmHg the retrolaminar tissue pressure stays at just below 4 mmHg when ONSAS pressure falls to 0 mmHg. In this region, experimental evidence from animals demonstrates that the small pressure differential is exerted by pia mater elastic compression of the optic nerve which reduces as the optic nerve subarachnoid space pressure increases, leading to some compression of the retrolaminar nerve. As ONSAS pressure falls towards 0 mmHg it is likely that the orbital tissue pressure compresses and sets a buffer floor (Fig. 2.11).

There is evidence that the intracranial pressure is lower in glaucoma patients (9.6 mmHg) compared to normals (12.7 mmHg) [73]. This has been confirmed in prospective studies [74], although some recent work suggests that there is no significant difference [75]. One problem with all these studies is the difficulty in taking orbital tissue and pia mater properties into account. An

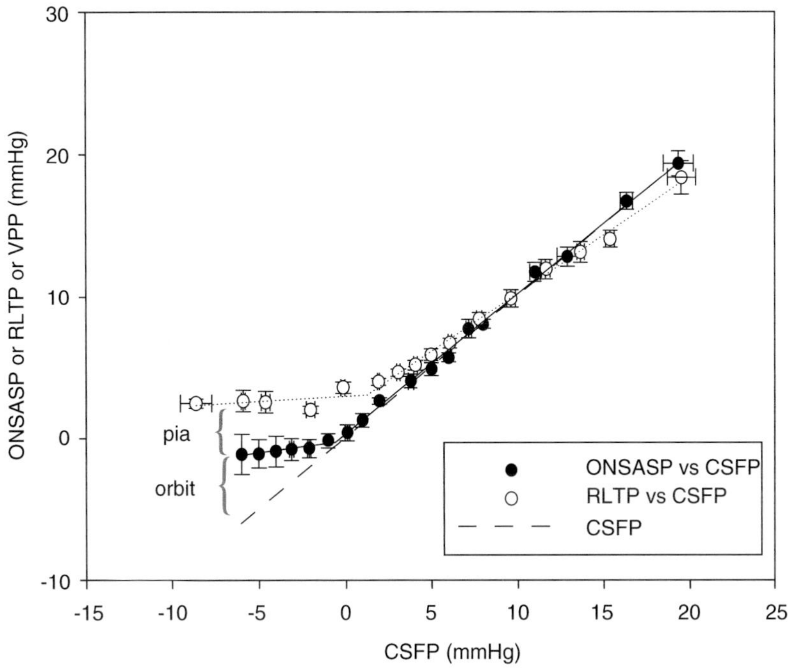

Fig. 2.11 The relationship of key pressures (±SE) to intracranial CSFP in the dog. A strong linear relationship is seen between ONSAS pressure (black circle), retrolaminar tissue pressure (RLTP (white circle) and intracranial CSFP (dashed line) above certain levels. Below these CSFP levels the pressures are constant. Lines of best fit are included. The difference between ONSAS and RLTP occurs across the pia mater (pia) and the difference between intracranial CSFP and ONSAS pressure is probably due to orbital pressure (orbit). Data from Morgan [72]

additional problem is the assumption that there is good hydraulic connection between the intracranial and optic nerve CSF, which may not be true in glaucoma [76]. It appears likely that the CSF pressure plays a significant role in producing the pressure gradient and forces across the optic disk, but this is modulated by other factors.

2.3.7 Pressure Gradient

2.3.7.1 Gradient in Dog and Human

Within the retrolaminar tissue the tissue pressure remains constant. Likewise, within the prelaminar tissue the tissue pressure remains constant as demonstrated in experiments using small micropipettes connected to sensitive pressure transducers manipulated across the optic disk [68]. However, across the lamina cribrosa a significant and quite large pressure gradient exists between the prelaminar and retrolaminar tissue pressures. Figure 2.12 shows typical tissue pressure measurements from a dog optic nerve at various depths from the optic disk surface and at various IOP and CSFP. Typically, the lamina cribrosa lies at a depth from 200 to 600 μm, and it is across this range that the pressure is seen to fall. In the normal dog with IOP 15 mmHg and CSFP 0 mmHg this pressure gradient averages some 20 mmHg/mm of lamina cribrosa tissue. In this animal the translaminar pressure gradient was significantly steeper when IOP is raised to 28 mmHg (60 mmHg/mm), and lower when CSFP rises to 10 mmHg with IOP of 20 mmHg (24 mmHg/mm) compared to 27 mmHg when IOP was 15 mmHg and CSFP was 0 mmHg. Within the human due to differences between the collagenous lamina cribrosa it has been estimated that this pressure gradient is between 20 and 30 mmHg/mm laminar tissue [2]. This is the highest pressure gradient recorded across a neural tissue anywhere in the body, and is also higher than pressure gradients known to exist along blood vessels [77]. The greatest pressure gradient along blood vessels is

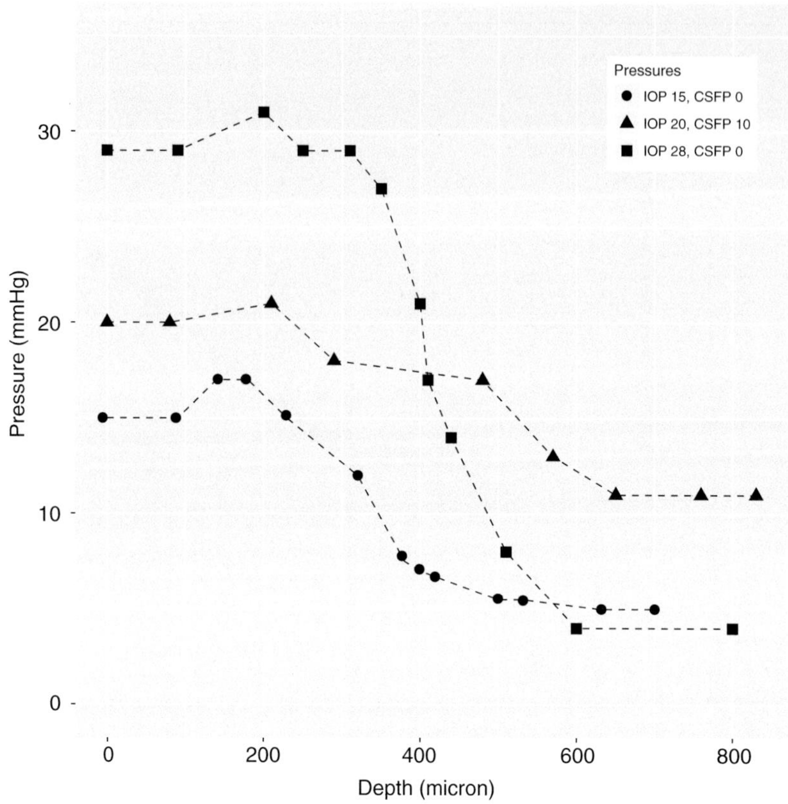

Fig. 2.12 Servo-null optic nerve tissue pressure measurements in a dog at various depths from the optic disk surface at set IOP and CSFP. Data from Morgan [72]

within the precapillary terminal arteriolar region where it averages 9 mmHg/mm tissue. This contrasts with approximately 1 mmHg/mm tissue in larger arterioles and venules such as the retinal arteries and veins (Fig. 2.13).

Forces acting across tissue are generated by differences between pressures not by absolute pressure. Most physiological processes like axonal transport are not altered by absolute changes in pressure [78]. An example is a subject travelling by aeroplane, which is de-pressurized to 3000 m. The absolute IOP may fall, but like other body fluid pressures, does not fall relative to surrounding air pressure. Likewise, a patient going scuba diving to 32 m water depth will experience an additional 760 mmHg hydrostatic pressure across their entire body. However, this does not change the pressure differentials within the body such as the blood pressure or the IOP with respect to surrounding environmental pressures.

It is also worth noting that a pressure differential exists across the sclera roughly equivalent to the translaminar pressure difference. However, the sclera is a very closely knit, densely packed, largely collagenous connective tissue structure which has strong physical properties to easily withstand the forces generated. That is the scleral physical properties generally can withstand the force load applied by standard IOP orbital tissue pressure differentials. This is not strictly the case in patients with high myopia who have significantly thinned and altered sclera, which tends to balloon posteriorly creating a so-called posterior staphyloma. It is interesting to note that posterior staphylomata in high myopes are particularly prominent where the optic nerve subarachnoid space termination has broadened out to involve much of the posterior sclera and so in those subjects the posterior sclera is tending to sink into the underlying subarachnoid space (Fig. 2.5).

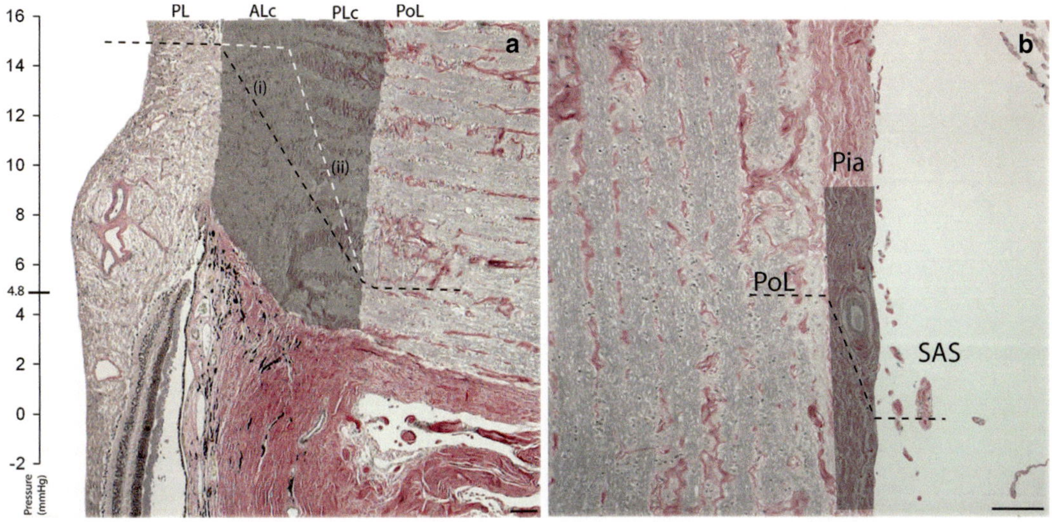

Fig. 2.13 Predicted pressure distributions in the human optic nerve. Schematic diagrams illustrate the predicted distributions of tissue pressure across the optic nerve head (**a**) and pia mater (**b**) of a normal human eye with an IOP of 15 mmHg and a CSF pressure of 0 mmHg. It remains unknown if pressure changes in the optic nerve head fall across the total thickness of the lamina cribrosa or the posterior lamina cribrosa only so an estimated plot for tissue pressure distribution across each of these regions is provided as plots (i) and (ii), respectively. Total lamina cribrosa thickness and pia mater thickness have been shaded in (**a**) and (**b**), respectively. Prelaminar (PL), anterior lamina cribrosa (ALc), posterior lamina cribrosa (PLc), postlaminar (PoL) and subarachnoid space (SAS) have also been identified where relevant. Scale bar = 100 μm. Reproduced with permission from Balaratnasingam et al. [2]

2.3.7.2 Effect of Gradient upon Neural Tissue

Physiologically, the major differentiating feature of the lamina cribrosa from surrounding tissues is the presence of this high pressure gradient. This increases with IOP elevation and also increases if retrolaminar tissue pressure decreases; as may occur when intracranial pressure falls depending upon orbital tissue pressure and pia mater characteristics within an individual. Figure 2.14 demonstrates the effect of 12 h IOP elevation to 43 mmHg within one pig eye compared to control at 13 mmHg where rapid axonal transport has been stained with an intravitreal injection of rhodamine tracer dye. One can see the accumulation in transport at the level of the lamina cribrosa in these animals (Fig. 2.14).

This work was pioneered in the 1970s by Anderson and others showing that not only is orthograde rapid axonal transport inhibited but also retrograde axonal transport [13, 80]. Curiously, when intracranial pressure is markedly elevated, leading to a rise in optic nerve subarachnoid space pressure and retrolaminar tissue pressure with a reversal in the pressure gradient across the lamina cribrosa, it is common to see a clinical syndrome of papilloedema. In this syndrome the optic disk swells from axoplasm accumulation in the prelaminar region leading to optic disk swelling [81]. One can clinically witness the interruption of orthograde axonal transport in this setting by seeing the optic disk swelling.

Axonal transport is highly energy dependent and requires the active functioning of molecular motors like kinesin and dynein traversing healthy microtubules within the setting of stable axonal environment partly determined by neurofilaments and actin constituents. In pig experiments after 3 h of elevated IOP there are decreased levels of neurofilament medium, neurofilament heavy and phosphorylated neurofilament detectable in the laminar and prelaminar regions. At 6 h reduced

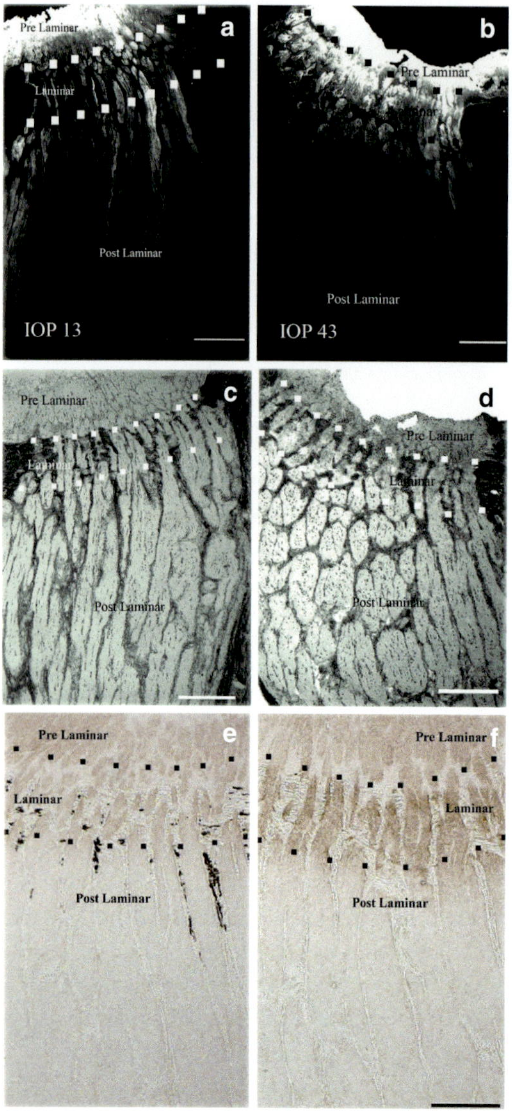

Fig. 2.14 Axonal transport in the control and high-IOP eyes. Confocal images of Rhodamine-B-isothiocyanate (RITC) transport after 12 h of raised IOP. Control eye, IOP 13 mmHg (**a**); High-IOP eye, IOP 43 mmHg (**b**). RITC travelled well past the lamina cribrosa in the control eye, whereas there was accumulation of tracer in the prelaminar and lamina cribrosa regions of the high-IOP eye, with little transport past the lamina cribrosa. Van Gieson–stained sections taken from similar regions of the RITC-labelled optic nerve are provided for reference; control eye—(**c**); high-IOP eye (**d**). Adjacent sections stained with cytochrome oxidase showing marked increase in mitochondrial activity in the high-IOP eye (**f**) compared to control (**e**). *Dotted lines*: lamina cribrosa region in each image. Scale bar, 400 m. Reproduced with permission from Balaratnasingam et al. [28, 79]

orthograde axonal transport is seen. At 12 h there are decreased levels of microtubules and microtubule associated proteins detectable in the laminar and prelaminar regions. These structures are vital for rapid axonal transport. In other studies where IOP is elevated, rapid axonal transport is inhibited with accumulation of organelles like mitochondria. Mitochondrial activity increases in the lamina cribrosa region with elevated IOP (Fig. 2.14 E and F) and is thought to be a sign that there is an increased energy requirement for the molecular motors: dynein and kinesin. Dynein is required to drive retrograde axonal transport up the translaminar pressure gradient. Energy depletion resulting in loss of adenosine triphosphate phosphorylation may affect surrounding processes like kinesin mediated orthograde transport and also alter phosphorylation of neurofilaments. Reduced blood flow into the anterior lamina region may compound this energy supply problem.

Early work on rabbit vagus nerve demonstrated that pressure gradients of approximately 45 mmHg/mm can inhibit axonal transport [82]. The vagus is myelinated and myelinated axons are known to be more resilient than unmyelinated axons. These experiments are complicated by the fact that the pressure gradient could not be measured at the same time that the nerve was being assessed.

Axons subjected to stretch and strain injury undergo cytoskeletal collapse with neurofilament compaction associated with calcium entry into the cells. Increasing IOP from 6 to 30 mmHg with CSFP remaining at 0 mmHg can induce 20% compressive strain and 5% tensile strain within the lamina cribrosa [83]. Significant strain variations are likely to occur within different laminar regions particularly around pores or holes, where local pressure gradients are likely to be much higher than surrounding gradients [23]. Measurements of neural injury effect tend to focus upon tensile strain and demonstrate neurofilament changes and axonal transport inhibition with more than 10% strain in rat dorsal root nerves [84]. In cultured cortical neural axons a strain of 2–10% can cause intracellular calcium release, neural sprouts and secondary axotomy [10]. Axonal transport is inhibited with organelle accumulation then axonal swelling leading to secondary axotomy. It is unclear whether the translaminar pressure gradient exerts its effect upon the axons only by inducing strain. There may be viscoelastic flow effects acting directly against retrograde axonal transport as well as leading to axonal strain [85, 86].

Pig optic nerve astrocytes within the laminar region become activated with altered morphology after just 6 h of IOP elevation. Such activation appears to be a protective response because mice without such a response experience greater axonal loss when IOP is elevated [87].

2.3.7.3 Effect of Gradient upon Retinal Vessels

Arteries and arterioles are not subject to direct influence of surrounding tissue pressure because their intraluminal pressure is significantly greater than the surrounds leading to maintenance of the vessel expansion. This does not hold true when surrounding tissue pressure increases so much that it can compress the arterioles in question. This can occur when IOP rises towards 60 or 70 mm/Hg with direct arteriolar compression. In this situation blood supply to the ciliary body is compromised reducing aqueous production and limiting further IOP rise. This situation can occur in acute angle closure.

However, veins are subject directly to surrounding tissue pressure because their intraluminal vascular pressure is generally equivalent to the surrounding tissue pressure. Studies of veins in other regions as well as on the retinal surface reveal that the pressure differential between the inside (intraluminal) vein and surrounding tissue pressure is approximately 1.3 mmHg only [88, 89]. The special case of the central retinal vein presents a physiological problem because it passes directly from a higher IOP compartment through the centre of the optic disk into the retrolaminar optic nerve at a much lower retrolaminar tissue pressure [5]. The simplest physiological model to explain the pressure consequence is that the central retinal vein would have the same or similar intraluminal pressure as its surrounding tissue and, hence, would have a similar pressure gradient, i.e. approaching 30 mmHg/mm tissue in the laminar region. Almost certainly this is not quite the case due to Starling resistor mechanisms which are beyond the scope of this manuscript to describe [5]. It is likely that this pressure gradient is stretched along the central retinal vein such that the pressure gradient partly exists within the prelaminar as well as retrolaminar region, in effect reducing the overall gradient but maintaining the pressure differential. This would mean that the intraluminal venous pressure at the prelaminar portion of the central retinal vein could become lower than surrounding IOP leading to a negative transmural pressure. This has been measured in pig eyes and does partially explain the phenomenon of spontaneous retinal venous pulsation seen in some 95% of normal subjects.

However, in spite of this likely expansion of the gradient zone with reduction in overall gradient, the pressure gradient along the vein is likely to be high, in the order of 15–20 mmHg/mm tissue. This probably explains why the central retinal vein endothelial cell morphology is spindle-shaped and identical to that seen in arteries rather than other veins where normal venous endothelial cell morphology is polygonal [90]. The higher pressure differential is likely to have haemodynamic effects with increased sheer stress and shear stress gradients along the central retinal vein. This is likely to explain part of the reason why central retinal vein occlusion is more commonly seen in glaucoma and also subjects with raised IOP [91]. In analogous Starling resistor engineering models the transmural pressure oscillates. Such oscillation in time with the cardiac cycle may provide the endothelial cells with some relief from an otherwise constant shear stress.

In glaucoma patients only some 50% have visible retinal venous pulsation [92]. This suggests that their central retinal vein is subject to more constant shear stress with a higher flow resistance and may explain some of the proclivity towards venous occlusion. Modelling work suggests that their retinal venous pressure is elevated, reducing perfusion pressure to the retina and anterior optic nerve [93].

2.3.7.4 Effect of Gradient upon Connective Tissue

The connective tissue most affected by glaucoma is that within the lamina cribrosa. The lamina cribrosa is normally comprised of collagen and elastin and other connective tissue subtypes forming connective tissue beams, which aggregate to form fenestrated sheets layered across approximately 450 μm tissue in the normal subject. This acts to stretch the distance over which the pressure differential acts and, hence, reduce the slope and magnitude of the translaminar pressure gradient. This forms a sieve with the superior and inferior regions having least connective tissue support with the largest pore size [94]. These are the regions of prime sensitivity for initial nerve loss in glaucoma.

The blood vessels pass through the centre of these connective tissue beams and are subject to the induced forces. The effect is not clear but likely to be significant. Optic disk rim haemorrhages are significantly associated with glaucoma and are also significantly associated with acquired focal lamina cribrosa defects [95].

With age and during glaucoma the connective tissue quality changes with loss of elastin and changes in the collagen [96, 97] resulting in a stiffer, less compliant lamina cribrosa [98]. The exact effect of these changes upon applied forces is not known but it appears likely that it may reduce the ability of the optic disk to absorb transient IOP changes like with blinking or eye rubbing [23, 99].

As the disease progresses the greater forces induced tend to act preferentially upon the peripheral lamina cribrosa pushing it posteriorly and peripherally as well as compressing the lamina, making it thinner [100]. The end result is posterior shift of the laminar attachment to the surrounding scleral rim with sheering of peripheral laminar attachments [101]. Additionally, laminar disruption occurs at the junction with sclera which can be seen using modern optical coherence tomography (OCT). Holes can occur within the lamina cribrosa which also become visible with OCT technology [95]. Laminar compression can result in the laminar thickness reducing from 450 μm down towards 200 μm [100]. A by-product of this compression is that the translaminar pressure gradient will be amplified by this reduction in separation distance. So, the effect of the forces upon the lamina cribrosa results in laminar distortion, compression and also sheering with the development of laminar disinsertion and holes. A common sign of glaucoma is the occurrence of optic disk rim haemorrhages: small flame or blot haemorrhages within the prelaminar tissue. Their origin is not known but may occur due to pathological changes in the lamina cribrosa. Their location has some association with lamina defects [102].

It has been surmised that laminar sheering and laminar stress, which would be passed on to the ganglion cell axons within that region, result directly in damage to those ganglion cell axons. It is unclear how ganglion cell axons bear the load generated within these pathological regions and it is difficult to model physical changes occurring.

On a more global scale analysing simple displacement of the central optic disk surface induced by changes in translaminar pressure gradient can be assessed with scanning laser tomography. This has been done in dogs where intracranial pressure and IOP were sequentially monitored and modified to generate particular pressure differentials and hence gradients across the laminar and optic disk regions. Figure 2.15 is a graph of the dog central optic disk displacement from baseline versus the difference between IOP and intracranial pressure (crude translaminar pressure difference) [11]. One can see that significant movement in optic disk occurred between the translaminar pressure difference of 3–15 mmHg with very little movement occurring thereafter. This non-linear axial compliance characteristic is seen in pigs albeit with reduced displacement above 30 mmHg [103] and may be present in the human situation as well. The mean IOP in various populations is 16 mmHg, indicating that half the population has an IOP less than this level and even with daily fluctuations in IOP, subjects at this range are at less risk of developing glaucoma but may be experiencing greater movement of their optic disk central cup region and likely greater fluctuations in axonal movement. It is possible that simple movement

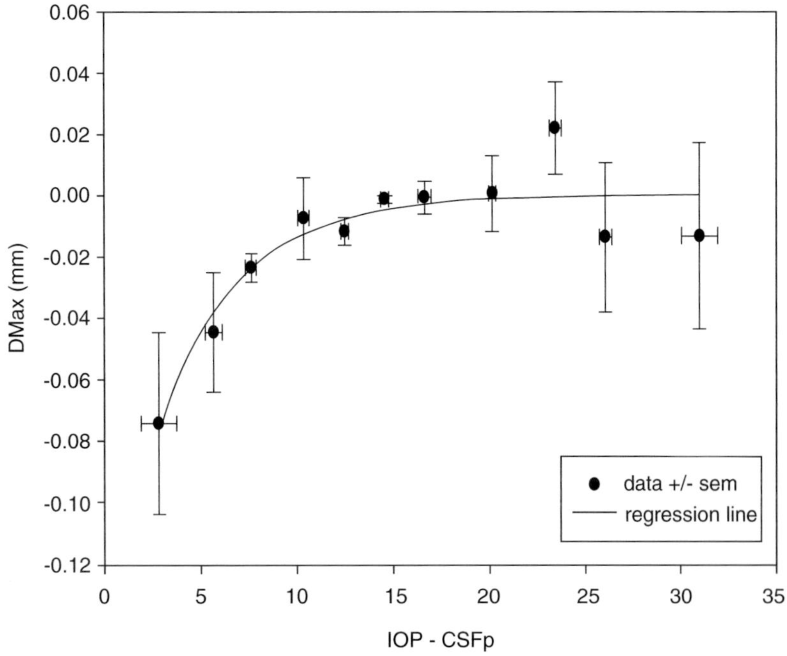

Fig. 2.15 Depth of the central optic disk surface (mm) vs. the difference between IOP and CSFP (mmHg), which is related to translaminar pressure difference. The line of best fit (regression) was an exponential function. Reproduced with permission from Morgan [11]

of ganglion cell axons is not enough to explain the resultant death and interruption of ganglion cell axons. These effects are complicated by the three dimensional nature of the forces produced [104, 105], and by the non-linear compliance of the eye itself, wherein IOP fluctuations tend to be greater as IOP increases.

2.3.7.5 Modelling Pressure Gradient in Glaucoma

It is useful to consider the translaminar pressure gradient in a variety of conditions. Figure 2.16 demonstrates the pressure gradient occurring in a typical human with IOP of 15 mmHg, intracranial pressure zero and retrolaminar tissue pressure of 4 mmHg with a gradient approximating 20 mmHg/mm tissue. Note that this gradient occurs across some 450 μm of laminar width and that this laminar width along with the pressure differential determines the gradient. Let us suppose that this subject over the course of some years develops an elevation in IOP to 25 mmHg. This will have the effect of increasing the pressure gradient across the same laminar width to approximately 40 mmHg/mm tissue. This is close to levels known to inhibit rapid axonal transport as well as having other physiological effects. Let us suppose that this individual is not diagnosed with the problem nor treated and that secondary changes occur in the connective tissue such that the lamina cribrosa is compressed to 250 μm in width as supported by histological data from moderate to severe glaucoma eyes [100]. Under this circumstance the translaminar pressure gradient now increases to 80 mmHg/mm tissue with pathological changes in axonal transport and supporting axonal elements. Let us suppose that at this point diagnosis of glaucoma is made and treatment instituted with IOP reduction to 15 mmHg. The treating clinician would normally consider this a success but examination of the effect upon the TPLG reveals that the pressure gradient in this situation would reduce from 80 mmHg/mm to approximately 40 mmHg/mm of tissue, still higher much higher than the initial physiological value because of the laminar compression and reduced distance across which the gradient operates. This may partly explain why patients with more severe glaucoma tend to progress even though IOP is brought well within a so-called normal physiological range. The problem therapeutically is that we cannot restore the normal supportive thickness and properties of a now compressed lamina cribrosa.

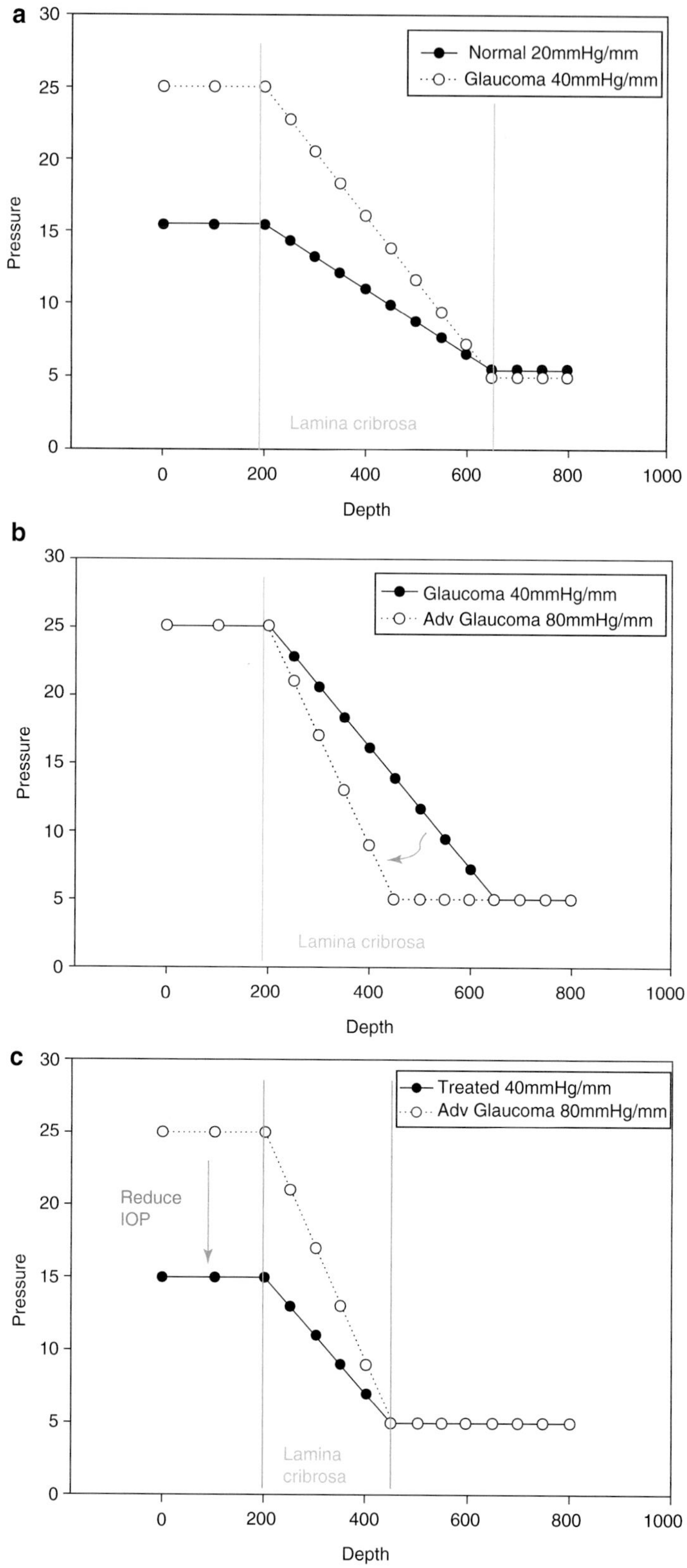

Fig. 2.16 Example of possible translaminar pressure gradient (TPLG) changes during glaucoma development. The IOP may increase from 15 to 25 mmHg in (**a**) with the subject going from normal to early glaucoma. Glaucoma advances further in (**b**) with lamina cribrosa compression, amplifying the TLPG. The glaucoma is recognized and treated in (**c**) with IOP lowering to 15 mmHg, but the TLPG remains elevated. Pressure is in mmHg, depth in μm from the surface across the optic disk tissue

Let us suppose that our individual is not normal to start with, but rather has high myopia. In this situation it has been shown that the normal high myope lamina cribrosa measures just 250 μm in width. Hence, the translaminar pressure gradient is going to be high to begin with at some 50 mmHg/mm of tissue. This places that individual at a much greater chance of glaucoma because the forces acting across the lamina cribrosa and ganglion cell axons are much higher with secondary compressive and other effects likely to occur. Over time this individual may experience and develop glaucomatous optic neuropathy with compression of the lamina down to 150 μm, as is seen histologically in high myopes with glaucoma [100]. This will again amplify the pressure gradient leading to a gradient in excess of 100 mmHg/mm of tissue assuming that the IOP has risen to just 22 mmHg. This subject with glaucoma is clearly at much higher risk of progressing even if the IOP is brought down towards 15 mm/Hg. One can see from this simple example of high myopia how optic disk vulnerability factors may operate to increase the likelihood of glaucoma development in subjects with apparently normal or mildly elevated IOP. There are almost certainly other properties within the connective tissue, glial cells and ganglion cell axons which increase vulnerability (Sect. 2.5.2). These factors are likely to not just be dependent upon laminar thickness.

2.4 Vascular Changes

2.4.1 Venous Changes

Venous changes have been largely described above. However, in relation to perfusion pressure venous pressure in the normal situation is only 1 mmHg greater than IOP just at the edge of the optic disk (in pigs and dogs). This means that in the normal situation perfusion pressure, which is determined by the difference between arterial and venous pressures, is in fact largely determined by the difference between arterial pressure and IOP. Unfortunately, in glaucoma this relationship may differ because the central retinal vein appears to change and undergo increased resistance to flow within the optic disk region leading to an elevation in retinal venous pressures significantly above IOP [5]. This has not been empirically measured because of the inability to directly measure retinal venous pressures in human eyes. It is indirectly estimated using ophthalmodynamometry.

2.4.2 Arterial Changes

The retinal artery morphology is not significantly altered by glaucoma. Retinal arterial pressure, however, is most important as a major determinant of perfusion pressure to the retina and anterior optic nerve. In dogs retinal artery pressure is approximately 72% of aortic pressure, indicating that some 28% pressure reduction occurs along the carotid and ophthalmic arteries [89]. The perfusion pressure in the anterior optic nerve and retina is likely to be significantly lower than that within the posterior laminar and retrolaminar regions because the venous pressure in the posterior laminar and retrolaminar regions is almost certainly significantly lower than that of the retinal venous pressure. Accordingly, most investigators of blood flow and pressure effects upon glaucoma are concerned with anterior optic nerve and retinal perfusion pressure [106].

Major arterial (carotid artery) pressure at eye level can be directly estimated by measuring brachial artery pressure at eye level by using sphygmomanometry with the cuff and arm held at eye level. Ophthalmodynamometry is performed by applying a contact lens to the eye with increasing force until central retinal artery pulsation (diastolic) or full arterial closure (systolic) is seen. Because occlusion of the retinal artery is induced these pressures are in fact closer to ophthalmic artery pressures rather than actual retinal artery pressures [31]. As patients age it is likely that atherosclerotic and other pathological processes increase the pressure drop along the major arteries and reduce the actual perfusion pressure within the eye. A low diastolic blood pressure is a well-known risk factor for glaucoma progression and it is likely that this is implicated because it results in a lower retinal and anterior optic nerve perfusion pressure [107]. However, elevated perfusion pressure with reduced blood flow is more commonly seen in glaucoma [108], which suggests a greater role for venous pathology.

An example of the importance of blood pressure is in the young, healthy individual situation with a blood pressure of 120/70 mmHg, which equates approximately to a mean arterial blood pressure of 87 mmHg. Blood pressure is typically measured in the seating posture with a sphygmomanometry cuff at heart level. Typically this is some 40 cm below eye level and when this gravitational effect is taken into account this means that some 30 mmHg is required simply to pump the blood up to eye level and, hence, the mean arterial pressure in the young, healthy person will be some 57 mm/Hg at eye level. If we subtract average 15 mm/Hg IOP (and presumed venous pressure) this reduces the perfusion pressure to 42 mmHg. Note that this does not take into account the pressure drop along the ophthalmic artery of approximately 28%. Large epidemiological studies have shown that diastolic pressures <30 mmHg greater than IOP are associated with increased rates of glaucoma progression [107].

It is also worth noting that a typical brachial artery blood pressure of 120/70 mmHg corresponds to carotid artery systolic pressure of 90 mmHg and with a 28% pressure drop suggests a likely 65 mmHg retinal artery pressure. Ciliary artery pressure is probably similar and this provides the reason why IOP can rise no higher than a similar 70 mmHg. Also, once the IOP reaches 70 mmHg almost total blood flow is cut off from the eye including the anterior optic nerve.

Perfusion pressure changes during the day and in particular with posture. An example is when a subject goes from sitting to lying down. The blood pressure at eye level will actually increase and in our example from above with a mean systemic blood pressure of 87 mmHg the blood pressure at eye level will increase from 57 mmHg to close to 87 mmHg if the subject lies down. However, there are also changes in IOP with the IOP tending to rise slightly with a supine posture. Additionally, some patients, particularly those prone to sleep apnoea or those with cardiovascular pathologies may experience reductions in cardiac output and blood pressure whilst sleeping and these may pose some effect upon perfusion pressure affecting the optic nerve. This is a complex area and is complicated by not only by the variability in cardiovascular pressure parameters over the course of time but also by the effect of postural changes upon those parameters. This largely explains why it is currently unclear how much affect nocturnal change in blood pressure actually has upon glaucoma progression or aetiology [109, 110].

Blood flow to the retina with presumed similar changes in blood flow to the optic nerve is reduced in patients with glaucoma. It had been assumed that this was due to changes in the arterial system but more recent evidence suggests in fact that this is largely due to changes in the venous system during the course of the disease [5, 93]. There is some evidence that regulation of blood flow to the retina and anterior optic nerve is reduced in glaucoma [111]. The changes in presumed retinal venous pressure are most strongly associated with glaucoma severity and rates of progression.

2.4.3 Disk Rim Haemorrhage

Disk rim haemorrhage is a known risk factor for glaucoma occurrence and progression. Disk haemorrhages are often flame shaped on the optic disk margin and are transient lasting an average 6 weeks (Fig. 2.1). Subsequent loss of adjacent nerve fibre layer and development of corresponding visual field loss is frequently observed [112]. The presence of disk rim haemorrhage increases the risk fourfold for subsequent development of primary open angle glaucoma [113]. Additionally, eyes with disk rim haemorrhage progress twice as rapidly compared to those without haemorrhage [114]. Recurrent haemorrhage in the same location does not appear to significantly elevate the progression risk beyond one haemorrhage [115]. Although, in other studies disk haemorrhage frequency was associated with increased progression [38]. Multiple haemorrhages in separate regions of the optic disk do increase the risk of progression above a single haemorrhage [116]. One problem with these studies is that some use more sensitive photography and others use clinical observation for haemorrhage detection.

The cause of disk haemorrhage is not known. They are associated with and found close to lamina cribrosa defects, although this is not invariate [102]. This does raise the possibility that smaller vessel such as venules within the lamina beam core are sheared by the connective tissue changes. A link to venular pathology related to the occurrence of venous occlusion has been suggested by some [117]. Central and hemi retinal vein occlusions are more common in glaucoma and in subjects with elevated IOP [91]. Studies measuring retinal venous pulsation pressure, related to larger vein resistance, have found no relationship or only a weak relationship with disk rim haemorrhage [118]. One can see that their cause is unclear and it is not known if the majority emanate from arteriolar, capillary or venular pathology.

2.5 Causes of Tissue Vulnerability

2.5.1 Age

Age is a major risk factor for primary open angle and angle closure glaucoma. Figure 2.17 demonstrates that the prevalence of primary open angle glaucoma increases with age across racial groups. There appears to be two prime reasons for age being such a risk for primary open angle glaucoma. One involves changes to the trabecular meshwork and other, optic disk structures. With ageing there are changes in the trabecular meshwork extracellular matrix with increased fibrosis and loss of trabecular meshwork cells [119]. Consequently the phagocytic ability of the meshwork appears to reduce which may have consequences downstream in the canal of Schlemm and collector channels. Extracellular matrix changes occur in glaucoma and are thought to be a major factor increasing trabecular meshwork resistance

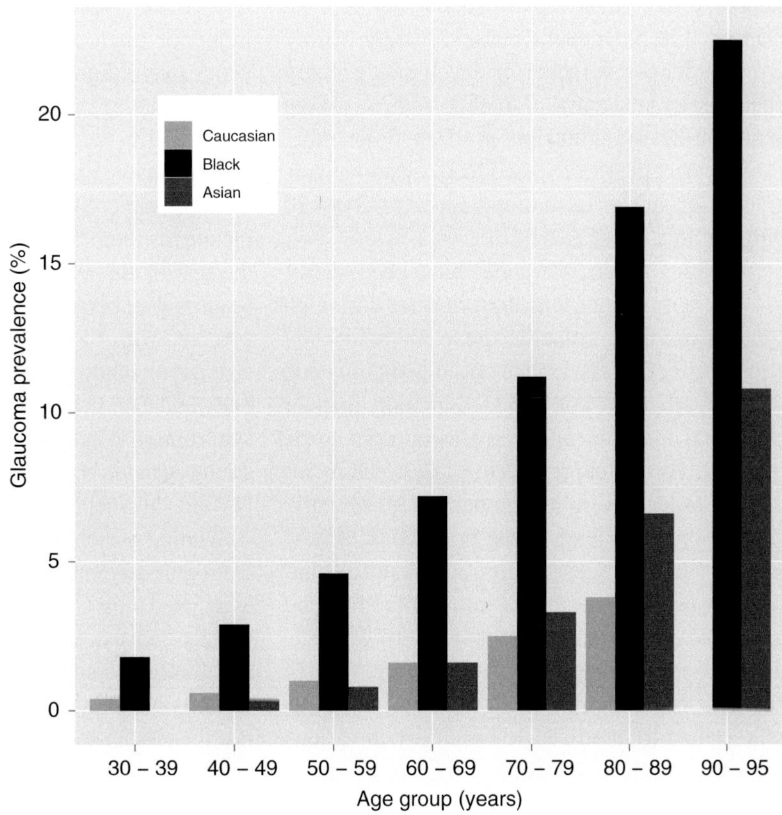

Fig. 2.17 The prevalence of primary open angle glaucoma (%) vs. age group for different racial groups. Blacks were those of predominant sub-Saharan African descent. Asians were those from south and east Asia. Data from Rudnicka [121]

[41, 57]. Outflow facility is reduced as one ages, but this tends to be balanced by reduced aqueous humour production with relatively constant IOP in most people [120].

The optic nerve connective tissue, particularly within the lamina cribrosa changes with age leading to increased stiffness with less elastin and altered collagen [119]. This may increase the susceptibility of the lamina structures to pressure gradient induced damage. The lens continues to grow during life leading to its expansion and tendency to cause increased pupil/iris and ciliary flow resistance, with an increased tendency to angle closure.

2.5.2 Genetic Susceptibility

Glaucoma has a strong genetic influence. It can be seen from Fig. 2.17 that certain racial groups, like sub-Saharan African descendants are much more likely to develop primary open angle glaucoma [121]. Certain groups like the Inuit and Mongolians are more likely to develop angle closure [122]. Such racial predilection is most likely due to polygenetic causes. Family history is a significant risk factor for developing primary open angle glaucoma. Subjects with a sibling or parent having glaucoma are four times more likely to develop the disease [123]. Genome wide association studies have shown links to at least 20 different loci [124].

Two high penetrance genes have been shown to be inherited in a Mendelian manner with high penetrance. The myocilin gene is associated with 3–4% of primary open angle glaucoma and is inherited in an autosomal dominant manner [125]. Myocilin encoded protein appears to be important for protein trafficking across cell membranes, especially in the trabecular meshwork. Genetic mutation leads to the production of misfolded proteins released into the extracellular space may cause decreased outflow facility and high IOP. This possible mechanism of effect is disputed and mutant myocilin protein may have effects upon trabecular meshwork cell mitochondria leading to increased vulnerability to various insults. Nevertheless, it commonly causes a juvenile onset open angle glaucoma.

More recently, optineurin gene mutations have been found to be strongly associated with primary open angle glaucoma in which the IOP is not elevated above 20 mmHg, the so-called normal tension glaucoma [126]. This mutation accounts for 0.4% of primary open angle glaucoma cases. The gene product is important for transport of endosomes along microtubules and for promoting autophagy. Autophagy is particularly important in neural cells, which don't divide and are required to live for a long period. It is the mechanism by protein aggregates and damaged mitochondrion are degraded. It is likely that this makes the ganglion cell axon more vulnerable within the lamina cribrosa region, due to the higher protein and mitochondria turnover required in this region. Mutations in the optineurin gene appear to render the optic nerve axons more vulnerable to pressure gradients that other eyes would tolerate.

There are other genes being discovered which are associated with increased likelihood of glaucoma occurrence. It is likely that these genes will have various effects, from altering the anterior chamber depth and lens size which could influence angle closure occurrence [47]. Other genes may influence elements along the aqueous outflow pathway and others add to optic nerve vulnerability factors.

Congenital glaucoma is uncommon but has a strong genetic component. In primary congenital glaucoma there are no other disease features in the rest of the eye or body, where elevated IOP, scalloped trabecular meshwork and an enlarging eye are seen. In secondary congenital glaucoma a range of other problems are seen involving the body and eye, frequently forming parts of unusual syndromes. Many of these syndromes have a strong genetic cause, but a full description is beyond the scope of this chapter [127]. Primary congenital glaucoma frequently occurs in children from consanguineous marriages, and is strongly associated with CYP1B1 gene mutation. The form of inheritance is autosomal recessive although it is usually sporadic. It occurs in approximately 1 in 10,000 births but is more common in some societies. It is associated with delayed or arrested maturation of the angle structures and hence the odd appearance commonly seen on gonioscopy.

2.5.3 Internal Environment: Factors Within the Eye

There are several properties that can change within an eye to promote glaucoma. The eye can produce large particles that may block the trabecular meshwork or produce harmful factors toxic to the meshwork and other parts of the outflow pathway. Their continued production adversely affects the effectiveness of therapy.

Pseudoexfoliation material is commonly found amongst certain racial groups, like north Europeans with a strong association with the LOXL1 gene [128, 129]. In this condition, cells in various parts of the body produce an abnormal basement membrane. In the eye this material flakes off from the ciliary body, and iris to float around with aqueous and accumulate within the trabecular meshwork. The trabecular meshwork has phagocytic ability but becomes overwhelmed by this material. This results in failure of the trabecular meshwork with elevated IOP. The pseudoexfoliation material can be released in showers with relatively rapid rises in IOP causing this form of glaucoma to be unpredictable.

Pigment from the posterior iris can be liberated by rubbing on the zonules under certain circumstances. This tends to occur in young myopic patients where the iris is bowed backwards (posterior pupil block) leading to contact with the zonules. It is thought that constant pupil contraction and dilation rubs off pigment granules from the posterior iris. This causes pigment dispersion syndrome, where the liberated pigment flows with aqueous humour and blocks the trabecular meshwork, with IOP elevation, like pseudoexfoliation [130]. With age and growth of the lens, the posterior pupil block may reduce and pigment release may stop. If the meshwork phagocytic capacity is still relatively intact the pigment may be phagocytosed and the process reversed with lowering of IOP. This is the only form of glaucoma that can occasionally heal by itself.

The eye, in particular the retina, can produce various factors that affect tissue growth. Rubeosis iridis (iris new vessels) is a common condition caused by vasoproliferative factors like the vascular endothelial growth factors produced in the retina [131]. This passes forward in the aqueous humour to reach the anterior chamber where it comes into contact with the trabecular meshwork. Here, it can stimulate growth of blood vessels and fibrous tissue across the trabecular meshwork and iris. If left untreated, this fibro-vascular tissue will block the trabecular meshwork leading to IOP elevation. Various causes of retinal ischaemia will induce the release of these angioproliferative factors and include diabetic retinopathy, ischaemic retinal vein and artery occlusions as well as forms of retinal vasculitis.

Chronic forms of uveitis, whereby inflammatory material is produced and enters the aqueous humour and/or cause direct inflammation of the trabecular meshwork and iris can cause glaucoma. Adhesions between the iris and trabecular meshwork (synechiae) or inflammatory debris within the trabecular meshwork can block meshwork function leading to elevation in IOP.

The retina normally produces various growth factors which enter the vitreous. Some of this diffuses anteriorly to the lens where they bind and are responsible for stimulating lens epithelial cell growth and differentiation [132]. If the lens and capsule are removed, termed "aphakia", these growth factors enter the aqueous humour in greater concentration and affect the trabecular meshwork. Glaucoma is significantly more common in aphakic patients. This phenomenon partially explains the high rates of childhood glaucoma that occur when congenital cataracts are removed. The lens also absorbs and uses oxygen from the aqueous and when it is removed, aqueous with greater oxygen concentration, reactive oxygen species, and altered glutathione and ascorbate levels reaches the trabecular meshwork [41].

Ideally, the aqueous humour should be free of particulates and clean of various toxic factors. Their presence makes glaucoma therapy more difficult because these forms of glaucoma often prove more resistant to medical therapy. Surgical drainage procedures tend to fail more commonly as well due to persistence of this "toxic" aqueous.

2.5.4 External Environment: Factors Outside the Eye

The commonest external factor leading to glaucoma is trauma, with a force hitting the eye leading to a compression/expansion injury. This may often injure the trabecular meshwork with visible signs of meshwork cleavage from the scleral spur (angle recession) or increased pigment deposition [133]. The trabecular meshwork may fail immediately or gradually with increased fibrotic change leading to a rise in IOP.

Another common external factor is topically applied steroid eye drops. They diffuse into the eye and pass through the trabecular meshwork, where they stimulate changes in the meshwork extracellular matrix. This can lead to a rise in IOP and secondary glaucoma [134].

Patients often ask if diet or other external factors contribute to glaucoma. There is no evidence that diet contributes to glaucoma aetiology. Caffeine intake has been questioned but again there is no evidence that it adds to the risk of getting glaucoma except with the possible exception of those with a family history of glaucoma [135].

Several infections may cause glaucoma. The commonest are ones that cause chronic uveitis, like herpes zoster and simplex viruses. Their mechanism is the same as with uveitis. Congenital rubella acquired in utero via the mother in the third trimester commonly infects the eye and affects differentiation of the trabecular meshwork, as well as lens and retina. This commonly leads to glaucoma with elevated IOP as well as cataract and a retinopathy [136].

2.6 Conclusion

There are many factors that contribute to one person developing glaucoma. The final common pathways involve mechanisms that elevate IOP and or increase the vulnerability of the optic disk to a pressure gradient. The actual neural loss appears to be via a combination of mechanisms affecting the neural tissue, supporting connective tissue and vascular supply. The most common IOP elevating mechanisms are those that affect trabecular meshwork function or lead to angle closure. In the optic nerve, factors that affect neural function and support in the lamina cribrosa part of the optic nerve are critical.

Acknowledgments National Health and Medical Research Council Australia.

References

1. Quigley HA, Green WR. The histology of human glaucoma cupping and optic nerve damage: clinicopathologic correlation in 21 eyes. Ophthalmology. 1979;86:1803–30.
2. Balaratnasingam C, Morgan WH, Johnstone V, Pandav SS, Cringle SJ, Yu DY. Histomorphometric measurements in human and dog optic nerve and an estimation of optic nerve pressure gradients in human. Exp Eye Res. 2009;89:618–28.
3. Jonas JB, Berenshtein E, Holbach L. Anatomic relationship between lamina cribrosa, intraocular space, and cerebrospinal fluid space. Invest Ophthalmol Vis Sci. 2003;44:5189–95.
4. Quigley HA, Addicks EM, Green WR, Maumenee AE. Optic nerve damage in human glaucoma. II. The site of injury and susceptibility to damage. Arch Ophthalmol. 1981;99:635–49.
5. Morgan WH, Hazelton ML, Yu DY. Retinal venous pulsation: expanding our understanding and use of this enigmatic phenomenon. Prog Retin Eye Res. 2016;55:82–107.
6. Vrabec F. Glaucomatous cupping of the human optic disk. Graefes Arch Clin Exp Ophthalmol. 1976;198:223–34.
7. Bradke F, Fawcett JW, Spira ME. Assembly of a new growth cone after axotomy: the precursor to axon regeneration. Nat Rev Neurosci. 2012;13:183–93.
8. Chung RS, Staal JA, Mccormack GH, Dickson TC, Cozens MA, Chuckowree JA, Quilty MC, Vickers JC. Mild axonal stretch injury in vitro induces a progressive series of neurofilament alterations ultimately leading to delayed axotomy. J Neurotrauma. 2005;22:1081–91.
9. Maxwell WL, Povlishock JT, Graham DL. A mechanistic analysis of nondisruptive axonal injury: a review. J Neurotrauma. 1997;14:419–40.
10. Staal JA, Dickson TC, Gasperini R, Liu Y, Foa L, Vickers JC. Initial calcium release from intracellular stores followed by calcium dysregulation is linked to secondary axotomy following transient axonal stretch injury. J Neurochem. 2010;112:1147–55.
11. Morgan WH, Chauhan BC, Yu DY, Cringle SJ, Alder VA, House PH. Optic disk movement with variations in intraocular and cerebrospinal fluid pressure. Inv Ophthalmol Vis Sci. 2002;43:3236–42.

12. Levy NS. The effects of elevated intraocular pressure on slow axonal protein flow. Investig Ophthalmol. 1974;13:691–5.
13. Minckler DS, Bunt AH, Johanson GW. Orthograde and retrograde axoplasmic transport during acute ocular hypertension in the monkey. Inv Ophthalmol Vis Sci. 1977;16:426–40.
14. Quigley H, Broman AT. The number of people with glaucoma worldwide in 2010 and 2020. Br J Ophthalmol. 2006;90:262–7.
15. Quigley HA, Addicks EM, Green R. Optic damage in human glaucoma III. Quantitative correlation of nerve fiber loss and visual field defect in glaucoma, ischaemic neuropathy, papilledema, and toxic neuropathy. Arch Ophthalmol. 1982;100:135–46.
16. Turpin A, Sampson GP, Mckendrick AM. Combining ganglion cell topology and data of patients with glaucoma to determine a structure-function map. Invest Ophthalmol Vis Sci. 2009;50:3249–56.
17. Harwerth RS, Wheat JL, Fredette MJ, Anderson DR. Linking structure and function in glaucoma. Prog Retin Eye Res. 2010;29:249–71.
18. Quigley HA, Dunkelberger GR, Green WR. Chronic human glaucoma causing selectively greater loss of large optic nerve fibres. Ophthalmology. 1988;95:357–63.
19. Sample PA, Bosworth CF, Weinreb RN. The loss of visual function in glaucoma. Semin Ophthalmol. 2000;15:182–93.
20. Nelson P, Aspinall P, Papasouliotis O, Worton B, O'brien C. Quality of life in glaucoma and its relationship with visual function. J Glaucoma. 2003;12:139–50.
21. Yun SC, Hahn IK, Sung KR, Yoon JY, Jeong D, Chung HS. Lamina cribrosa depth according to the level of axial length in normal and glaucomatous eyes. Graefes Arch Clin Exp Ophthalmol. 2015;253:2247–53.
22. Burgoyne CF, Downs JC. Premise and prediction-how optic nerve head biomechanics underlies the susceptibility and clinical behavior of the aged optic nerve head. J Glaucoma. 2009;17:318–28.
23. Downs JC. Optic nerve head biomechanics in aging and disease. Exp Eye Res. 2015;133:19–29.
24. Anderson DR. Ultrastructure of human and monkey lamina cribrosa and optic nerve head. Arch Ophthalmol. 1969;82:800–14.
25. Stowell C, Burgoyne CF, Tamm ER, Ethier CR. Biomechanical aspects of axonal damage in glaucoma: a brief review. Exp Eye Res. 2017;157:13–9.
26. Ohno-Matsui K, Akiba M, Moriyama M, Ishibashi T, Tokoro T, Spaide RF. Imaging retrobulbar subarachnoid space around optic nerve by swept-source optical coherence tomography in eyes with pathologic myopia. Invest Ophthalmol Vis Sci. 2011;52:9644–50.
27. Saxton WM, Hollenbeck PJ. The axonal transport of mitochondria. J Cell Sci. 2012;125:2095–104.
28. Balaratnasingam C, Morgan WH, Bass L, Matich G, Cringle SJ, Yu DY. Axonal transport and cytoskeletal changes in the laminar regions after elevated intraocular pressure. Invest Ophthalmol Vis Sci. 2007;48:3632–44.
29. Emi K, Pederson JE, Toris CB. Hydrostatic pressure of the suprachoroidal space. Inv Ophthalmol Vis Sci. 1989;30:233–8.
30. Silver DM, Quigley HA. Aqueous flow through the iris-lens channel: estimates of differential pressure between the anterior and posterior chambers. J Glaucoma. 2004;13:100–7.
31. Morgan WH, Yu DY, Alder VA, Cringle SJ, Constable IJ. Relation between pressure determined by ophthalmodynamometry and aortic pressure in the dog. Br J Ophthalmol. 1998;82:821–5.
32. Goldmann H, Schmidt T. Über Applanationstonometrie. Ophthalmologica. 1957;134:221–42.
33. Kotecha A, White E, Schlottmann PG, Garway-Heath DF. Intraocular pressure measurement precision with the Goldmann applanation, dynamic contour, and ocular response analyzer tonometers. Ophthalmology. 2010;117:730–7.
34. Okafor KC, Brandt JD. Measuring intraocular pressure. Curr Opin Ophthalmol. 2015;26:103–9.
35. Moses RA, Hart WM. Intraocular pressure. In: Physiology of the eye, clinical application. St Louis: Mosby; 1987.
36. Hollows FC, Graham PA. Intra-ocular pressure, glaucoma, and glaucoma suspects in a defined population. Br J Ophthalmol. 1966;50:570–86.
37. Sommer A. Intraocular pressure and glaucoma. Am J Ophthalmol. 1989,107.186–8.
38. Leske MC, Heijl A, Hyman L, Bengtsson B, Dong L, Yang Z. Predictors of long-term progression in the early manifest glaucoma trial. Ophthalmology. 2007;114:1965–72.
39. Brubaker RF. Flow of aqueous humor in humans [The Friedenwald Lecture]. Invest Ophthalmol Vis Sci. 1991;32:3145–66.
40. Civan MM, Macknight AD. The ins and outs of aqueous humour secretion. Exp Eye Res. 2004;78:625–31.
41. Carreon T, Van Der Merwe E, Fellman RL, Johnstone M, Bhattacharya SK. Aqueous outflow - a continuum from trabecular meshwork to episcleral veins. Prog Retin Eye Res. 2017;57:108–33.
42. Alm A, Nilsson SF. Uveoscleral outflow--a review. Exp Eye Res. 2009;88:760–8.
43. Brubaker RF. The flow of aqueous humor in the human eye. Trans Am Ophthalmol Soc. 1982;80:391–474.
44. Chandler PA, Simmons RJ, Grant WM. Malignant glaucoma. Medical and surgical treatment. Am J Ophthalmol. 1968;66:495–502.
45. Ng WT, Morgan W. Mechanisms and treatment of primary angle closure: a review. Clin Exp Ophthalmol. 2012;40:e218–28.
46. Prata TS, Dorairaj S, De Moraes CG, Mehta S, Sbeity Z, Tello C, Liebmann J, Ritch R. Is preoperative ciliary body and iris anatomical configuration a predictor of malignant glaucoma development? Clin Exp Ophthalmol. 2013;41:541–5.
47. Sun X, Dai Y, Chen Y, Yu DY, Cringle SJ, Chen J, Kong X, Wang X, Jiang C. Primary angle closure glaucoma: what we know and what we don't know. Prog Retin Eye Res. 2017;57:26–45.

48. Ritch R, Shields MB, Krupin T. The glaucomas. St Louis: Mosby; 1996.
49. Maepea O, Bill A. The pressures in the episcleral veins, Schlemm's canal and the trabecular meshwork in monkeys: effects of changes in intraocular pressure. Exp Eye Res. 1989;49:645–63.
50. Johnstone M, Martin E, Jamil A. Pulsatile flow into the aqueous veins: manifestations in normal and glaucomatous eyes. Exp Eye Res. 2011;92:318–27.
51. Johnson M. What controls aqueous humour outflow resistance? Exp Eye Res. 2006;82:545–57.
52. Grant W. Further studies on facility of flow through the trabecular meshwork. AMA Arch Ophthalmol. 1958;60:523–33.
53. Ellingsen BA, Grant WM. The relationship of pressure and aqueous outflow in enucleated human eyes. Investig Ophthalmol. 1971;10:430–7.
54. Van Buskirk EM, Grant WM. Lens depression and aqueous outflow in enucleated primate eyes. Am J Ophthalmol. 1973;76:632–40.
55. Bill A. The aqueous humor drainage mechanism in the cynomolgus monkey (Macaca irus) with evidence for unconventional routes. Investig Ophthalmol. 1965;4:911–9.
56. Tamm ER. The trabecular meshwork outflow pathways: structural and functional aspects. Exp Eye Res. 2009;88:648–55.
57. Tektas OY, Lutjen-Drecoll E. Structural changes of the trabecular meshwork in different kinds of glaucoma. Exp Eye Res. 2009;88:769–75.
58. Liton PB. The autophagic lysosomal system in outflow pathway physiology and pathophysiology. Exp Eye Res. 2016;144:29–37.
59. Brubaker RF. Goldmann's equation and clinical measures of aqueous dynamics. Exp Eye Res. 2004;78:633–7.
60. Goldmann H. The aqueous veins and the Poiseuille law. Ophthalmologica. 1949;118:496–519.
61. Schiotz H. Et nyt tonometer, tonometri. Norsk Mag Lægevidensk. 1905;66:597–622.
62. Selvadurai D, Hodge D, Sit AJ. Aqueous humor outflow facility by tonography does not change with body position. Invest Ophthalmol Vis Sci. 2010;51:1453–7.
63. Sit AJ, Ekdawi NS, Malihi M, Mclaren JW. A novel method for computerized measurement of episcleral venous pressure in humans. Exp Eye Res. 2011;92:537–44.
64. Lim KS, Nau CB, O'byrne MM, Hodge DO, Toris CB, Mclaren JW, Johnson DH. Mechanism of action of bimatoprost, latanoprost, and travoprost in healthy subjects. A crossover study. Ophthalmology. 2008;115:790–795.e4.
65. Caprioli J, Coleman AL. Intraocular pressure fluctuation. A risk factor for visual field progression at low intraocular pressures in the advanced glaucoma intervention study. Ophthalmology. 2008;115:1123–9.
66. Mansouri K, Orguel S, Mermoud A, Haefliger I, Flammer J, Ravinet E, Shaarawy T. Quality of diurnal intraocular pressure control in primary open-angle patients treated with latanoprost compared with surgically treated glaucoma patients: a prospective trial. Br J Ophthalmol. 2008;92:332–6.
67. Killer HE, Laeng HR, Flammer J, Groscurth P. Architecture of arachnoid trabeculae, pillars, and septa in the subarachnoid space of the human optic nerve: anatomy and clinical considerations. Br J Ophthalmol. 2003;87:777–81.
68. Morgan WH, Yu DY, Alder VA, Cringle SJ, Cooper RL, House PH, Constable IJ. The correlation between cerebrospinal fluid pressure and retrolaminar tissue pressure. Invest Ophthalmol Vis Sci. 1998;39:1419–28.
69. Morgan WH, Yu DY, Balaratnasingam C. The role of cerebrospinal fluid pressure in glaucoma pathophysiology: the dark side of the optic disk. J Glaucoma. 2008;17:408–13.
70. Magnaes B. Body position and cerebrospinal fluid pressure. Part 2. Clinical studies on orthostatic pressure and the hydrostatic indifferent point. J Neurosurg. 1976;44:698–705.
71. Moller PM. The pressure in the orbit. Acta Ophthalmol Suppl. 1955;43:1–100.
72. Morgan WH. Pressure gradients across the optic disk. PhD, University of Western Australia; 1999.
73. Berdahl JP, Allingham R, Johnson DH. Cerebrospinal fluid pressure is decreased in primary open-angle glaucoma. Ophthalmology. 2008;115:763–8.
74. Ren R, Jonas JB, Tian G, Zhen Y, Ma K, Li S, Wang H, Li B, Zhang X, Wang N. Cerebrospinal fluid pressure in glaucoma: a prospective study. Ophthalmology. 2010;117:259–66.
75. Linden C, Qvarlander S, Johannesson G, Johansson E, Ostlund F, Malm J, Eklund A. Normal-tension glaucoma has normal intracranial pressure: a prospective study of intracranial pressure and intraocular pressure in different body positions. Ophthalmology. 2018;125(3):361–8.
76. Killer HE, Jaggi GP, Flammer J, Miller NR, Huber AR, Mironov A. Cerebrospinal fluid dynamics between the intracranial and the subarachnoid space of the optic nerve. Is it always bidirectional? Brain. 2007;130:514–20.
77. Zweifach BW. Quantitative studies of microcirculatory structure and function. I. Analysis of pressure distribution in the terminal vascular bed in cat mesentery. Circ Res. 1974;34:843–57.
78. Ochs S. Energy metabolism and supply of -P to the fast axoplasmic transport mechanism in nerve. Fed Proc. 1974;33:1049–58.
79. Balaratnasingam C, Pham D, Morgan WH, Bass L, Cringle SJ, Yu DY. Mitochondrial cytochrome C oxidase expression in the central nervous system is elevated at sites of pressure gradient elevation but not absolute pressure increase. J Neurosci Res. 2009;87:2973–82.
80. Anderson DR, Hendrickson A. Effect of intraocular pressure on rapid axoplasmic transport in monkey optic nerve. Inv Ophthalmol Vis Sci. 1974;73:771–83.
81. Tso MO, Hayreh SS. Optic disk edema in raised intracranial pressure. IV. Axoplasmic transport

in experimental papilledema. Arch Ophthalmol. 1977;95:1458–62.

82. Hahnenberger RW. Inhibition of fast anterograde axoplasmic transport by a pressure barrier. The effect of pressure gradient and maximal pressure. Acta Physiol Scand. 1980;109:117–21.
83. Feola AJ, Coudrillier B, Mulvihill J, Geraldes DM, Vo NT, Albon J, Abel RL, Samuels BC, Ethier CR. Deformation of the lamina cribrosa and optic nerve due to changes in cerebrospinal fluid pressure. Invest Ophthalmol Vis Sci. 2017;58:2070–8.
84. Singh A. Extent of impaired axoplasmic transport and neurofilament compaction in traumatically injured axon at various strains and strain rates. Brain Inj. 2017;31:1387–95.
85. Ahmed WW, Fodor E, Betz T. Active cell mechanics: measurement and theory. Biochim Biophys Acta. 2015;1853:3083–94.
86. Joanny JF, Prost J. Active gels as a description of the actin-myosin cytoskeleton. HFSP J. 2009;3:94–104.
87. Sun D, Moore S, Jakobs TC. Optic nerve astrocyte reactivity protects function in experimental glaucoma and other nerve injuries. J Exp Med. 2017;214:1411–30.
88. Lipowsky HH, Kovalsheck S, Zweifach B. The distribution of blood rheological parameters in the microvasculature of cat mesentery. Circ Res. 1978;43:738–49.
89. Morgan WH, Yu DY, Cooper RL, Alder VA, Cringle SJ, Constable IJ. Retinal artery and vein pressures in the dog and their relationship to aortic, intraocular, and cerebrospinal fluid pressure. Microvasc Res. 1997;53:211–21.
90. Kang MH, Balaratnasingam C, Yu PK, Morgan WH, Mcallister IL, Cringle SJ, Yu DY. Morphometric characteristics of central retinal artery and vein endothelium in the normal human optic nerve head. Invest Ophthalmol Vis Sci. 2011;52:1359–67.
91. The Eye Disease Case-Control Study Group. Risk factors for central retinal vein occlusion. Arch Ophthalmol. 1996;111:545–54.
92. Morgan WH, Hazelton ML, Azar SL, House PH, Yu DY, Cringle SJ, Balaratnasingam C. Retinal venous pulsation in glaucoma and glaucoma suspects. Ophthalmology. 2004;111:1489–94.
93. Pillunat KR, Ventzke S, Spoerl E, Furashova O, Stodtmeister R, Pillunat LE. Central retinal venous pulsation pressure in different stages of primary open-angle glaucoma. Br J Ophthalmol. 2014;98:1374–8.
94. Radius RL. Anatomy of the optic nerve head and glaucomatous optic neuropathy. Surv Ophthalmol. 1987;32:35–44.
95. Park SC, Hsu AT, Su D, Simonson JL, Al-Jumayli M, Liu Y, Liebmann JM, Ritch R. Factors associated with focal lamina cribrosa defects in glaucoma. Invest Ophthalmol Vis Sci. 2013;54:8401–7.
96. Hernandez MR, Andrzejewska WM, Neufeld AH. Changes in the extracellular matrix of the human optic nerve head in primary open-angle glaucoma. Am J Ophthalmol. 1990;1009:180–8.
97. Quigley HA, Brown A, Dorman-Pease ME. Alterations in elastin of the optic nerve head in human and experimental glaucoma. Br J Ophthalmol. 1991;75:552–7.
98. Albon J, Purslow PP, Karwatowski WSS, Easty DL. Age related compliance of the lamina cribrosa in human eyes. Br J Ophthalmol. 2000;84:318–23.
99. Burgoyne CF. A biomechanical paradigm for axonal insult within the optic nerve head in aging and glaucoma. Exp Eye Res. 2011;93:120–32.
100. Jonas JB, Berenshtein E, Holbach L. Lamina cribrosa thickness and spatial relationships between intraocular space and cerebrospinal fluid space in highly myopic eyes. Invest Ophthalmol Vis Sci. 2004;45:2660–5.
101. Yang H, Williams G, Downs JC, Sigal IA, Roberts MD, Thompson H, Burgoyne CF. Posterior (outward) migration of the lamina cribrosa and early cupping in monkey experimental glaucoma. Invest Ophthalmol Vis Sci. 2011;52:7109–21.
102. Sharpe GP, Danthurebandara VM, Vianna JR, Alotaibi N, Hutchison DM, Belliveau AC, Shuba LM, Nicolela MT, Chauhan BC. Optic disk hemorrhages and laminar disinsertions in glaucoma. Ophthalmology. 2016;123:1949–56.
103. Fatehee N, Yu PK, Morgan WH, Cringle SJ, Yu DY. The impact of acutely elevated intraocular pressure on the porcine optic nerve head. Invest Ophthalmol Vis Sci. 2011;52:6192–8.
104. Burgoyne CF, Downs JC, Bellezza AJ, Suh JKF, Hart RT. The optic nerve head as a biomechanical structure: a new paradigm for understanding the role of IOP-related stress and strain in the pathophysiology of glaucomatous optic nerve head damage. Prog Retin Eye Res. 2005;24:39–73.
105. Sigal IA, Flanagan JG, Tertinegg I, Ethier CR. Predicted extension, compression and shearing of optic nerve head tissues. Exp Eye Res. 2007;85:312–22.
106. Riva CE, Grunwald JE, Sinclair SH, Petrig BL. Blood velocity and volumetric flow rate in human retinal vessels. Inv Ophthalmol Vis Sci. 1985;26:1124–32.
107. Tielsh JM, Katz J, Sommer A, Quigley HA, Javitt JC. Hypertension, perfusion pressure, and primary open-angle glaucoma. Arch Ophthalmol. 1995;113:216–21.
108. Abegao Pinto L, Willekens K, Van Keer K, Shibesh A, Molenberghs G, Vandewalle E, Stalmans I. Ocular blood flow in glaucoma - the Leuven eye study. Acta Ophthalmol. 2016;94(6):592–8.
109. Caprioli J, Coleman AL. Blood pressure, perfusion pressure, and glaucoma. Am J Ophthalmol. 2010;149:704–12.
110. Costa VP, Harris A, Anderson D, Stodtmeister R, Cremasco F, Kergoat H, Lovasik J, Stalmans I, Zeitz O, Lanzl I, Gugleta K, Schmetterer L. Ocular perfusion pressure in glaucoma. Acta Ophthalmol. 2014;92:e252–66.
111. Grieshaber MC, Flammer J. Blood flow in glaucoma. Curr Opin Ophthalmol. 2005;16:79–83.

112. Drance SM, Begg IS. Sector haemorrhage--a probable acute ischaemic disk change in chronic simple glaucoma. Can J Ophthalmol. 1970;5:137–41.
113. Budenz DL, Anderson DR, Feuer WJ, Beiser JA, Schiffman J, Parrish RK, Piltz-Seymour JR, Gordon MO, Kass MA. Detection and prognostic significance of optic disk hemorrhages during the ocular hypertension treatment study. Ophthalmology. 2006;113:2137–43.
114. Medeiros FA, Alencar LM, Sample PA, Zangwill LM, Susanna R Jr, Weinreb RN. The relationship between intraocular pressure reduction and rates of progressive visual field loss in eyes with optic disk hemorrhage. Ophthalmology. 2010;117:2061–6.
115. De Beaufort HC, De Moraes CG, Teng CC, Prata TS, Tello C, Ritch R, Liebmann JM. Recurrent disk hemorrhage does not increase the rate of visual field progression. Graefes Arch Clin Exp Ophthalmol. 2010;248:839–44.
116. Park HY, Kim EK, Park CK. Clinical significance of the location of recurrent optic disk hemorrhage in glaucoma. Invest Ophthalmol Vis Sci. 2015;56:7524–34.
117. Sonnsjo B, Dokmob Y, Krakau T. Disc haemorrhages, precursors of open angle glaucoma. Prog Retin Eye Res. 2002;21:35–56.
118. An D, House P, Barry C, Turpin A, Mckendrick AM, Chauhan BC, Manners S, Graham SL, Yu DY, Morgan WH. The association between retinal vein pulsation pressure and optic disk haemorrhages in glaucoma. PLoS One. 2017;12:e0182316.
119. Liu B, Mcnally S, Kilpatrick JI, Jarvis SP, O'brien CJ. Aging and ocular tissue stiffness in glaucoma. Surv Ophthalmol. 2018;63:56–74.
120. Guo T, Sampathkumar S, Fan S, Morris N, Wang F, Toris CB. Aqueous humour dynamics and biometrics in the ageing Chinese eye. Br J Ophthalmol. 2017;101:1290–6.
121. Rudnicka AR, Mt-Isa S, Owen CG, Cook DG, Ashby D. Variations in primary open-angle glaucoma prevalence by age, gender, and race: a Bayesian meta-analysis. Invest Ophthal Vis Sci. 2006;47:4254–61.
122. Yip JLY, Foster PJ. Ethnic differences in primary angle-closure glaucoma. Curr Opin Ophthalmol. 2006;17:175–80.
123. Green CM, Kearns LS, Wu J, Barbour JM, Wilkinson RM, Ring MA, Craig JE, Wong TL, Hewitt AW, Mackey DA. How significant is a family history of glaucoma? Experience from the glaucoma inheritance study in Tasmania. Clin Exp Ophthalmol. 2007;35:793–9.
124. Gemenetzi M, Yang Y, Lotery AJ. Current concepts on primary open-angle glaucoma genetics: a contribution to disease pathophysiology and future treatment. Eye (Lond). 2012;26:355–69.
125. Stone EM, Fingert JH, Alward WL, Nguyen TD, Polansky JR, Sunden SL, Nishimura D, Clark AF, Nystuen A, Nichols BE, Mackey DA, Ritch R, Kalenak JW, Craven ER, Sheffield VC. Identification of a gene that causes primary open angle glaucoma. Science. 1997;275:668–70.
126. Minegishi Y, Nakayama M, Iejima D, Kawase K, Iwata T. Significance of optineurin mutations in glaucoma and other diseases. Prog Retin Eye Res. 2016;55:149–81.
127. Lewis CJ, Hedberg-Buenz A, Deluca AP, Stone EM, Alward WLM, Fingert JH. Primary congenital and developmental glaucomas. Hum Mol Genet. 2017;26:R28–36.
128. Grodum K, Heijl A, Bengtsson B. Risk of glaucoma in ocular hypertension with and without pseudoexfoliation. Ophthalmology. 2005;112:386–90.
129. Schlotzer-Schrehardt U. Molecular pathology of pseudoexfoliation syndrome/glaucoma--new insights from LOXL1 gene associations. Exp Eye Res. 2009;88:776–85.
130. Niyadurupola N, Broadway DC. Pigment dispersion syndrome and pigmentary glaucoma--a major review. Clin Exp Ophthalmol. 2008;36:868–82.
131. Aiello LP, Avery RL, Arrigg PG, Keyt BA, Jampel HD, Shah ST, Pasquale LR, Thieme H, Iwamoto MA, Park JE, Nguyen HV, Aiello LM, Ferrara N, King GL. Vascular endothelial growth factor in ocular fluid of patients with diabetic retinopathy and other retinal disorders. N Engl J Med. 1994;331:1480–7.
132. Lovicu FJ, Mcavoy JW, De Iongh RU. Understanding the role of growth factors in embryonic development: insights from the lens. Philos Trans R Soc Lond Ser B Biol Sci. 2011;366:1204–18.
133. Sihota R, Kumar S, Gupta V, Dada T, Kashyap S, Insan R, Srinivasan G. Early predictors of traumatic glaucoma after closed globe injury: trabecular pigmentation, widened angle recess, and higher baseline intraocular pressure. Arch Ophthalmol. 2008;126:921–6.
134. Razeghinejad MR, Myers JS, Katz LJ. Iatrogenic glaucoma secondary to medications. Am J Med. 2011;124:20–5.
135. Kang JH, Willett WC, Rosner BA, Hankinson SE, Pasquale LR. Caffeine consumption and the risk of primary open-angle glaucoma: a prospective cohort study. Invest Ophthalmol Vis Sci. 2008;49:1924–31.
136. Brooks AM, Gillies WE. Congenital rubella syndrome. Br J Ophthalmol. 1994;78:79.

3 Briefs on Evaluation Techniques for Glaucoma

Xiangmei Kong and Xinghuai Sun

Abstract

Accurate evaluation of glaucoma is the basis for effective control of this disease. The major parameters for glaucoma include intraocular pressure, anterior chamber angle, optic nerve head, and visual function. This chapter will focus briefly on the assessment of such parameters, including different tonometry and its influencing factors for IOP; gonioscopy, UBM, and AS-OCT for anterior chamber angle; ophthalmoscopy, fund photography, and OCT for optic nerve head and retina; and perimetry, contract sensitivity, ERG, and VEP for visual function.

Keywords

Intraocular pressure · Anterior chamber angle Optic nerve head · Visual function · Ultrasound biomicroscopy · Optical coherence tomography

3.1 Assessment of Intraocular Pressure (IOP)

The major risk factor for glaucomatous damage is elevated IOP, and the only clinical proven therapeutic intervention for glaucoma is to reduce IOP [1]. Epidemiologic studies have revealed that the alteration of 1 mmHg in the mean IOP may be vital enough to decide the visual field prognosis for glaucoma patients. Therefore, a precise assessment of IOP is of great importance for diagnosis and decision-making in terms of treatment modalities, especially for advanced stage glaucoma cases. IOP measurements can be classified into two categories in a broad sense, direct and indirect measurements. In terms of the direct/invasive approach, the sensor is implanted inside the eye which can provide an accurate representation of the true internal IOP. In the latter one,

X. Kong
Department of Ophthalmology & Visual Science, Eye & ENT Hospital, Shanghai Medical College, Fudan University, Shanghai, China

NHC Key Laboratory of Myopia (Fudan University), Key Laboratory of Myopia, Chinese Academy of Medical Sciences, Shanghai, China

Shanghai Key Laboratory of Visual Impairment and Restoration, Fudan University, Shanghai, China

X. Sun (✉)
Department of Ophthalmology & Visual Science, Eye & ENT Hospital, Shanghai Medical College, Fudan University, Shanghai, China

NHC Key Laboratory of Myopia (Fudan University), Key Laboratory of Myopia, Chinese Academy of Medical Sciences, Shanghai, China

Shanghai Key Laboratory of Visual Impairment and Restoration, Fudan University, Shanghai, China

State Key Laboratory of Medical Neurobiology, Institutes of Brain Science and Collaborative Innovation Center for Brain Science, Fudan University, Shanghai, China
e-mail: xhsun@shmu.edu.cn

X. Sun, Y. Dai (eds.), *Medical Treatment of Glaucoma*,
https://doi.org/10.1007/978-981-13-2733-9_3

IOP measurements depend on the related knowledge of the relationship between the true IOP and measured parameters such as applanation and corneal radius alteration of curvature. Nowadays, only noninvasive approaches are widely used clinically [2]. Palpation of the eyeball with the fingertips and estimating turgidity is also a form of the most crude level tonometry. However, different tonometry and its related factors might influence the accuracy of IOP measurements. An understanding of the different tonometers is important for clinician to diagnose, screen, and manage glaucomatous cases.

3.1.1 Tonometry

3.1.1.1 Goldmann Applanation Tonometer (GAT)

GAT is based on the modified Imbert–Fick principle and is universally accepted as the gold standard for IOP measurements till now. It is based on a corneal thickness of 520 μm together with an IOP of 1 mmHg equivalent to flatten the corneal surface with the area in the diameter of 3.06 mm by a force 0.1 g of the tonometer head. To obtain a correct IOP reading, it needs a skillful examiner to perform. GAT is relatively unaffected by ocular rigidity because the applanation does not substantially increase the pressure in the eye. However, corneal thickness, curvature, and tear film can interfere with the IOP readings, so it has poor accuracy in the eyes with irregular corneal surface [3]. GAT requires topical anesthetic and fluorescein dye in the tear film before measurements, and it is suitable for sitting positioned patients. While the Perkins tonometer is a portable applanation one, and it can be used with the patient either upright or supine position.

3.1.1.2 Schiotz Indentation Tonometry

Schiotz tonometer is based on the theory of indentation by gravity oppression eyeball. With a metal plunger of known weight, it calculates the amount and depth of corneal indentation and converts to mmHg by a line scale on the instrument. It is used in the clinic since 1905 and costs relatively low, so some primary care physicians still use it, especially in the primary medical units and underdeveloped area. However, the Schiotz tonometer needs to be calibrated and sterilized before use, and IOP measurements can be interfered by alterations of curvature and thickness of the cornea, particularly ocular rigidity [4].

3.1.1.3 Noncontact Tonometer (NCT)

This tonometer is to flatten (really to indent) a fixed point (area 3.06 mm in diameter) of the central cornea with a controllable air puff, and to record the time of receiving the reflected light from the corneal flattening surface through the monitoring system, and to convert it to measured IOP. The advantage of NCT includes noninvasive examination, avoids cross-infection because it does not need anesthetics, and no contact with the eyeball. It is measured quickly, even if repeatedly measured also does not cause IOP to drop, and automatically prints test results. So it is simply easy to operate even by non-ophthalmologists. Even the IOP values obtained with NCT are linear with the true IOP values, while they have widely greater bias of data in eyes with higher or lower IOP. Curvature and thickness of the cornea can affect the deviation IOP measurements as well, especially for patients with corneal abnormalities surface, as well as eyes with long eyelashes.

3.1.1.4 TonoPen Tonometer

TonoPen, one of Mackay-Marg type tonometer, different from GAT avoids the tear film's effect together with the force to deform the cornea. The diameter of the central plunger with the TonoPen is 1.02 mm. Electrical devices are used to detect the movement of the central plunger and also, the force to flatten the cornea consists of central plunger and a sleeve guard. Advantages of TonoPen tonometer include that it can be applied to eyes with irregular cornea and soft contact lens. It can also be measured at peripheral cornea and does not rely on patient position. Usually, the measurement results of TonoPen tonometer are higher than that of GAT.

3.1.1.5 Rebound Tonometer

The rebound tonometer does not require an anesthetic and does not applanate the cornea. The length for the stainless steel probe of this device (iCARE) is 50 mm and its diameter is 1.4/1.0 mm which is horizontally repelled by a two-coaxial magnet system. It hits the cornea from the distance of 4–8 mm. There is a voltage in the bounced probe's solenoid which is then transformed into a digital signal. It can be of great use for children and aged patients with poor cooperation because it is portable. And it can be measured at peripheral cornea.

3.1.1.6 Dynamic Contour Tonometer (DCT)

The concave plunger (10.5 mm) in DCT is contour-matched to patients' cornea with the appositional force as 9.81 mN (1 g). It is not influenced by the tear film or the deforming force to cornea. What's more, the safety range for the appositional force is wide, leading to less operator bias. The advantage of DCT is that it is not affected by CCT. Patients with poor fixation or nystagmus are not that suitable for DCT. A very flat or cliffy cornea or with an irregular scar may lead to reading bias of IOP [5, 6].

3.1.1.7 Ocular Response Analyzer (ORA)

ORA ejects 20 ms of air impulse as a new air-puff tonometer. It can supervise the time course changes, inward shift, applanation, slight concavity, second applanation, and the return to normal convex curvature using an electro-optical collimation detector system. The viscoelastic properties of the corneoscleral shells have an effect on the difference between "in" and "out" applanation pressure because of opposition forces absorbing energy from corneal hysteresis which is also known as the air impulse. Many corneal parameters can affect the measured IOP, but not CCT. The advantage of ORA is that it is noncontact and can measure corneal hysteresis. The ultra-high speed Scheimpflug camera (Corvis ST) is also a new device with precise, repeatable, and reproducible measurements of corneal biomechanical properties, which provides quantitative information, including the magnitude and direction of the displacement of the corneal apex [7, 8].

3.1.1.8 Continuous IOP Assessment

IOPs of glaucoma patients always have fluctuations. These fluctuations have been proved relevant to glaucoma progression and as a result, the need for continuous IOP measurements is pressing. Twenty-four hour IOP measurement by NCT or iCARE for 24 h at different intervals is a commonly used method [9, 10]. The IOP curve, peak IOP, trough IOP, and IOP fluctuation can be obtained. Its disadvantage is that an operator is needed and the patients should be awakened at night. With the help of a soft contact lens, a microstrain gauge is embedded that allows measurement of changes in corneal curvature. The system is based on the hypothesis that 1 mm Hg change in IOP leads to approximately 3 mm curvature change in central corneal radius. Their work has been improved to be a commercially available product such as SENSIMED Lausanne's wireless telemetric options at Switzerland [11].

3.1.2 Influencing Factors

3.1.2.1 Central Corneal Thickness (CCT)

The mean CCT in healthy human eyes is about 545 μm and a thin CCT is now regarded as a risk factor for glaucoma. CCT could affect the IOP readings measured by GAT, NCT, TonoPen, and rebound tonometer, but not affect the measurement with DCT, which documents the IOP without deforming the cornea. Several reports have revealed a positive relationship between CCT and measured IOP readings. The correlation coefficient varies from 1.1 to 14.2 mmHg per 100 μm CCT. While there is no standard nomogram correcting applanation IOP measurements for CCT has yet been validated. Even though, measuring CCT is important in terms of precise diagnosis as well as managing patients with glaucoma [3].

3.1.2.2 Corneal Topography

A study has reported a weak but significant correlation between IOP reading results and corneal curvature whose correlation coefficient $r = 0.1788$. One diopter change of corneal curvature leads to 0.34 mmHg changing in the IOP reading [3].

3.1.2.3 Ocular Rigidity

Ocular rigidity refers to the relationship between pressure and volume changes in the eyeball. Usually, ocular rigidity is higher in hyperopia and lower in myopia, and then might cause a higher or lower IOP measurement value. A scarred cornea might cause a higher IOP reading.

3.1.2.4 Tear Film

Tear film does have an influence on tonometric IOP readings. The range for effect is from 2 to 4.15 mmHg in reports. However, the impact of tear film can be relatively avoided by NCT, the rebound tonometer, and Mackay-Marg-type tonometers.

3.1.2.5 Refractive Surgery

Refractive surgery, especially surgeries on cornea such as laser in situ keratomileusis, could cause inaccurate IOP measurement, mainly by the reduction in CCT and partially by the radius of curvature and corneal rigidity. Instrument which is independent of cornea properties is ideal for IOP measurement in terms of patients with post-LASIK. So far, DCT measurements of IOP are correlated relatively well in both post-LASIK and pre-LASIK eyes.

3.1.2.6 Patient Cooperation

Patients' cooperation during IOP measurement is important for a more accurate result. If the patient is too nervous to cooperate, for example, winking too much, it will provide extra force to the eyeball by eyelids spasm and then lead to a higher IOP reading.

In conclusion, physicians should be aware that a correction algorithm for GAT may be inaccurate when estimating the true IOP in those subjects. New tonometer like DCT may improve GAT-related problems. Those new tonometers, on the other hand, may have difficulties in applying in diseased eyes to get accurate IOP values although with superiorities over GAT.

3.2 Assessment of Anterior Chamber Angle

Evaluation for anterior segment structures together with their relationships can be done with complementary skills such as gonioscopy, slit-lamp biomicroscopy, anterior segment OCT (AS-OCT), and ultrasound biomicroscopy (UBM). Slit-lamp biomicroscopy could provide a clear view of cornea, iris, and depth of peripheral anterior chamber, which could be graded by van Herick method. However, it doesn't allow direct observation of the anterior chamber angle. The other methods are interpreted below [12, 13].

3.2.1 Gonioscopy

The reasons for performing gonioscopy examination related to glaucoma are: estimation of the risk and extent of angle closure; identification of glaucomatous mechanism: open- or closed-angle, primary or secondary glaucoma induced by pseudoexfoliation, pigmentary dispersion, angle recession, uveitis, etc.; to monitor the changes of angle for glaucoma after laser-treatment manipulation: iridotomy, iridopasty, trabeculoplasty, etc.; and also learning the anatomical structure of normal angle (Fig. 3.1).

The association for International Glaucoma Societies promoted that the structure of anterior chamber angle should be observed by 1 mm beam with adequate illumination in a dark room when

Fig. 3.1 Normal angle viewed by gonioscopy

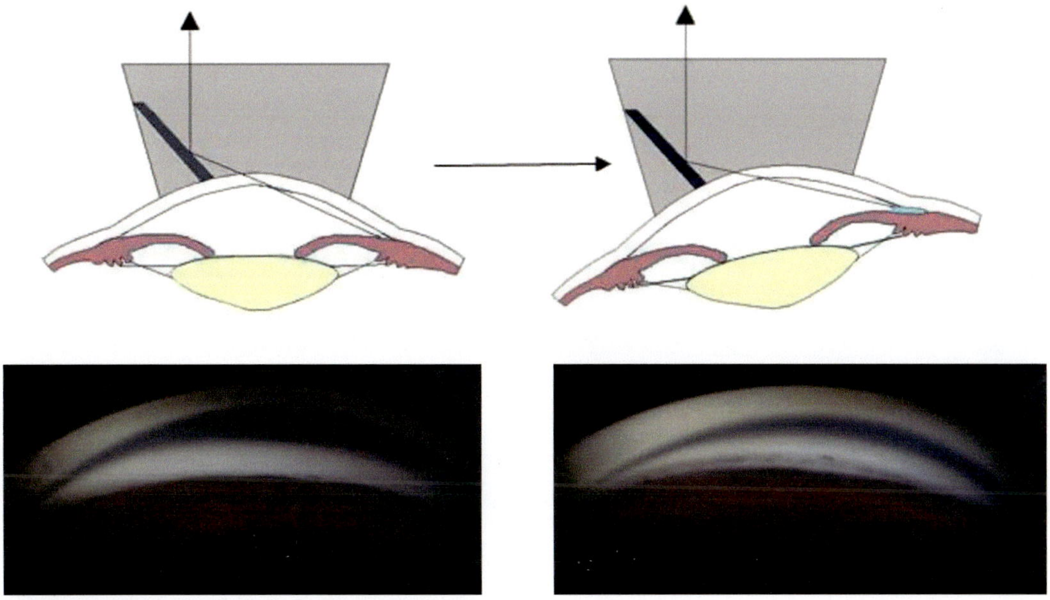

Fig. 3.2 Gonioscopy. Left column: appositional angle closure and iris bombe are present in static gonioscopy. Right column: in indentation gonioscopy, the angle opens with pigmentation

the patients look straight ahead. Comparison between static gonioscopy and indentation gonioscopy is important because it helps to differentiate between permanent synechiae and reversible appositive angle closure (Fig. 3.2) [14].

Instead of the compression gonioscopy method that the entire lens was pushed uniformly into the cornea, the recommended method is to "heel in" or indent the mirror we are examining. The mirror could push aqueous humor across the anterior chamber and then push the peripheral iris of the adverse direction backward. Releasing and reapplying pressure helps judge the relative pupillary block and whether synechial or appositional closure is present [15].

There are several critical points that are essential to keep in mind as gonioscopy was performed: (1) whether there is relative pupillary block (peripheral iris bowed anteriorly) and inverse pupillary block (peripheral iris bowed posteriorly); (2) evaluation of the angle in degrees, which extent of iris insertion (ciliary body, scleral spur, and trabecular meshwork), and the presence of plateau. Evaluation of ciliary body depth at the corresponding quadrants of both eyes helps identify traumatic angle recession; (3) angle pigmentation should not be neglected. The pigmentation feature of pseudoexfoliation is clumpier, while that of pigment dispersion syndrome is heavy and powder-like pigmentation; (4) if the anatomical structure of angle is covered by peripheral iris, note to distinguish the appositional closure and peripheral anterior synechiae; and (5) look for and distinguish normal (circumferential but not stretch to the scleral spur) and abnormal blood vessels (cross the scleral spur), which could be found in the very early stage of neovascular glaucoma (Fig. 3.3).

The Shaffer, Spaeth, and Scheie system were created to document the angle findings. The Scheie provides four grades to describe the degree of the angle closure: grade 1: narrow slightly; grade 2: invisible ciliary body band; grade 3: invisible trabecular meshwork; and grade 4: no structure of the angle is visible. The patients with angles defined as grades 3 and 4 were in danger of angle-closed glaucoma. The Shaffer system uses an opposite method of Scheie system, it also has four grades to evaluate the angle: 4 − 40°, 3 = 30°, 2 = 20°, and 1 = 10°, then slit and closed. The Spaeth system includes the extent of iris insertion (A–E represent the angle structure

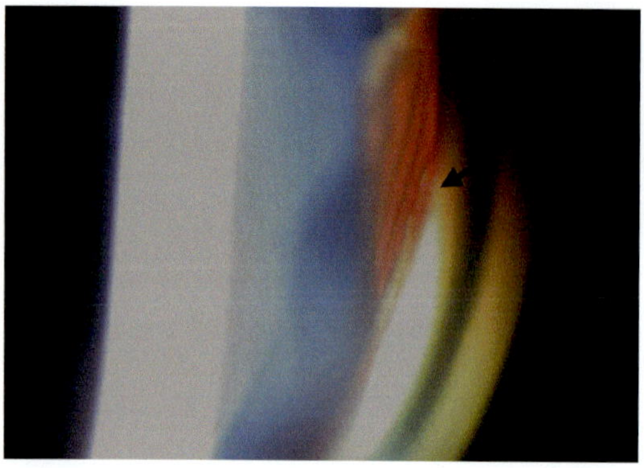

Fig. 3.3 The abnormal blood vessels were present across the scleral spur in the angle of neovascular glaucoma

exposed), angle width (in degree), and peripheral iris structure (steep, regular, or queer).

3.2.2 UBM

UBM's development can be dated back to early 1990s. A higher frequency use of transducer gives a chance for the acquisition of high-resolution and objective images of anterior segment anatomical structures including corneal, iris, anterior chamber, anterior chamber angle, posterior chamber, and ciliary body. The tissue resolution of this technique is up to approximately 50 μm, which provides a useful diagnostic tool for several anterior segmental diseases. Particularly, the scleral spur is vital landmark, the trabecular meshwork is located in front of this structure and behind the Schwalbe's line, and it is the key to do quantitative analysis of the angle [16].

The notes of observation of angle-closure glaucoma include: (1) anterior chamber: to measure the central anterior chamber depth and compare the binocular values, the difference between two eyes should be <0.2 mm, and the lens and zonule laxity should be noted if there is obvious difference; (2) the configuration of iris: to observe the degree of iridauxesis and iris bombe, and the position of iris inserted on the ciliary face (Fig. 3.4); (3) ciliary process: to observe the edema and anterior rotation of ciliary process, to evaluate the distance between ciliary body and the lens equator, and to measure its diameter size if there exists the ciliary cyst; (4) anterior chamber angle: to observe the iris–trabecular contact and involved range; and (5) lens: to evaluate the zonule laxity and to measure the thickness of the lens [17, 18].

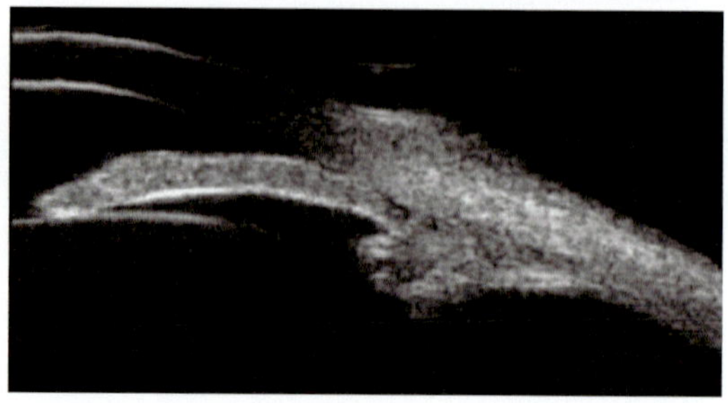

Fig. 3.4 UBM image depicts the relative pupillary block with the iris bombe and iris–trabecular contact in the eye with primary closed-angle glaucoma

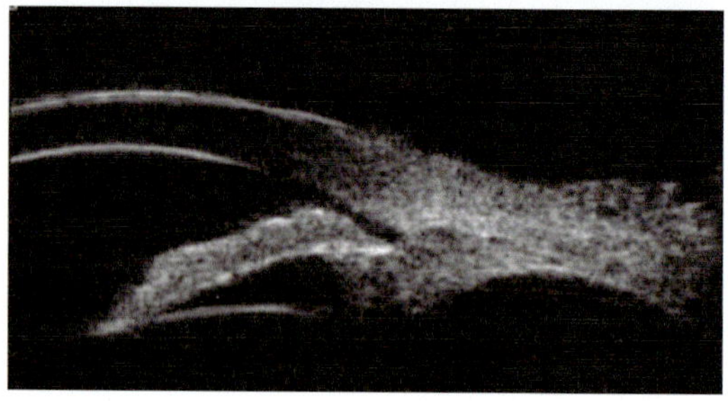

Fig. 3.5 The image of the plateau iris syndrome eye indicates an abnormal "kneeling change" of the peripheral iris, anterior insertion of iris to the ciliary body

In plateau iris syndrome, the root of iris is thicker and there is a steep bend near its point of insertion so that the narrower and even occluded angle is observed. However, the convex iris and extremely shadow central anterior chamber are not visible (Fig. 3.5).

In the congenital glaucoma, UBM found these features: (1) dysplasia of anterior chamber angle: the residual mesodermal tissue could be visible at the iridocorneal angle, the iris root insertion is parallel with the tip of scleral spur; (2) the base of iris is thinner and the shape of it is more rigid than normal control; and (3) the ciliary body is smaller, the ciliary processes are stretched out, and their placement are sparse and disorderly.

The characteristics of the malignant glaucoma include: (1) extremely shallow anterior chamber;

(2) anterior movement of lens–iris diaphragm; (3) anterior rotation of the ciliary body, together with the suprachoroidal fluid or not; (4) absence of the posterior chamber; and (5) absence of the distance between ciliary processes and lens equator margin.

Furthermore, UBM technique could be used to evaluate the function and failure of filtration bleb (diffuse, encapsulated, flattened, and cystic avascular thin-walled blebs) (Fig. 3.6). The internal ostium, the height, and the wall thickness of the bleb could be evaluated. And UBM is also able to assess the tube shunts placed under the sclera or in the chamber, drainage area around shunt plate, and to identify the obstruction of tube shunts with iris, vitreous, blood clots, and so on.

Furthermore, the technique realizes the identification of posttraumatic eyes including angle recession, cyclodialysis cleft, and ciliary choroid detachment (Fig. 3.7).

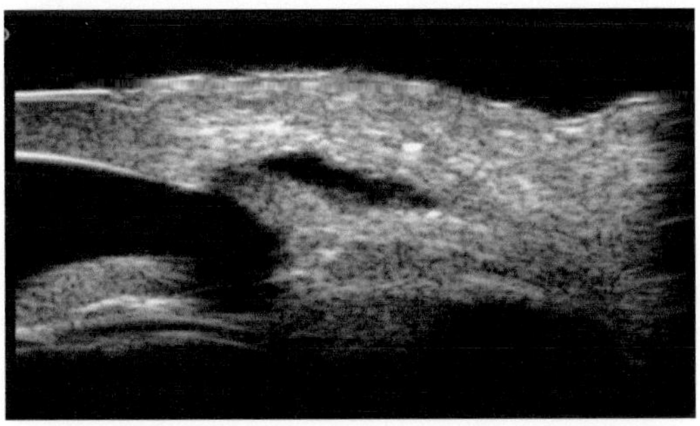

Fig. 3.6 The post-trabeculectomy image by UBM. The space beneath the scleral flap still exists. But the filtration bleb is flattened due to scarring

3.2.3 AS-OCT

AS-OCT is a noncontact imaging technology using low-coherence light to acquire the cross-section of biological structures of anterior segment with high resolution. It is capable to monitor and document the occludable angles and to assess the level of the peripheral anterior closure [19–21]. The closed anterior chamber is defined as the status of contact between iris and angle anterior to the scleral spur, which is valuable for diagnosing primary angle-closure glaucoma (Figs. 3.8 and 3.9).

And the technique could be used to monitor the changes in the angle morphology after laser peripheral iridotomy (LPI). Clinical reports demonstrated that LPI caused the deepening of anterior chamber, widening of the angle, and the amelioration of iris convexity. AS-OCT is also useful in certifying different forms of secondary glaucoma. In pigment dispersion syndrome, AS-OCT could reflect the increased irido-lenticular contact and reverse pressure difference between anterior and posterior chamber AS-OCT allows the visualization of bleb morphology and assessment of its function after glaucoma scleral fistulizing surgery. Cystic blebs are noted to have multiple hyporeflective spaces with fluid collection covered by

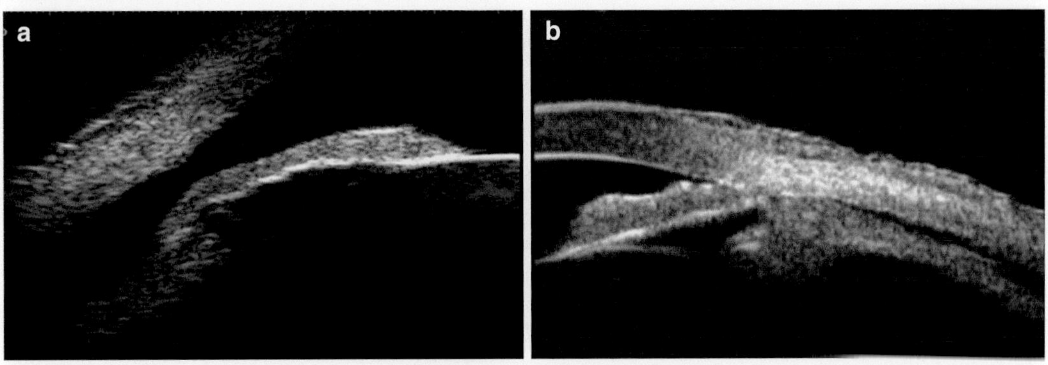

Fig. 3.7 The UBM images show: (**a**) the cyclodialysis cleft was certified by avulsion of the ciliary body from the scleral spur which is its normal location. (**b**) Ciliochoroidal effusion in one eye with acute angle-closure attack which has the detachment of the ciliary body from the sclera (does not include the scleral spur)

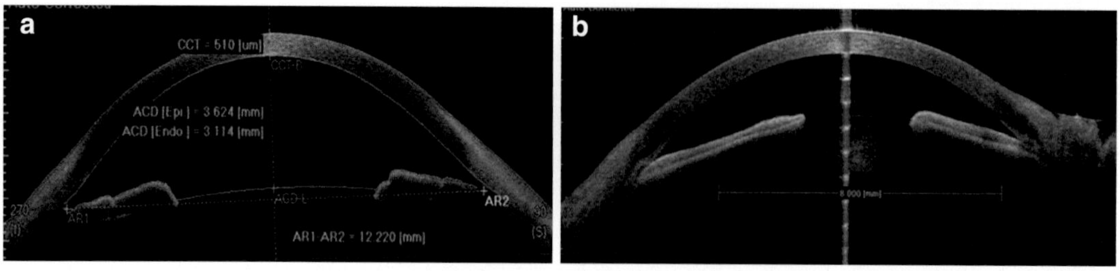

Fig. 3.8 AS-OCT images: (**a**) a normal eye with deep anterior chamber and an open angle; (**b**) an eye with PACG which has shallow anterior chamber, closed angle in two quadrants of an eye, and a relative pupillary block

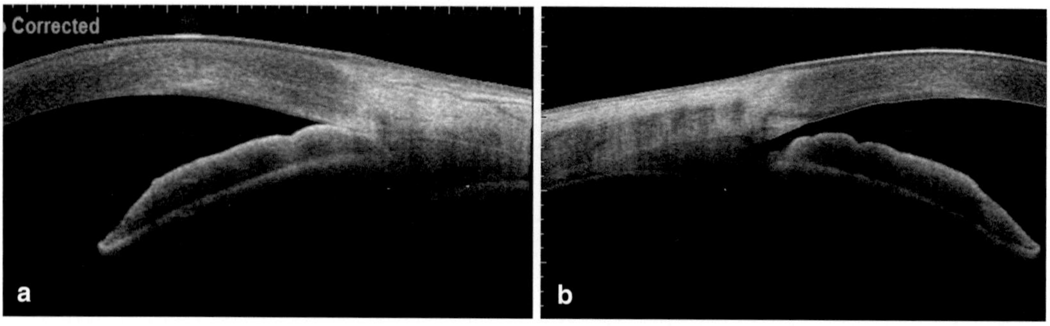

Fig. 3.9 AS-OCT images: (**a**) occludable angle that has iris–trabecular contact with slight convex iris; (**b**) narrow angle in a quadrant of an eye with PACG

thin conjunctiva. Diffuse blebs are characterized by the presence of supra-scleral fluid space and subconjunctival fluid collections. Flat blebs are regarded as the failed blebs, which have occluded ostium, apposition of conjunctiva–episclera to sclera flap, and absence of bleb. Encapsulated blebs are observed to have thicker bleb walls with high reflectivity [19, 22, 23].

3.3 Assessment of Optic Nerve Head and Retina

Monitoring optic disc and retinal nerve fiber layer (RNFL) damage and alteration is the cornerstone of glaucoma management. The assessment of the optic disc might be subjective or objective by different ways. Clinical examination by ophthalmoscopy and fundus photography were still the "gold standard" for assessing glaucomatous optic disc and RNFL damage, but they might be limited by the subjective and qualitative evaluation. Written descriptions and drawings for optic disc are necessary to extract information from the clinical examination, making it difficult to detect accurate change over time. Photography provides objective documentation for comparison during follow-up, but subjective assessment is still needed, and variation in interpretation of photographs is well documented. Recently, computer-based imaging instruments provide reproducible, quantitative information on optic disc and RNFL. Optical coherence tomography (OCT), using the principles of low-coherence interferometry, could acquire high-resolution images of ocular structures.

3.3.1 Ophthalmoscopy and Photography

Fundus examination for optic disc and surrounding retina is essential for glaucoma diagnosis and glaucoma progression monitoring [24]. Clinically, there are several evaluation methods including direct ophthalmoscopy, indirect ophthalmoscopy, and slit-lamp biomicroscopy with handheld lens (90 or 120 diopter lens), while the last method is preferred because it could provide with good stereoscopic and larger scope view.

Despite slit-lamp and ophthalmoscopy examination, optic disc photography offers more clinical information and documents. The optical principle of ophthalmoscopy is based on Gullstrand india ophthalmoscope, in which the exit pupil of the illumination system and the entrance pupil of the observation system are imaged in the pupillary zone, preventing the reflection of light from cornea and lens into the observation system. In general, fundus ophthalmoscopy requires the pupil diameter maintained at 4–5 mm so as to realize the illumination and fundus photograph. Now, nonmydriatic fundus cameras have been developed to provide a low-power infrared focusing system avoiding reflective miosis. It is more convenient and efficient to operate and examine without mydriasis. However, some patients whose pupil diameters are <3 mm may not be suitable for the nonmydriatic cameras.

Fundus photograph as a fast and noninvasive method could offer morphological information for glaucoma patients including color, size, rim, and abnormal ridges or concavities of optic nerve head, together with the defect of the nerve fiber layer. It is one of the gold standards for diagnosing glaucoma and more importantly evaluates glaucoma patients at risk of vision loss. Patients developed glaucoma diseases are often accompanied with pathological changes including optic disc neuroretinal rim narrow, RNFL defect, and optic disc linear hemorrhages.

We will refer to several core points of clinical assessment for the optic disc using the ophthalmoscopy or photography as follows: Firstly, the optic disc size should be evaluated at the start of observation because it is critical in the explanation of other optic nerve head findings. The discs are small, average, or large in size (Fig. 3.10).

There are several methods to evaluate the disc size. The disc edge is defined as the internal margin of the white scleral ring, which is easily visible in most cases. However, identification of the border of optic disc is very challenging in the following conditions: crowded disc, tilted disc, or high myopic disc embraced by retinal and choroidal atrophic ring (Fig. 3.11). The scanning laser ophthalmoscopy (SLO), which consists of a low-powered laser light and a confocal raster scanning technique, could offer higher quality of images in those cases.

During the slit-lamp biomicroscopy with handheld lens, the slim beam can be regulated to coincide with the edge of the disc and measure its size by reading the scale. Another option, Heidelberg retinal tomography (HRT) analysis of SLO also allows accurate evaluation of optic disc size. And the optic cup size varies between normal eyes and it is associated with the optic disc size.

Secondly, identification of cup-to-disc ratio of optic nerve head is critical to judge the occurrence and severity of the glaucomatous disease. However, determining the cup border is sometimes not easy. The border of the optic cup is best determined by the acute bending of the circumlinear blood vessels as they lost the support of neuroretinal rim. There are several appearances of circumlinear blood vessels including: bayoneting, baring, and nasalization. Bayoneting means the sharp turn (90° or <90°) of a blood

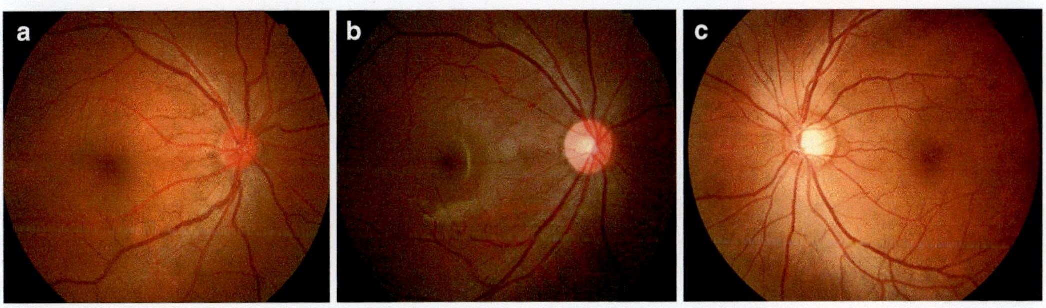

Fig. 3.10 Images of a small optic disc (**a**), average optic disc (**b**), and a large optic disc (**c**)

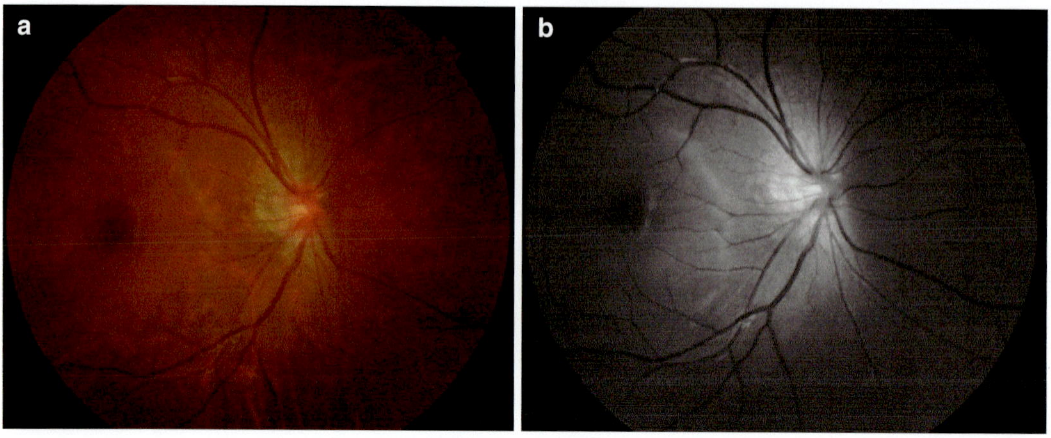

Fig. 3.11 The photography image of an eye with POAG. (**a**) A crowded disc, the optic C/D is approximately 0.4 which seems like a normal disc. (**b**) SLO image provides the high quality image showing RNFL defect in the inferior part

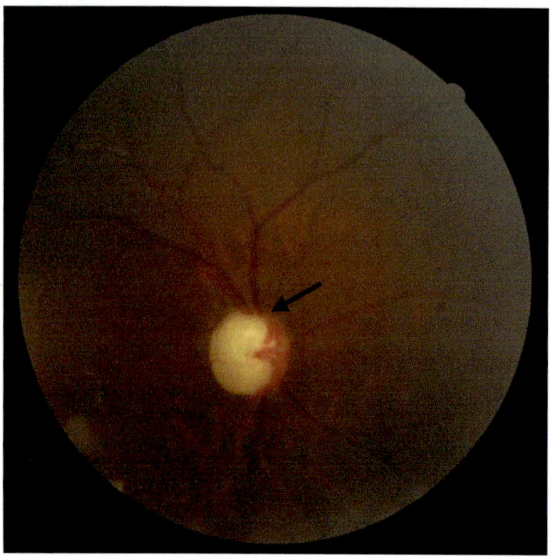

Fig. 3.12 Optic disc of late-stage of glaucomatous eye. In this optic nerve head, the branch of the retinal vessels in both superior and inferior quadrants marked by arrow exhibits bayoneting and there is nasalization of the vessels as well

vessel as they emerge out the pit due to the neuroretinal rim loss. Baring refers to the unsupported blood vessels appearance when no neuroretinal rim is contacted with them. Nasalization occurs as the diffuse neuroretinal rim loss and as a result major blood vessels emerging more nasal than central (Fig. 3.12).

However, the large cup-to-disc ratio doesn't necessarily mean the occurrence of the glaucoma. It is better to combine the analysis of neuroretinal rim including looking for thinning, notching,

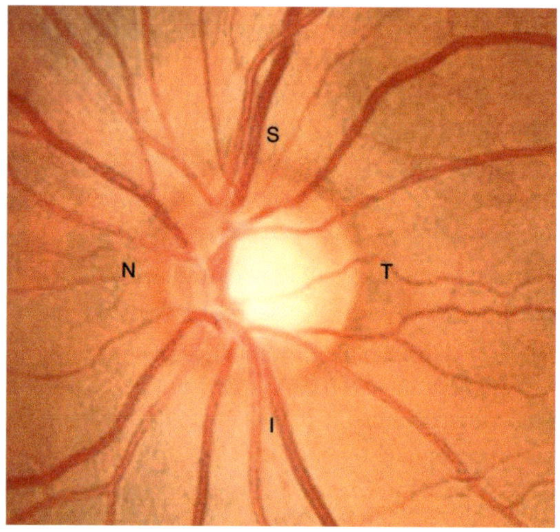

Fig. 3.13 The photography shows the physical macro cup, which obeys the ISNT rule

and disc hemorrhages areas. There is a useful rule concluded from the normal disc called ISNT rule, which describes that the inferior neuroretinal rim is thickest, then the thickness of them decreases in the following order: superior, nasal, and temporal direction. Therefore, there is a need to judge whether the optic disc obeys the ISNT rule particularly when the cup-to-disc ratio is large. Figure 3.13 represents a large cup-to-disc ratio (0.8); however, the neuroretinal rim of four directions is in accordance with the ISNT rule. Therefore, the optic disc in this figure is called physical macro cup rather than glaucomatous occurrence.

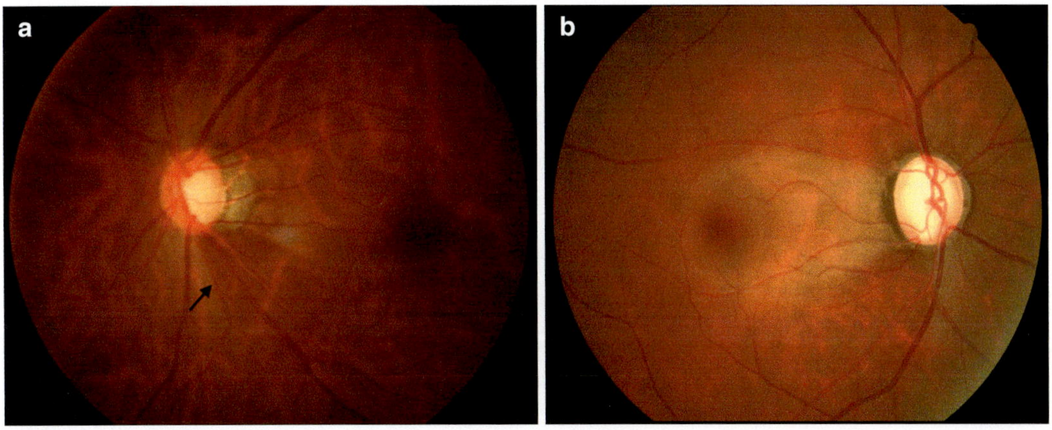

Fig. 3.14 The photography of the eyes with POAG. (**a**) Arrow refers to the wedge-shaped RNFL loss; (**b**) the diffuse RNFL loss in the inferior and superior quadrants

In fundus photograph of high quality, normal retinal nerve fiber layer shows bright reflections and therefore thinness in retinal nerve fiber layer, which shows relative darkening area, is easy to observe and record with it. Figure 3.14 showed a typical wedge-shaped RNFL thinning in glaucomatous disease. However, not like the wedge-shaped RNFL thinning, it is difficult to judge the diffuse RNFL thinning (Fig. 3.14).

Furthermore, the C/D ratio asymmetry of 0.2 or greater between both eyes has been an indicator of the glaucoma. However, whether there is asymmetry of the optic disc size should be observed before evaluating asymmetry of the cup or neuroretinal rim. And asymmetry of C/D should be correlated with the other asymmetric findings such as IOP and visual field measurement.

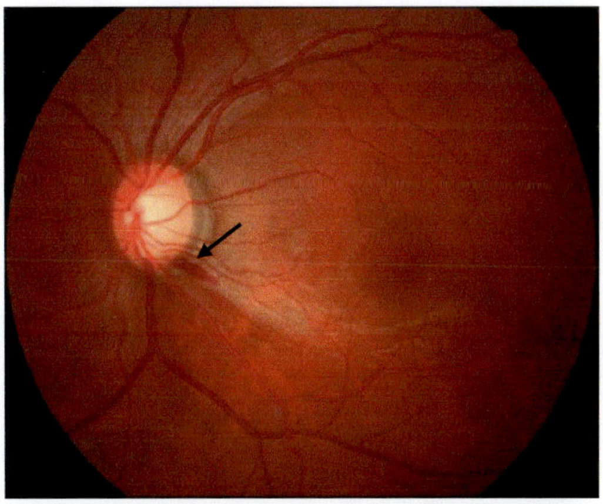

Fig. 3.15 The photography of optic disc hemorrhage. Linear hemorrhage is observed in the inferotemporal quadrant of the optic rim

Additionally, looking for the optic disc hemorrhages is critical because they are common in the optic nerves head with established glaucoma. The optic disc hemorrhages usually appear in the inferotemporal or superotemporal regions (Fig. 3.15).

Previous studies showed that the disease will progress in 50–80% of patients with glaucoma within median 2–3 years after suffering an optic disc hemorrhage. In OHTS study, 14% of glaucomatous patients following disc hemorrhages demonstrated progressive neuroretinal rim loss after 13 months of follow-up. The novel study showed that RNFL thinning was faster in a disc hemorrhage quadrant than non-disc hemorrhage quadrant. Therefore, the photodocumentation or automated devices is a good way to monitor the changes of optic nerve head [25].

3.3.2 OCT

Over the recent years, the imaging technologies for glaucoma detection have evolved rapidly. From time domain optical coherence tomography (TD-OCT) to spectral-domain OCT (SD-OCT), the scan speed and the image resolution have been significantly improved. Thus, the analysis of optic nerve head and retinal structure changes for glaucoma with OCT is burgeoning. OCT is a helpful tool for the diagnosis and long-term monitoring of glaucomatous changes [26, 27]. At present, several SD-OCT devices are commercially available and each has unique advantages. The software in the devices automatically analyzes the acquired images and compares them to normal databases and then gives reminder with different color sections. The green section indicates that the data is within the 5th to 95th percentile of the normal range. The yellow section is regarded as a "borderline" value (1th to 5th percentile of the normal population range). The red section represents "outside normal limits" (<1th percentile value).

The RNFL protocol provides total RNFL thickness, average superior and inferior hemisphere thickness, and average thickness of sections by clock hours, which is expressed in a wheel-like format. A "double hump" presence is a typical feature of RNFL thickness pattern in a healthy individual, because RNFL is thicker at the superior and inferior quadrants than other quadrants. We will interpret the indexes and the significance of them for detecting disease using the example of RTVue (Optovue Inc., Fremont, CA) device (Fig. 3.16).

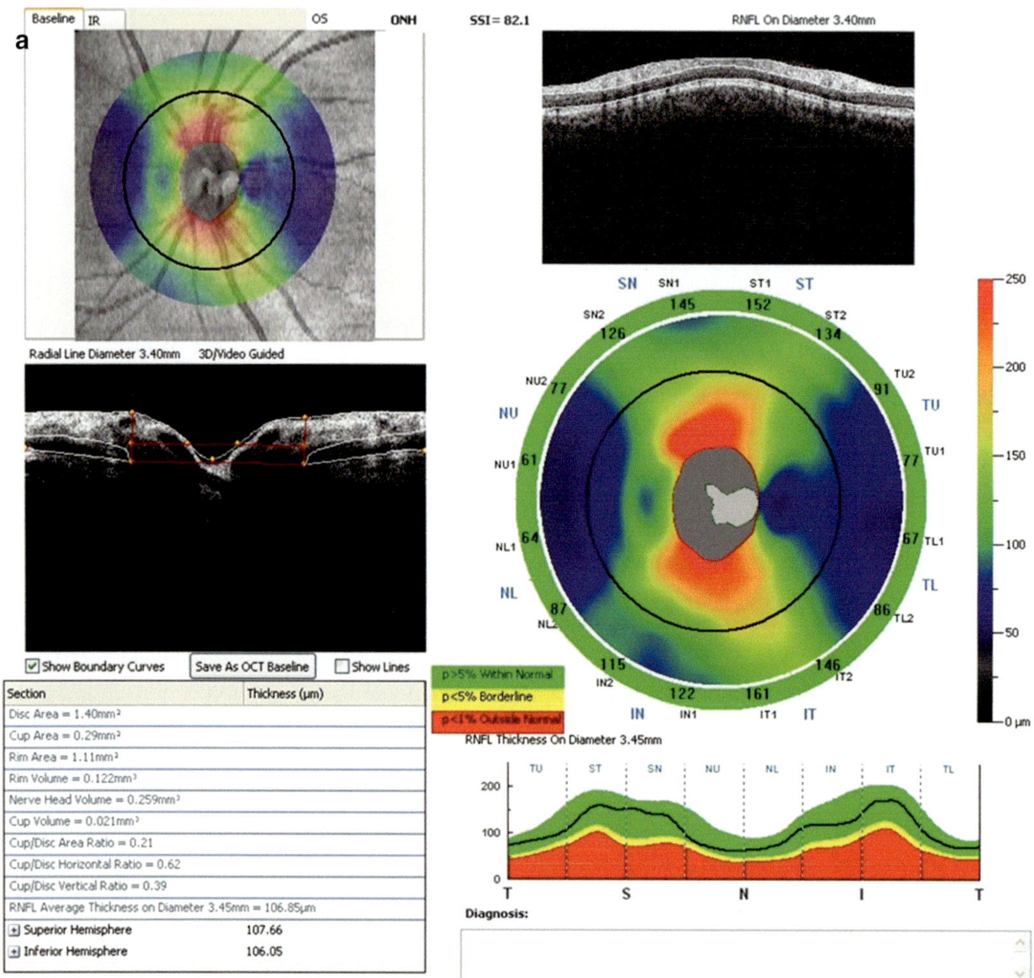

Fig. 3.16 The RNFL map from normal eye (**a**) and glaucoma eye (**b**)

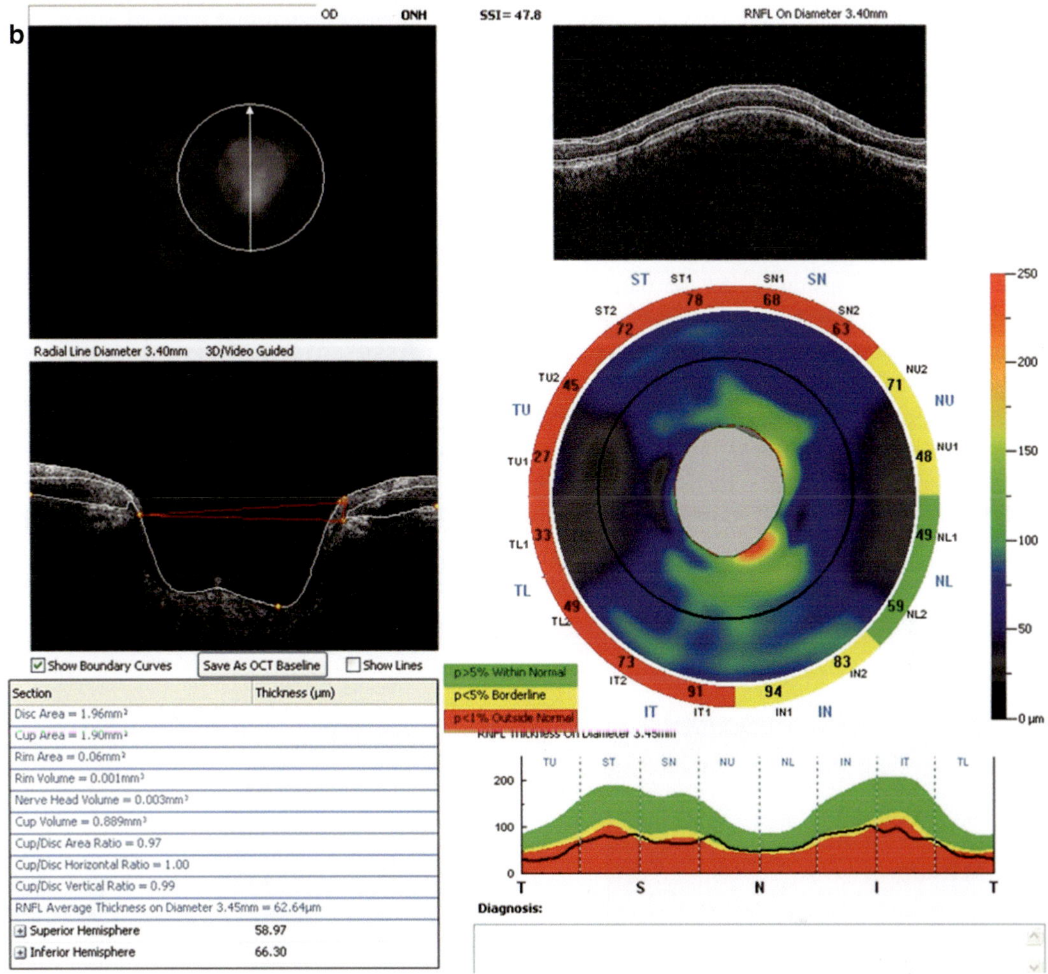

Fig. 3.16 (continued)

The GCC protocol provides total ganglion cell complex (GCC = macular retinal nerve fiber layer + ganglion cell layer + inner plexiform layer) thickness, superior and inferior GCC thickness, and two other parameters including global loss volume (GLV) and focal loss volume (FLV). GLV and FLV, respectively, refer to the average and focal GCC loss over the entire GCC map, much alike with the total and pattern deviation map used in visual fields (Fig. 3.17) [28, 29].

In the optic nerve head analysis result, several parameters could be read in the form including cup/disc area ratio, cup/disc vertical and horizontal ratio, rim area, disc area, and cup volume. The identification of the RPE/Bruch's membrane by the algorithm is critical because its termination determines the edge of the disc margin. Thus, the disc diameter is measured by the distance of the two points of RPE termination. Another line is drawn above (about 250 μm) and parallel to the connection line between the two termination points. And the intersection points with the inner limited membrane of optic nerve head determine the cup margin. The diameter of the cup is defined as the distance between two intersections. The rim area is calculated by the area of disc minus that of the cup.

A large number of research studies have showed that RNFL and GCC thickness are excellent predictors for diagnosing glaucoma. And for detecting the preperimetric glaucomatous changes, RNFL thickness performed significantly better than macular and optic nerve head parameters. The quantitative and reliable measurements of structural damage of glaucoma provide the possibility of monitoring the disease progression over time [30]. The software is also available for longitudinal assessment of the parameters. The algorithm of the software is capable of performing the trend-based and event-based analyses. Recent report demonstrated that the parameters in OCT are more sensitive than the visual field index for monitoring the early-glaucoma progression. And GCC is a better parameter than RNFL for detecting the progression from early to advanced stage of glaucoma [31].

At present, OCT angiography has been developed [32, 33]. Using it, the retinal vasculature to the capillary level could be visualized and quantified (Fig. 3.18). It is invasive and fast imaging. It has been demonstrated that reduced retinal perfused micro-vessel density at both the peripapillary and parafoveal region was closely positively correlated with the retinal structure [34, 35] and visual function damage of glaucoma [36].

It is hoped that the further improvement of these techniques will bring more messages to the clinician.

3.4 Assessment of Visual Function

Except for the structural changes detection, visual function examination is also an important part for glaucoma diagnosis and treatment, which includes perimetry, contrast sensitivity, ERG, and VEP.

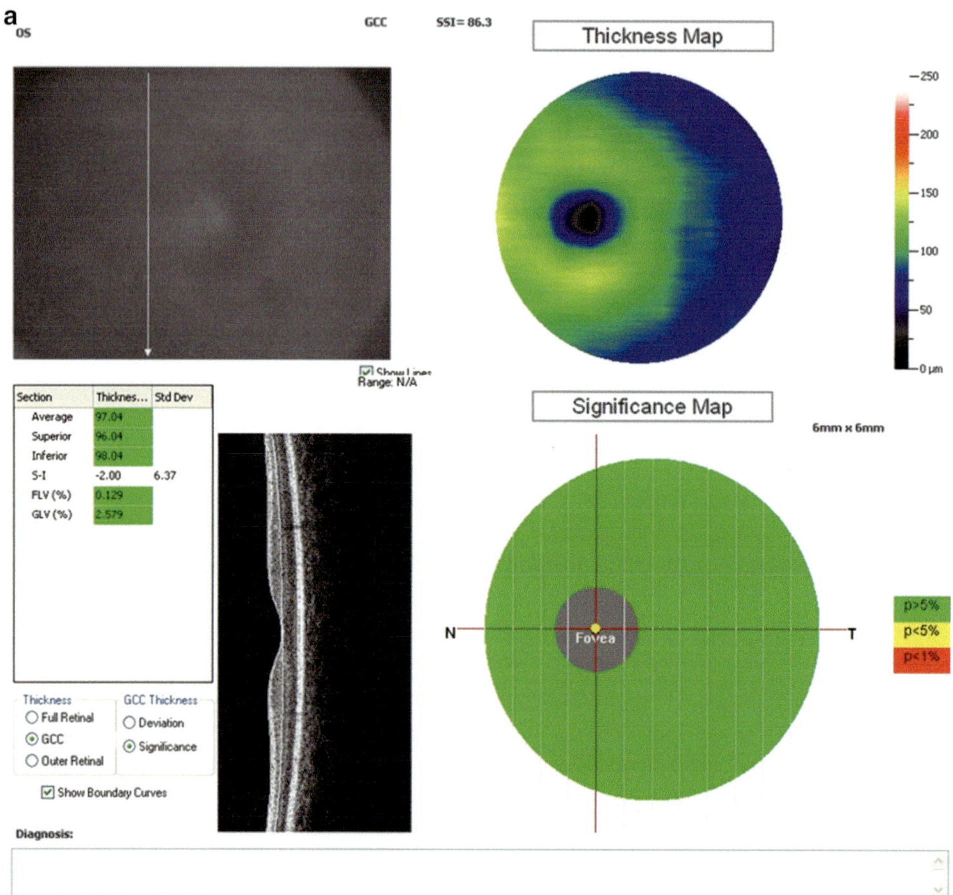

Fig. 3.17 The GCC protocol map from normal eye (**a**) and glaucoma eye (**b**)

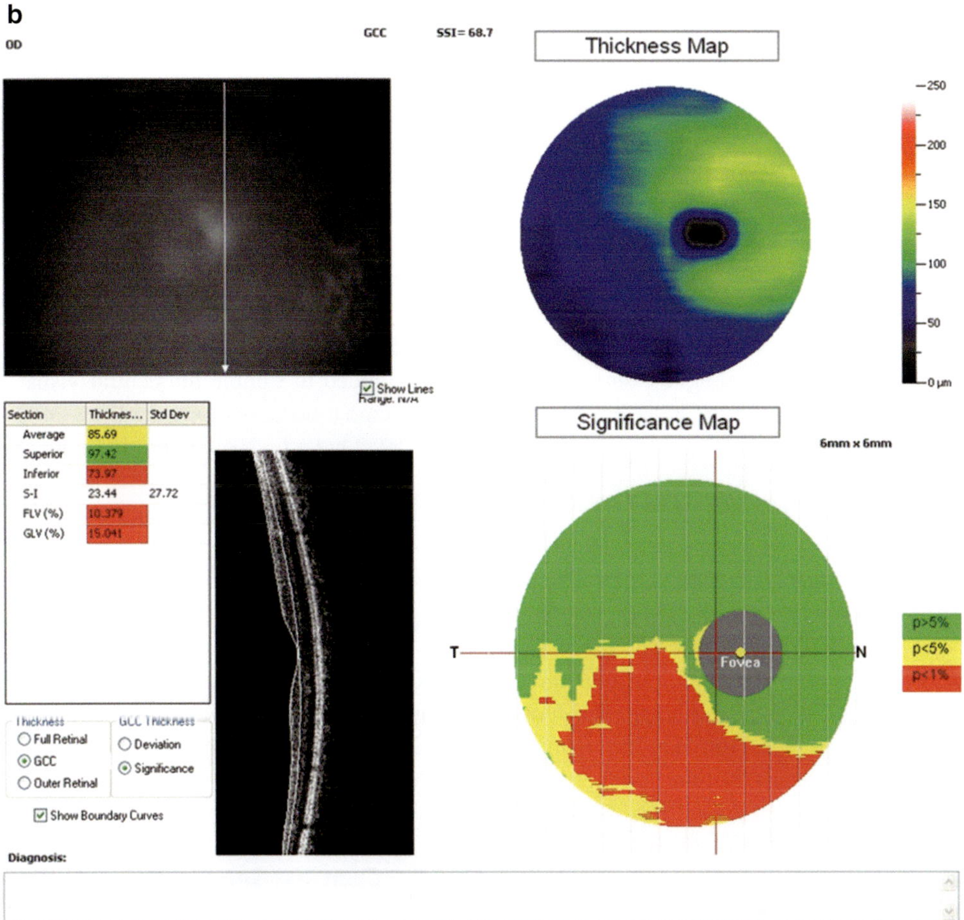

Fig. 3.17 (continued)

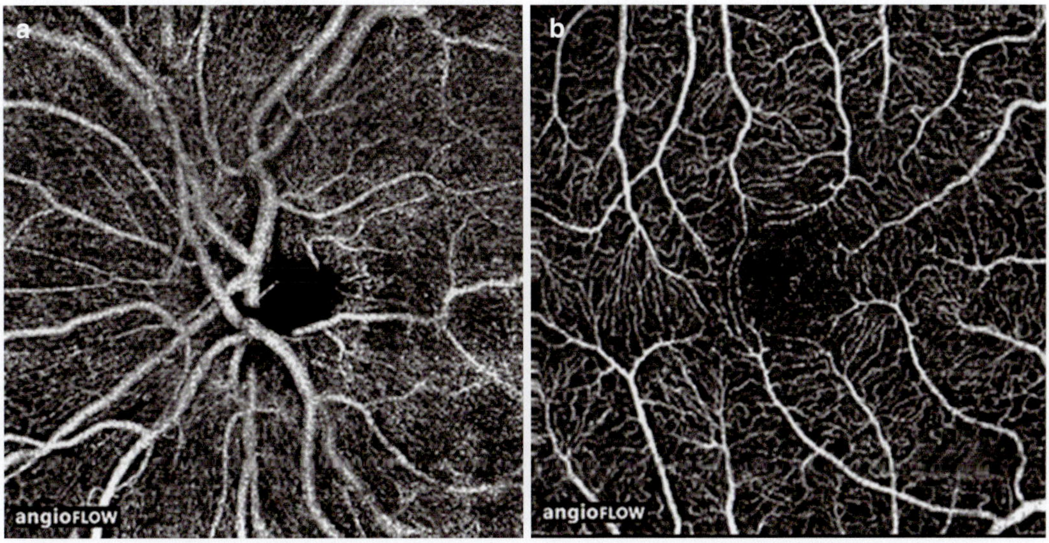

Fig. 3.18 OCT angiography images show the micro-vessels at the papillary area (**a**) and macular area (**b**)

3.4.1 Perimetry

The standard method of testing the visual disfunction with glaucoma has been assessment of the visual field by perimetry for long times. The perimetry measures differential light sensitivity or the ability of patient to distinguish a stimulus from a uniform background. The purposes of perimetry for glaucoma are identification and quantification of abnormal visual fields, and assessment of the glaucomatous progression as follow-up. Regular visual field testing in clinic are automated static perimetry and kinetic perimetry [37].

Kinetic perimetry, which has manual or automated testing, may be considered as an anachronism in glaucoma diagnostics nowadays. But it is especially helpful and efficient for differentiating advanced visual field defects via "edge detection." And also in patients who are unable to perform the automated test, manual kinetic perimetry may be suitable and helpful for monitoring their visual fields. However, the technique of manual kinetic perimetry relies on the skill of examiners to rather great extent (Fig. 3.19).

Static perimetry, which is known as standard automated perimetry (SAP), uses a stationary test object of a constant size with variable intensity to measure the visual threshold at a specific location in the visual field. Automated techniques related with stimulus presentation are especially suitable for measurement. There are two techniques including suprathreshold technique and threshold technique. Suprathreshold technique employs a stimulus intensity which should be seen in every place of the visual field. The stimulus intensity is kind of likely constant over the entire field or may also accord with the slope of the visual hill. Suprathreshold technique may be employed to perform qualitative estimates of visual fields and the screening is very fast. However, it could not detect some early abnormalities including shallow localized depressions of increased variability of localized areas' responses. Threshold technique is very sensitive to shallow depressions of the visual field in case of the stimuli located together closely enough, which could lead to an increased detection rate of early-glaucomatous defects and enhance our competence to compare successive visual field examinations with meaning.

Grid patterns examining visual field defects eventually became widely used and standardized owing to the majority of them occur in central 30 degrees from fixation,, for example, there are 30–2, 24–2 and 10–2 test grids on the Humphrey field analyzer. The role of each test pattern and density for a series of diseases has been examined, for instance, the use of the 10–2 pattern is recommended to sample the central visual field in glaucoma because compared to 24–2 and 30–2, 10–2 has a finer point density; moreover, it is able to better sample the central papillomacular bundle. It is noted that the influence of ocular media, retinal pathology, and other optic nerve pathologic condition should be considered and excluded before judging the effect of glaucoma (Fig. 3.20).

Generally, static perimetry within central 30° is recommended for normal and early glaucoma, while kinetic perimetry is chosen for those severely damaged eyes with advanced glaucoma.

3.4.2 Contrast Sensitivity

For glaucoma suspect subjects, who are with an absence of visual field defects on SAP, frequency-doubling technology (FDT), or short-wavelength automated perimetry (SWAP), the use of contrast sensitivity test may be some helpful for detecting very early changes of visual function [38]. Contrast sensitivity serves an important role in many aspects of vision, specifically visual field, motion detection, dark adaptation, pattern recognition, as well as visual acuity. Several contrast sensitivity tests can be used, and each one has advantages and disadvantages. The contrast sensitivity function (CSF) curve could test multiple spatial frequencies. It has been proven that peak contrast sensitivity ranging from 3 to 6 cpd is the most crucial feature of CSF for predicting performance in daily tasks including driving, mobility, and reading. Testing peak CSF and standard visual acuity might be the best pattern to evaluate patients in clinical practice. But for glaucoma

Fig. 3.19 Manual kinetic perimetry reports show normal (**a**), moderate damage (**b**), and severe damage (**c**)

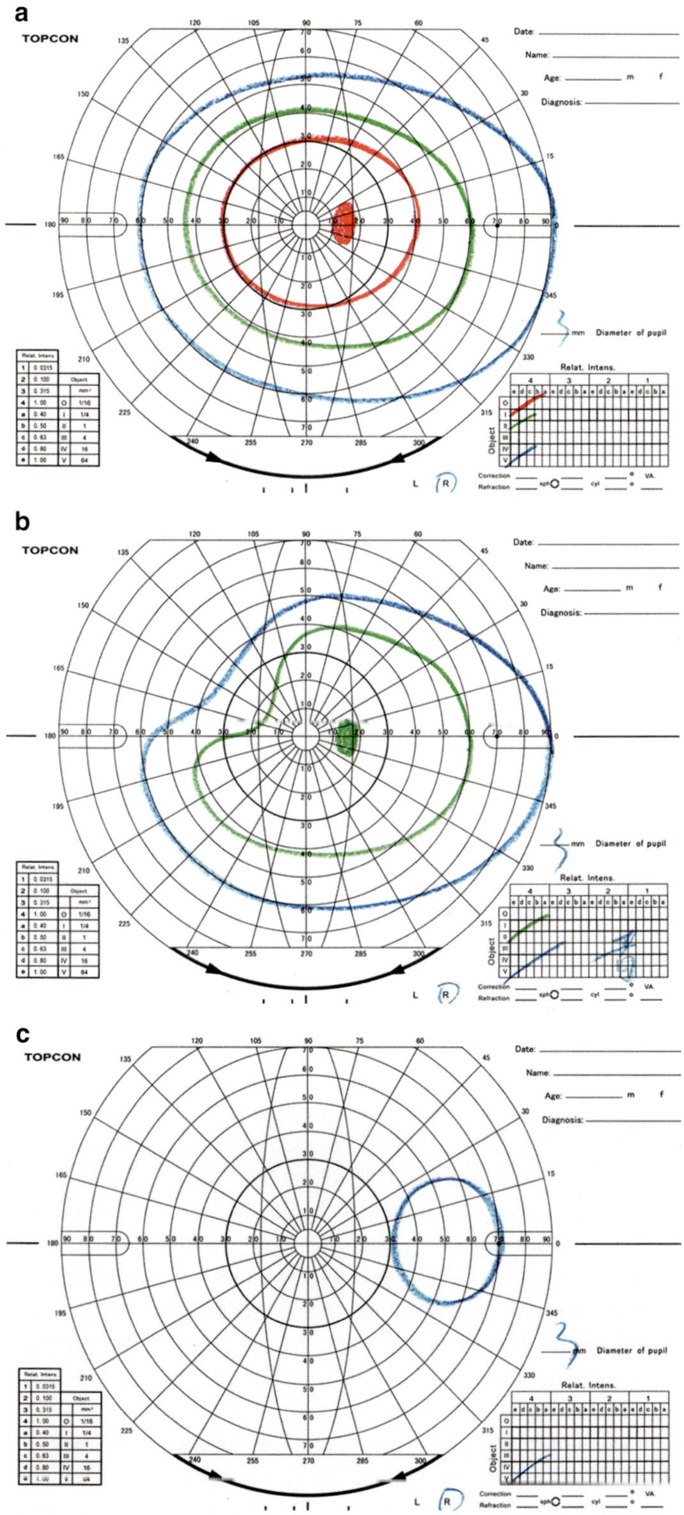

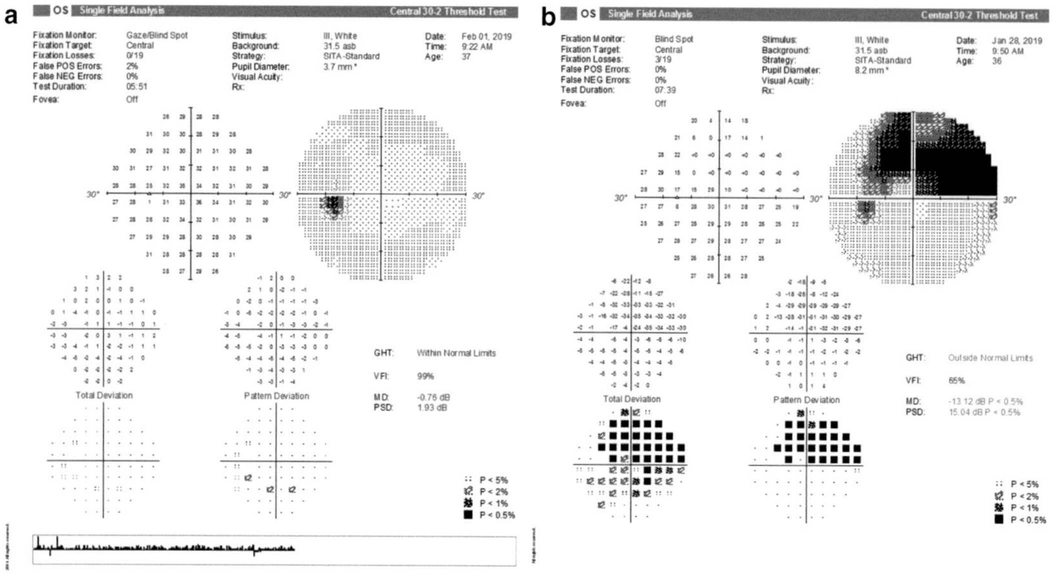

Fig. 3.20 Static perimetry reports show normal (**a**) and moderately damaged (**b**) visual field

diagnosis in clinic, this testing will need further evaluation and more research work.

3.4.3 ERG and VEP

Electrophysiological measures of vision function are objective testing, so glaucoma researchers and physicians have interests to use them for years [39]. There is potential to help clarify pathophysiological processes of glaucomatous damage as well as to provide a potential supplementary metric of function which is more sensitive than standard automated perimetry. The pattern reversal ERG (PERG) together with the photopic negative response (PhNR) of the cone-driven focal, multifocal, or full-field ERG offers objective measures of retinal ganglion cells' function which are sensitive to glaucomatous damage. Recent studies show that a reduced PERG amplitude is predictive of progressive retinal nerve fiber layer thinning and normal visual field converting to glaucomatous changes, which may indicate PERG having a potential role in risk stratification. What's more, converging evidence shows that some parts of PERG and PhNR abnormality are on behalf of a reversible aspect of dysfunction in glaucoma [39].

Visual evoked potential (VEP), especially pattern VEP (PVEP) is a vital visual electrophysiological tool used for the assessment of visual field defects in glaucoma. It has an added advantage of objectivity. In comparison with psychophysical tests, VEP is a more objective measurement of optic nerve function because it is not affected by the motor skills or cognitive factors of the subject. The correlation between those electrophysiological PVEP parameters and mean defect (MD) of Humphrey static perimetry implies that the damaged visual cortical responses observed in patients with glaucoma can be explained by psychophysical and electrophysiological methods. What's more, the significant correlation between MD and PVEP latencies indicates that the severity of global glaucomatous impairment proven by reduction in MD could rely on the delay in neural conduction from retina to the visual cortex.

However, there is no clear consensus on whether the changes of PERG, PhNR, and PVEP are closely related with the early damage of visual function in glaucoma. It is reasonable to develop new strategies for sensitive detection and objective measurements of glaucomatous visual dysfunction in glaucoma suspect and progression of visual function impairment in patients with glaucoma.

References

1. Gordon MO, Beiser JA, Brandt JD, et al. The Ocular Hypertension Treatment Study: baseline factors that predict the onset of primary open-angle glaucoma. Arch Ophthalmol. 2002;120(6):714–720. discussion 829–30.
2. Leonardi M, Leuenberger P, Bertrand D, Bertsch A, Renaud P. First steps toward noninvasive intraocular pressure monitoring with a sensing contact lens. Invest Ophthalmol Vis Sci. 2004;45(9):3113–7. https://doi.org/10.1167/iovs.04-0015.
3. Damji KF, Muni RH, Munger RM. Influence of corneal variables on accuracy of intraocular pressure measurement. J Glaucoma. 2003;12(1):69–80.
4. Ravin JG, Higginbotham EJ. Are we there yet? Celebrating the centennial of the Schiøtz tonometer. Arch Ophthalmol. 2006;124(9):1337–8. https://doi.org/10.1001/archopht.124.9.1337.
5. Hoffmann EM, Grus F-H, Pfeiffer N. Intraocular pressure and ocular pulse amplitude using dynamic contour tonometry and contact lens tonometry. BMC Ophthalmol. 2004;4(1):4. https://doi.org/10.1186/1471-2415-4-4.
6. Kanngiesser HE, Kniestedt C, Robert YCA. Dynamic contour tonometry: presentation of a new tonometer. J Glaucoma. 2005;14(5):344–50.
7. Luce DA. Determining in vivo biomechanical properties of the cornea with an ocular response analyzer. J Cataract Refract Surg. 2005;31(1):156–62. https://doi.org/10.1016/j.jcrs.2004.10.044.
8. Medeiros FA, Weinreb RN. Evaluation of the influence of corneal biomechanical properties on intraocular pressure measurements using the ocular response analyzer. J Glaucoma. 2006;15(5):364–70. https://doi.org/10.1097/01.ijg.0000212268.42606.97.
9. Cheng J, Kong X, Xiao M, Sun X. Twenty-four-hour pattern of intra-ocular pressure in untreated patients with primary open-angle glaucoma. Acta Ophthalmol. 2016;94(6):e460–7. https://doi.org/10.1111/aos.12963.
10. Cheng J, Xiao M, Xu H, et al. Seasonal changes of 24-hour intraocular pressure rhythm in healthy Shanghai population. Medicine (Baltimore). 2016;95(31):e4453. https://doi.org/10.1097/MD.0000000000004453.
11. Kakaday T, Hewitt AW, Voelcker NH, Li JSJ, Craig JE. Advances in telemetric continuous intraocular pressure assessment. Br J Ophthalmol. 2009;93(8):992–6. https://doi.org/10.1136/bjo.2008.144261.
12. Friedman DS, He M. Anterior chamber angle assessment techniques. Surv Ophthalmol. 2008;53(3):250–73. https://doi.org/10.1016/j.survophthal.2007.10.012.
13. Maslin JS, Barkana Y, Dorairaj SK. Anterior segment imaging in glaucoma: an updated review. Indian J Ophthalmol. 2015;63(8):630–40. https://doi.org/10.4103/0301-4738.169787.
14. Sun X, Dai Y, Chen Y, et al. Primary angle closure glaucoma: what we know and what we don't know. Prog Retin Eye Res. 2017;57:26–45. https://doi.org/10.1016/j.preteyeres.2016.12.003.
15. Forbes M. Gonioscopy with corneal indentation. A method for distinguishing between appositional closure and synechial closure. Arch Ophthalmol. 1966;76(4):488–92.
16. Pavlin CJ, Harasiewicz K, Sherar MD, Foster FS. Clinical use of ultrasound biomicroscopy. Ophthalmology. 1991;98(3):287–95.
17. Dada T, Gadia R, Sharma A, et al. Ultrasound biomicroscopy in glaucoma. Surv Ophthalmol. 2011;56(5):433–50. https://doi.org/10.1016/j.survophthal.2011.04.004.
18. Salim S, Dorairaj S. Anterior segment imaging in glaucoma. Semin Ophthalmol. 2013;28(3):113–25. https://doi.org/10.3109/08820538.2013.777749.
19. Smith SD, Singh K, Lin SC, et al. Evaluation of the anterior chamber angle in glaucoma: a report by the American academy of ophthalmology. Ophthalmology. 2013;120(10):1985–97. https://doi.org/10.1016/j.ophtha.2013.05.034.
20. Wang D, Pekmezci M, Basham RP, He M, Seider MI, Lin SC. Comparison of different modes in optical coherence tomography and ultrasound biomicroscopy in anterior chamber angle assessment. J Glaucoma. 2009;18(6):472–8. https://doi.org/10.1097/IJG.0b013e31818fb41d.
21. Dada T, Sihota R, Gadia R, Aggarwal A, Mandal S, Gupta V. Comparison of anterior segment optical coherence tomography and ultrasound biomicroscopy for assessment of the anterior segment. J Cataract Refract Surg. 2007;33(5):837–40. https://doi.org/10.1016/j.jcrs.2007.01.021.
22. Angmo D, Nongpiur ME, Sharma R, Sidhu T, Sihota R, Dada T. Clinical utility of anterior segment swept-source optical coherence tomography in glaucoma. Oman J Ophthalmol. 2016;9(1):3–10. https://doi.org/10.4103/0974-620X.176093.
23. Dorairaj S, Tsai JC, Grippo TM. Changing trends of imaging in angle closure evaluation. ISRN Ophthalmol. 2012;2012:597124. https://doi.org/10.5402/2012/597124.
24. Spaeth GL, Reddy SC. Imaging of the optic disk in caring for patients with glaucoma: ophthalmoscopy and photography remain the gold standard. Surv Ophthalmol. 2014;59(4):454–8. https://doi.org/10.1016/j.survophthal.2013.10.004.
25. Akagi T, Zangwill LM, Saunders LJ, et al. Rates of local retinal nerve fiber layer thinning before and after disc hemorrhage in glaucoma. Ophthalmology. 2017;124(9):1403–11. https://doi.org/10.1016/j.ophtha.2017.03.059.
26. Bussel II, Wollstein G, Schuman JS. OCT for glaucoma diagnosis, screening and detection of glaucoma progression. Br J Ophthalmol. 2014;98(Suppl 2):ii15–9. https://doi.org/10.1136/bjophthalmol-2013-304326.
27. Leung CK-S. Diagnosing glaucoma progression with optical coherence tomography. Curr

Opin Ophthalmol. 2014;25(2):104–11. https://doi.org/10.1097/ICU.0000000000000024.
28. Greenfield DS, Bagga H, Knighton RW. Macular thickness changes in glaucomatous optic neuropathy detected using optical coherence tomography. Arch Ophthalmol. 2003;121(1):41–6.
29. Wong JJ, Chen TC, Shen LQ, Pasquale LR. Macular imaging for glaucoma using spectral-domain optical coherence tomography: a review. Semin Ophthalmol. 2012;27(5–6):160–6. https://doi.org/10.3109/08820538.2012.712734.
30. Mwanza J-C, Budenz DL. Optical coherence tomography platforms and parameters for glaucoma diagnosis and progression. Curr Opin Ophthalmol. 2016;27(2):102–10. https://doi.org/10.1097/ICU.0000000000000231.
31. Zhang X, Dastiridou A, Francis BA, et al. Comparison of glaucoma progression detection by optical coherence tomography and visual field. Am J Ophthalmol. 2017;184:63–74. https://doi.org/10.1016/j.ajo.2017.09.020.
32. Wan KH, Leung CKS. Optical coherence tomography angiography in glaucoma: a mini-review. F1000Res. 2017;6:1686. https://doi.org/10.12688/f1000research.11691.1.
33. Jia Y, Morrison JC, Tokayer J, et al. Quantitative OCT angiography of optic nerve head blood flow. Biomed Opt Express. 2012;3(12):3127–37. https://doi.org/10.1364/BOE.3.003127.
34. Jia Y, Wei E, Wang X, et al. Optical coherence tomography angiography of optic disc perfusion in glaucoma. Ophthalmology. 2014;121(7):1322–32. https://doi.org/10.1016/j.ophtha.2014.01.021.
35. Xu H, Yu J, Kong X, Sun X, Jiang C. Macular microvasculature alterations in patients with primary open-angle glaucoma: a cross-sectional study. Medicine (Baltimore). 2016;95(33):e4341. https://doi.org/10.1097/MD.0000000000004341.
36. El Beltagi TA, Bowd C, Boden C, et al. Retinal nerve fiber layer thickness measured with optical coherence tomography is related to visual function in glaucomatous eyes. Ophthalmology. 2003;110(11):2185–91. https://doi.org/10.1016/S0161-6420(03)00860-1.
37. Phu J, Khuu SK, Yapp M, Assaad N, Hennessy MP, Kalloniatis M. The value of visual field testing in the era of advanced imaging: clinical and psychophysical perspectives. Clin Exp Optom. 2017;100(4):313–32. https://doi.org/10.1111/cxo.12551.
38. Richman J, Spaeth GL, Wirostko B. Contrast sensitivity basics and a critique of currently available tests. J Cataract Refract Surg. 2013;39(7):1100–6. https://doi.org/10.1016/j.jcrs.2013.05.001.
39. Wilsey LJ, Fortune B. Electroretinography in glaucoma diagnosis. Curr Opin Ophthalmol. 2016;27(2):118–24. https://doi.org/10.1097/ICU.0000000000000241.

Medical Treatment Strategy for Glaucoma

4

Yuhong Chen, Kuan Jiang, Gang Wei, and Yi Dai

Abstract

Glaucoma physicians frequently face dilemmas generated by atypical or complicated cases and must answer questions such as "yes or no," "treat or wait," "medication or surgery," and "switch or add." There are no gold standard answers to these questions. Treatment decisions are usually based on comprehensive evaluation of the type and stage of the disease, medical history, general condition, life habits, and life expectancy of the particular patient. Because glaucoma is a chronic, progressive disease that persists throughout patients' lives, therapy should be always considered from long-term and holistic views.

Primary open-angle glaucoma and primary angle-closure glaucoma are the two most important types of primary glaucoma. Although they share characteristics, especially in the relatively advanced stages, they have completely different pathogeneses, leading to different treatment strategies. In the first part of this chapter, we discuss basic questions about the principles of medical treatment for glaucoma, such as the goals for therapy, when to start treatment, how to choose medications, and to what extent we should treat.

Due to the particular anatomical and physiological structure of the eye, ocular drug delivery remains a significant challenge because of various barriers that protect the eye from harmful exterior substances and also therapeutics. Currently, drug delivery methods for ocular diseases can be divided into topical and systemic administration. Topical delivery is used more common than systemic delivery in glaucoma treatment, mainly because of its convenience and high level of patient compliance. In the second part of this chapter, we discuss barriers and absorption routes for ocular drug delivery. More importantly, we summarize delivery methods for various glaucoma therapy drugs in clinic settings, both topical and systemic methods.

Y. Chen and K. Jiang made equal contributions to this chapter.

Y. Chen · Y. Dai (✉)
Department of Ophthalmology & Visual Science, Eye & ENT Hospital, Shanghai Medical College, Fudan University, Shanghai, China

NHC Key Laboratory of Myopia (Fudan University), Key Laboratory of Myopia, Chinese Academy of Medical Sciences, Shanghai, China

Shanghai Key Laboratory of Visual Impairment and Restoration, Fudan University, Shanghai, China
e-mail: ydai@fudan.edu.cn

K. Jiang · G. Wei
Key Laboratory of Smart Drug Delivery (Fudan University), Ministry of Education, Shanghai, China

Department of Pharmaceutics, School of Pharmacy, Fudan University, Shanghai, China

X. Sun, Y. Dai (eds.), *Medical Treatment of Glaucoma*,
https://doi.org/10.1007/978-981-13-2733-9_4

Keywords
Primary open-angle glaucoma (POAG)
Primary angle-closure glaucoma (PACG)
Ocular hypertension (OHT) · Normal-tension glaucoma (NTG) · High-tension glaucoma (HTG) · Secondary glaucoma · Target intraocular pressure (IOP) · Drug therapy
Topical · Systemic

4.1 Goals for Therapy

The general goal of managing patients with glaucoma is to maintain the patient's visual function and related quality of life [1].

4.1.1 POAG

Primary open-angle glaucoma (POAG) is the most common type of glaucoma around the world. To maintain the patient's visual function and related quality of life, medical treatment is implemented to slow the progression of glaucoma as much as possible and to avoid visual function loss by preventing further damage to the optic nerve. Currently, the only available objective of medical treatment for POAG is lowering the intraocular pressure (IOP) [2].

4.1.2 PACG

The final goal of therapy for primary angle-closure glaucoma (PACG) is also to maintain the patient's useful visual function during his or her lifetime. However, the detailed goals for therapy targeting PACG differ from those for POAG. Besides IOP-lowering medication, the underlying cause also must be addressed. With respect to PACG, protecting the anterior chamber angle from closing, avoiding temporary iris trabecular contact from permanent synechia, and reversing the closed anterior chamber angle are more important than lowering the IOP only, since the IOP will be out of control eventually if no proper treatment stops the anterior chamber angle from closing.

4.2 When to Start

Although treatment of glaucoma includes lasers and surgery, medical therapy is typically initiated first. Since glaucoma is incurable and it needs lifelong follow-up, once patients begin medical treatment, they most likely will continue using certain eye drops for years or even decades. Side effects affecting the ocular surface are unavoidable after long-term use of anti-glaucoma eye drops. Thus, over-treatment brings unnecessary discomfort and risks harming the ocular surface. On the other hand, glaucoma patients may lose some visual function irreversibly if they are treated too late, so being too conservative in treatment decisions could also be risky. Therefore, determining the best timing for glaucoma intervention affects patients' life quality and sometimes can be difficult.

Furthermore, glaucoma is a chronic, progressive disease. Glaucoma treatment must be individualized. Physicians should clearly discuss with patients and glaucoma suspects their diagnoses, current treatment, and potential outcomes before starting treatment in order to maximize its efficacy. After evaluating all available information, physicians and patients must decide whether treatment is necessary and what treatment regimen should be followed. Patients are more likely to follow their treatment regimen if they fully understand glaucoma [3].

4.2.1 POAG

Theoretically, any patient with evidence of optic nerve deterioration based on optic nerve head (ONH) appearance, such as retinal nerve fiber layer (RNFL) defects or visual field (VF) changes consistent with glaucomatous damage, should be treated for POAG [4]. In practice, however, judgments can be difficult to make when the patient only has minimal RNFL thinning on optic coherence tomography (OCT) without any VF defects and has normal IOP in the mid- or low-teens range. In this situation, it is helpful to evaluate other existing risk factors, such as family history of glaucoma, myopia, lower ocular perfusion pressure, thinner central cornea, disc hemorrhage, and larger cup disc ratio.

Although the best timing for intervention is not fully clear, the treatment decision mainly rests on whether the IOP is related, or partly related, to the RNFL loss and VF defects, since for POAG, there is nothing else medical treatments could help except for lowering IOP. When the observed IOP level is higher the retinal ganglion cells (RGCs) could endure, judged from both the objective and subjective examination results of optic nerve, then treatments should be initiated.

Prior to the initiation of treatment, a comprehensive ocular examination is required. Unless the damage is severe and the IOP is very high, it is not recommended to begin treatment before all appropriate baseline data has been collected. At least three independent records of IOP should be recorded at different times before treatment in order to have an accurate estimate of the baseline IOP level to use for judging the treatment's effect. In addition, for glaucoma suspects, 24-h IOP monitoring is suggested if multiple records of diurnal IOP are under 21 mmHg. Histories of ocular diseases, injuries, drug allergies, and disease need to be recorded. Best corrected visual acuity, maximum IOP, corneal thickness, axial length, optic nerve photographs, VFs, and RNFL measurements should also be obtained.

4.2.2 PACG

The timing of treatment for PACG is different from that for POAG, since with PACG, the IOP is usually elevated after a certain proportion of the anterior chamber angle is closed, typically 180°. Treatment is much less effective for eyes with a wide range of peripheral anterior synechia (PAS). As we mentioned at the beginning of this chapter, the main goal of therapy for PACG is to prevent the anterior chamber angle from further synechial closure. Thus, waiting until the IOP became elevated or VF defect occurred would probably be too late. It is important to recognize the early stages of appositional angle closure in the absence of PAS. Eyes with occludable angles are indicated to be intervened [1, 5].

Although evidence from clinical trials does not yet sufficiently support whether and when to intervene primary angle-closure suspect (PACS) eyes (with 180° or more of iridotrabecular contact, no PAS, and normal IOP) [6]. Laser peripheral iridotomy (LPI) is still often considered because it is a relatively safe procedure that potentially benefits the roughly 20% of PACS patients who would progress to primary angle closure (PAC) (with elevated IOP or PAS compared to PACS) in 5 years [7, 8].

There is consensus that the fellow eye of a patient with acute angle-closure attack should be treated because it is at high risk for a similar event. Half of such fellow eyes develop acute angle closures within 5 years [9, 10]. Long-term miotic therapy is not an appropriate alternative for prophylaxis of the fellow eye because pilocarpine is not as effective as it was initially believed to be, and side effects develop from long-term use. Instead, prophylactic LPI is recommended to be promptly scheduled [5, 11, 12]. Evidence shows that about 40% of fellow eyes treated with miotics can still suffer from an acute attack within 5 years, and eyes with angle closure can still develop progressive formation of synechial angle closure even with miotic use [10]. Compared to miotic therapy, prophylactic LPI is more effective in preventing acute angle closure in the fellow eye [11, 12].

Again, comprehensive evaluation and effective communication with patients are needed before initiating treatment for PACG. In addition to the anatomical structures of the eye, other risk factors including age, gender, family history, status of the contralateral eye, and compliance should be considered before the decision is made on "when to start."

4.2.3 OHT

Ocular hypertension (OHT) is defined as having documented IOP levels greater than the normal range without evidence of glaucomatous optic neuropathy (GON) [13]. Does OHT need to be treated? From the results of The Ocular Hypertension Treatment Study (OHTS), we know

9.5% of OHT patients develop POAG in 5 years, while the probability decreases to 4.4% if treated [14]. Thus, OHT patients do benefit from IOP-lowering treatment. However, a US study found that it was not cost effective to treat all OHT patients as the incremental cost-effectiveness ratio (ICER) for the entire population of OHT patients to prevent one case from progressing to POAG was $89,072 [15].

In principle, treatment should be initiated when the IOP is high enough to cause optic nerve damage or VF loss. Since the amount of pressure the ganglion cells can endure differs from case to case, the decision to treat patients with OHT is difficult in actual clinical situations. Ocular hypertension patients can display a wide range of IOPs. Obviously, the patients with an IOP in the low twenties have lower risks compared to patients with an IOP in the thirties. Furthermore, evaluating other glaucoma risk factors is helpful in making the decision. For example, if the patient also has an enlarged cup disc ratio, high myopia, or a family history of glaucoma, a relatively aggressive decision needs to be made.

Apart from the disease itself, multiple factors such as a patient's compliance, economic condition, and psychological status should also be considered. Patients with OHT can be left untreated if they can be well-monitored, and treatment could be initiated when signs of GON begin to develop. In contrast, the threshold for treatment should be lower in patients who cannot be regularly monitored. That is also the case for some anxious patients; lower IOP records provide them peace and comfort no matter whether there is loss of RNFL and VF or not.

4.2.4 NTG

Although elevated IOP is recognized as the most significant risk factor for glaucoma, not all glaucoma patients present IOP higher than the normal range. Normal-tension glaucoma (NTG) is defined as having evidence of GON but consistently normal IOP levels [16]. The VF of NTG patients usually deteriorates slowly over time, despite IOP being in the normal range. The natural course of NTG varies widely. Some patients are quite stable, while others progress relatively rapidly to the very late stage. Although evidence from the Collaborative Normal Tension Glaucoma Study (CNTGS) illustrated that 50% of NTG patients who received no treatment did not have VF progression over 5 years' observation [17], a substantial reduction in IOP was beneficial in the course of the disease for approximately 60% of the NTG patients [16]. Especially for those who have advanced VF loss or VF defects close to fixation at presentation, a more aggressive treatment is needed to achieve low to normal IOP levels.

The lower the measured IOP where damage has occurred, the lower the target IOP that is required. Thus, the target IOP for NTG is lower than that for high-tension glaucoma (HTG). Medical treatments might not work on a minority of NTG patients who present with an IOP in the low teens with normal central cornea thickness. If VF progression does occur, the treatment is still to lower the IOP, attempting to consistently achieve low IOP levels around 10 mmHg. However, chances are low that such a target IOP can be achieved for this category of patients. Thus, generally speaking, medically treating NTG is relatively more difficult than treating HTG. In contrast, if a patient's VF function is stable, simple follow-up is recommended. Fortunately, most NTG patients tend to progress more slowly than HTG patients [18].

Great care needs to be taken in diagnosing NTG. A diagnosis cannot be made solely on the basis of normal-range IOP. Physicians must also carefully review the retina, optic nerve, central nerve system diseases, transient ocular hypertension diseases, and systemic diseases. It is not uncommon for patients with an NTG diagnosis to undergo years of medical treatment and then discover they suffer from other non-glaucomatous neurological or vascular diseases that could mimic the VF defects and optic nerve head atrophy of glaucoma. Therefore, simple observation without medical treatment is an option if the VF seems stable and hidden causes are highly suspected.

4.2.5 24-h IOP

Intraocular pressure is a dynamic parameter that fluctuates during the day (diurnal fluctuation) as well as over a 24-h period (circadian fluctuation). Currently, we rely on in-office measurements of IOP to diagnose glaucoma and determine treatment. However, it has been reported that more than 50% of POAG patients display peak IOP outside of office time [19, 20]. Thus, a single measurement is insufficient to identify peak IOP or mean diurnal IOP obviously. The measurements of IOP only reflect a fraction of a patient's circadian IOP pattern and may frequently miss IOP peaks.

Circadian fluctuation in glaucoma eyes is demonstrated to be greater (>8 mmHg) than in healthy eyes (2–6 mmHg), and it has been suggested that fluctuation >10 mmHg indicates glaucoma [18]. Because IOP is one of the most important risk factors for glaucoma, a complete profile is optimal; such a profile should include the amplitude of peak and trough IOP, the frequency of spontaneous spikes, and the magnitude and duration of the nocturnal IOP rise. Continuous 24-h IOP data may guide our treatment for glaucoma patients.

Monitoring IOP for 24 h is technically and logistically difficult, even in a sleeping laboratory where patients need to be awakened, potentially introducing stress-related artifacts [21]. Although various devices for IOP self-tonometry have been developed in recent years, many issues remain unresolved, including inaccuracy, technical challenges for elderly patients, and obtaining IOP measurements without sleep disturbance. Currently, the contact lens sensor (CLS) is the only commercially available device that provides continuous information on IOP fluctuations over 24 h. By monitored with CLS, the peak IOP was found to occur during the nocturnal period in 69% of patients [22].

Therefore, if a patient presents typical GON and VF defects, before making a treatment decision, physicians should conduct a 24-h IOP check to gain a more accurate impression of the circadian curve. Similarly, multiple measurements of IOP in the daytime or a 24-h IOP monitor may be required when patients appear to be progressing even though IOP measurements are satisfactory during a routine office examination.

4.3 How to Choose

Currently, the only approach proven to be effective at preserving visual function is lowering the IOP [2]. The Early Manifest Glaucoma Trial (EMGT) indicated that each 1 mmHg reduction in IOP was associated with an approximately 10% reduction in the risk of glaucoma progression [23]. Since a proportion of glaucoma patients can continue to deteriorate despite an apparently well-controlled IOP, it is widely acknowledged that effective non-IOP related treatments are needed. Some possible treatments, including ocular blood flow enhancement and neuroprotection, have been investigated. However, to date there is no conclusive evidence to support the effectiveness of treatments other than IOP reduction.

4.3.1 POAG

Certain glaucoma treatment trials (the Scottish Glaucoma Trial [24] and the Moorfields Primary Treatment Trial [25]) have suggested that filtering surgery may be more successful prior to medical therapy, and the Glaucoma Laser Trial concluded that initial treatment with laser trabeculoplasty was at least as effective as initial treatment with timolol [26]. However, these studies were conducted before the introduction of prostaglandin analogues (PGAs), which are potent and generally well-tolerated. Meanwhile, the Collaborative Initial Glaucoma Treatment Study (CIGTS) showed that medically treated patients with a 35% reduction in IOP had similar rates of glaucoma stabilization over 5 years compared to the surgically treated group [27]. Therefore, the most common approach is still to begin with medical treatment for POAG rather than laser or surgery.

The basic principle of medical treatment for glaucoma is to use the fewest number of drugs to achieve the intended IOP. Thus, treatment should begin with a single drug unless the initial IOP is very high. Currently, topical PGAs or beta-blockers are the first-line medical treatment for glaucoma. The PGAs are more effective than beta-blockers in lowering IOP and require only once-daily dosages [28–30]. Several other factors also need to be considered in drug selection, including cost, the patient's age, and concomitant diseases.

Monotherapy aimed at lowering the IOP can usually achieve up to a 35% reduction in IOP. If the IOP target is not achieved by the initial monotherapy, as is the case in more than 50% of patients [31], then either adding a drug or substituting a different drug should be considered. If a demonstrable response (i.e., at least a 20% reduction) in IOP has been achieved with the first drug, then it may be appropriate to add a second drug. If there is no demonstrable response to the first drug, then replacement with a different drug is suggested. In this situation, switching to a drug from a different class is the most logical option.

Combination therapy with multiple drugs may achieve up to a 50% reduction of IOP. Although it is a common practice to use multiple drugs in patients whose IOPs are not well-controlled, it is believed that more than three drugs are not likely to achieve additional pressure lowering. Thus, little additional benefit would be gained by treating a patient with more than three classes of agents.

Long-term use of multiple eye drops causes significant discomfort in symptoms as burning, stinging, foreign body sensation, tearing, dry eye sensation, and eyelid itching. Moreover, using multiple eye drops significantly reduces adherence to the treatment regime and quality of life, especially if more than three eye drops are used. Thus, three different eye drops are usually the maximum medical therapy; with more than that number, few patients can follow the physician's advice and strictly use the eye drops on time daily. Greater topical side effects may also occur.

4.3.2 PACG

Medical treatment for PACG is different from that for POAG because the mechanism differs between these two types of glaucoma. The severity of PACG is roughly proportionate to the degree of angle closure. Thus, to open the closed anterior chamber angle and to protect the open angle from closure are the most important objectives. As stated in Preferred Practice Pattern (PPP) from the American Academy of Ophthalmology (AAO) [5], the first goal of managing a PAC patient is to reverse or prevent the angle-closure process. Pilocarpine, the only eye drop that can contract the root of the iris and ciliary muscle, is usually prescribed to open the angle and prevent recurrence of angle closure. However, pilocarpine can also cause many ocular side effects, such as myopic shifts, decreased vision at night, eye pain, headaches, hastening the progression of cataracts, and development of posterior synechia [5]. Therefore, pilocarpine is not recommended for long-term use by PACG patients or suspects. Instead, iridotomy should be considered to reduce the risk of developing angle closure if a pupillary block exists.

Acute primary angle closure (APAC) is a medical emergency. Immediate medical management is required to reverse the attack and prevent severe permanent damage to the affected eye, including the optic nerve, trabecular meshwork, iris, lens, and cornea. The principle for treating APAC is to use aggressive medical intervention involving systemic hyperosmotic agents and carbonic anhydrase inhibitors (CAI), accompanied by the high frequency use of miotics and other topical IOP-lowering eye drops, including beta-adrenergic antagonists, alpha2-adrenergic agonists, and carbonic anhydrase inhibitors. A topical corticosteroid should simultaneously be used to help release the inflammation and injection of the anterior segment. If there is no response, laser iridotomy, laser iridoplasty, anterior chamber paracentesis, and surgical intervention are other procedures often used to stop an attack.

The fellow eye of a patient with an acute attack should be evaluated at the same time because it is also at high risk for developing such attacks [5]. Pilocarpine is usually not a primary choice due to its limited effectiveness in preventing acute attacks or progression in the fellow eye, as well as its side effects when used in the long-term.

Prophylactic LPI is recommended to prevent acute angle closure in the fellow eye [12].

Various mechanisms are involved in the development of PACG, mainly pupillary block and non-pupillary block. Currently, iridotomy is the only treatment available to relieve pupillary block. However, iridotomy is not helpful on non-pupillary block factors and may be insufficient for preventing the recurrence of angle closure with mixed mechanism, especially when a non-pupillary block mechanism is dominant. An extreme example is plateau iris syndrome, which is defined as continuing to have iridotrabecular contact (ITC) after iridotomy, with a gonioscopic appearance of the peripheral iris closely apposed to the angle despite a deep central anterior chamber [13]. Such patients might need to use pilocarpine to prevent angle synechial closure after LPI.

Generally speaking, glaucoma surgery is more often required for PACG than for POAG. In PACG, medical therapy is often used in acute patients to lower pressure and in chronic patients after treatment with laser iridotomy. However, the mainstays of treatment for PACG are laser iridotomy, laser iridoplasty, phacoemulsification, and trabeculectomy [5].

4.3.3 Secondary Glaucoma

The concept of secondary glaucoma refers to the glaucoma type with an identifiable underlying ocular or systemic disorder [18]. Although a heterogeneous group of conditions can cause secondary glaucoma, elevated IOP with complex pathomechanisms is the leading pathological factor [13]. Secondary glaucoma can also be divided into secondary open-angle glaucoma and secondary angle-closure glaucoma, which have treatments similar to POAG and PACG, respectively. However, secondary glaucoma tends to present with higher IOP, which is often more difficult to control with an active primary disease. The underlying causes also must be identified and treated. The main types of secondary glaucoma and their underlying causes, treatment strategies, and alternative medication options are listed in Table 4.1.

4.4 To What Extent?

After we initiate treatment for patients, the next question regards the extent to which we should treat. The decision should be made primarily based on the stage of disease, degree of IOP elevation, rate of progression, age of onset, and the patient's life expectancy [18]. It is important to fully discuss the risks and benefits of treating or not treating with the patients or suspects.

Stage of Disease In general, more advanced disease requires more aggressive treatment. For example, a patient with a severe VF defect or a VF defect close to fixation is at a high risk of further VF loss. Aggressive treatments are required to achieve a lower target IOP, and surgery is suggested if medical treatments are not effective. On the other hand, mild disease may be left untreated unless there is demonstrable progression or a high risk of progression.

Rate of Progression

The rate of progression of POAG varies widely among patients, from very fast to very slow [32, 33]. With a more rapid rate of progression, more aggressive treatment should be considered because the patients are more likely to experience significant visual impairment over the rest of their lives. Adding more IOP-lowering eye drops or switching to surgery is often advised when the VF exhibits steady deterioration, even if the IOP is in the normal range. On the other hand, patients with a very slow rate of deterioration will not benefit from unnecessarily excessive treatments (Fig. 4.1).

Life Expectancy

In some situations where the glaucomatous damage at diagnosis is mild and progression is slow, the chances of significant visual impairment need to be weighed against the disadvantages of treatment, especially for the elderly. However, in patients younger than 50 years old, even slow progression could cause visual disability in their lifetime. This means a lower target pressure and closer VF monitoring are required. For example, a 40-year-old patient with mild bilateral visual

Table 4.1 Main types of secondary glaucoma and their therapeutic principles

Secondary glaucomas	Underlying mechanism	Principles/aims of medical treatment	Alternative medication
Pigmentary glaucoma	Pigment from abrasion of posterior surface of the peripheral iris and zonules during accommodation deposits on trabecular meshwork	Eliminate iridozonular contact, break reverse pupillary block, improve aqueous flow, lower IOP	Miosis, PGA, β-blocker, α-agonist, CAI
Exfoliative glaucoma	Fibrillar material accumulated with pigment liberated from iris deposit on trabecular meshwork	Lower IOP, alleviate iridolenticular contact	PGA, β-blocker, α-agonist, CAI, miosis
Uveitic glaucoma	Obstruction and edema of the trabecular meshwork, pupillary block, angle synechial closure	Alleviate uveitis, break pupillary block, lower IOP	Corticosteroids, cycloplegics, mydriatics, β-blocker, α-agonist, CAI
Lens-induced glaucoma	Pupillary block or angle closure caused by phacomorphic lens or ectopia lentis, obstruction of the trabecular meshwork by lens material	Extract lens or lens fragments, break pupillary block, reduce inflammation, lower IOP	Cycloplegics, β-blocker, α-agonist, CAI
Traumatic glaucoma	Inflammation, obstruction, and scarring of the trabecular meshwork	Reduce inflammation, break pupillary block, clean up debris, lower IOP	Corticosteroids, cycloplegics, mydriatics, β-blocker, α-agonist, CAI
Neovascular glaucoma	Trabecular meshwork obstruction caused by angle neovascularization	Eliminate neovascular, protect anterior chamber angle, lower IOP	Anti-VEGF agent, β-blocker, α-agonist, CAI, corticosteroid
Malignant glaucoma	Aqueous humor misdirection due to ciliary block	Relieve ciliary block, suppress aqueous production, lower IOP	Atropine, corticosteroid hyperosmotic agent, β-blocker, α-agonist, CAI
Corticosteroid-induced glaucoma	Changes in the trabecular extracellular matrix due to corticosteroid exposure cause increased resistance to aqueous outflow	Discontinue or reduce corticosteroid exposure, lower IOP	PGA, β-blocker, α-agonist, CAI
Elevated episcleral venous pressure-induced glaucoma	Reduction of trabecular outflow due to elevation of episcleral venous pressure	Treat original disease to lower episcleral venous pressure, lower IOP	β-blocker, α-agonist, CAI

PGA prostaglandin analogue, *CAI* carbonic anhydrase inhibitor, *α-agonist* α2 receptor agonist, *β-blocker* β-receptor blocker, *VEGF* vascular endothelial growth factor

function damage is at higher risk for blindness than an 80-year-old patient with a similar amount of damage. However, we need to be very cautious in practice, since the life expectancy of older patients is difficult to predict.

Degree of IOP Elevation

The higher the IOP, the faster the progression [34]. Thus, it is obvious that the higher the initial IOP, the larger the extent of IOP needs to be decreased. For patients presented with an untreated IOP level that is more than double the estimated target IOP, the likelihood that the target pressure will be achieved with medical therapy alone is <50% [18]. Both patients and physicians need to be prepared for aggressive medical treatment or surgery in such cases.

4.4.1 Target IOP

The target IOP is described as the IOP range at which damage is least likely to occur or progress. Once medical treatment starts, follow-up is required to ensure that the target IOP has been achieved and the VF remains stable. The target

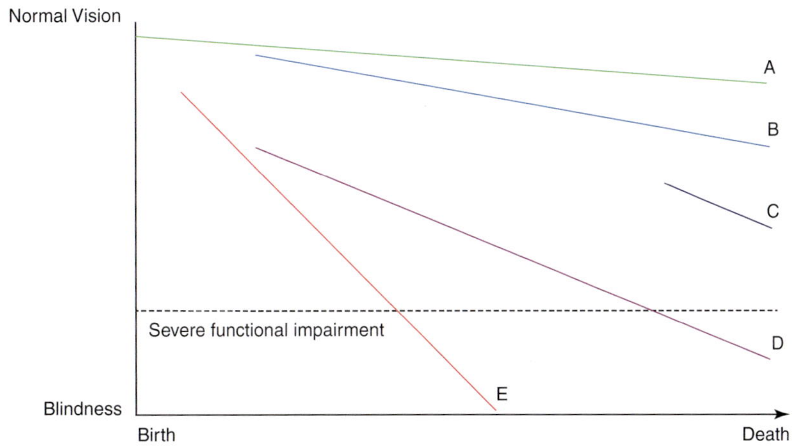

Fig. 4.1 Different rates of progression over lifetime. Line A represents the effect of aging alone. Line B represents a POAG patient with slow lifetime VF progression. Line C represents a POAG patient with late onset, who preserves the functional VF before the end of life despite a relatively faster rate of progression than with line B. Line D represents a POAG patient with severe functional impairment before the end of life, although with the same onset age as line B and the same decreasing slope as line C. Line E represents a rapid rate of progression in a very early diagnosed POAG patient who has blindness early in life

IOP varies from patient to patient and from eye to eye, so it needs to be estimated individually for each eye of each patient. In most cases, the treatment target is a compromise between reducing the risk of vision loss and the consequences of therapy. Primary factors including stage of glaucoma, baseline IOP, age, and rate of progression need to be considered when the target IOP is set. In addition, lower target pressures are associated with increased financial costs and treatment-related side effects. If the potential benefit of reaching the target IOP is outweighed by the potential risks of further treatment, the target IOP may be re-adjusted upward.

The greater the glaucoma damage, the lower the IOP at which damage has occurred; the younger the age and the faster the rate of progression, the lower the target IOP that is required. The target IOP for NTG is lower than that for HTG. The target IOP also depends on the presence of additional risk factors for progression, such as ocular or systemic comorbidities. Patients' preferences need to be taken into account as well [35]. Since IOP fluctuates and VF progression is a long time behind initial treatment, precisely estimating the target IOP is challenging. For newly diagnosed patients, there is no particular algorithm to set the target IOP. Generally, in early glaucoma, an IOP <21 mmHg with a reduction of at least 20% may be sufficient, in moderate glaucoma, an IOP <18 mmHg with a reduction of at least 30% may be required, and in severe glaucoma a reduction of 35–40% may be appropriate [1].

It is important to remember that the target IOP needs to be revised and adjusted regularly. If the VF is worsening rapidly enough to threaten a patient's quality of life, then the target IOP should be lowered. In general, the target IOP should be revised downward in light of demonstrated consistent VF progression on repeat VF tests. The target IOP could also be revised upward if the patient's therapy proves excessive.

4.4.2 Progression of VF

Progression of glaucoma is normally diagnosed by detecting a significant change in the VF. However, the VF appearance may fluctuate quite significantly from one office visit to the next. Therefore, it is important not to diagnose progression based on only two VF tests. The European Glaucoma Society (EGS) recommends three VF tests per year for the first 2 years after diagnosis; this approach allows physicians to identify rapidly progressing patients [1].

VF progression is primarily recognized with two methods: (1) the protocol of the Early Manifest Glaucoma Trial (EMGT) [36, 37], an event-based analysis in which VF progression is deemed to be present when at least three test point locations show significant change compared with the baseline examination in at least three consecutive tests, and (2) the point-wise linear regression (PLR) criterion [37, 38], a trend-based analysis in which VF progression is deemed to be present when at least three contiguous locations show a significant negative trend in the linear regression analysis at $P < 0.01$. To date, the evaluation of glaucoma progression in all landmark glaucoma clinical trials has been largely predicated on VF assessment (Fig. 4.2). Alternatively, optical imaging technologies, such as optic coherence tomography (OCT), can also objectively measure the thinning of the retinal nerve fiber layer (RNFL) to reflect the progressive loss of the retinal ganglion cell axons. Optic coherence tomography systems' trend analyses of the RNFL thickness and inner macular retinal thickness parameters are reported to be particularly useful in detecting glaucoma progression [39, 40], especially in relatively early to mid-stage glaucoma (Fig. 4.3).

Many risk factors have been demonstrated with VF progression. They are higher IOP [23, 41], older age [23, 34, 42–44], an increased cup disc ratio [45, 46], baseline mean deviation or mean defect (MD) [2], and disc hemorrhage [23, 34, 44, 47, 48]. Other factors include thinner central cornea [49–51], decreased corneal hysteresis [52], parapapillary atrophy [53], and lower ocular perfusion pressure [54]. Of these risk factors, IOP has the greatest impact and is the only one that is amenable to treatment.

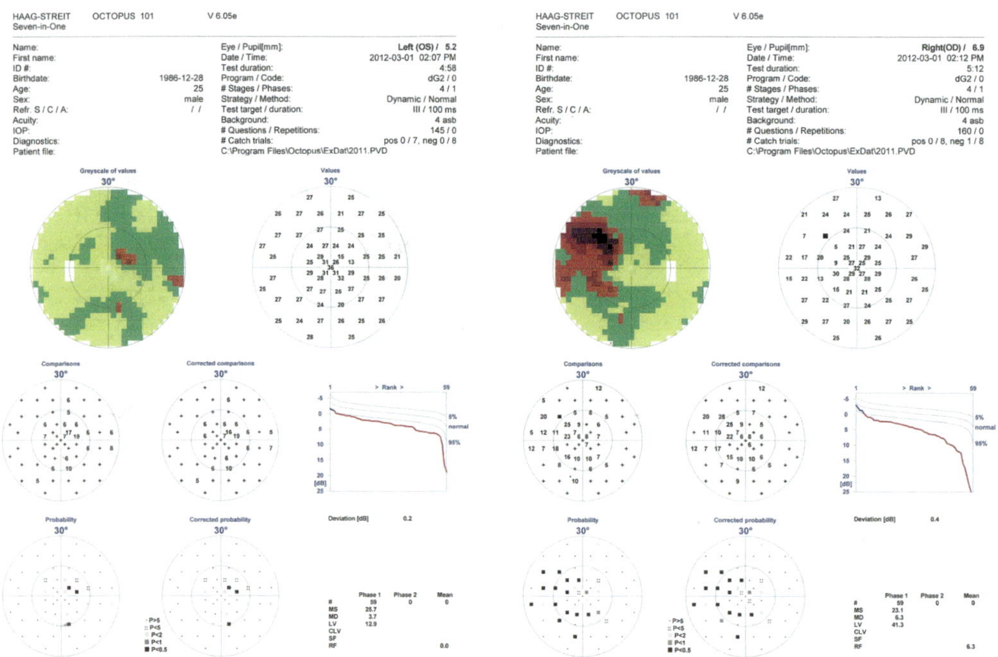

Fig. 4.2 An example of rapid VF progression detected by Octopus perimeter. The upper left and upper right boxes depict the Octopus VFs of the left and right eyes, respectively, of a patient examined in March 2012. The lower left and lower right boxes show the VFs of the left and right eyes of the same patient, examined in December 2012. Significant progression occurred in both eyes

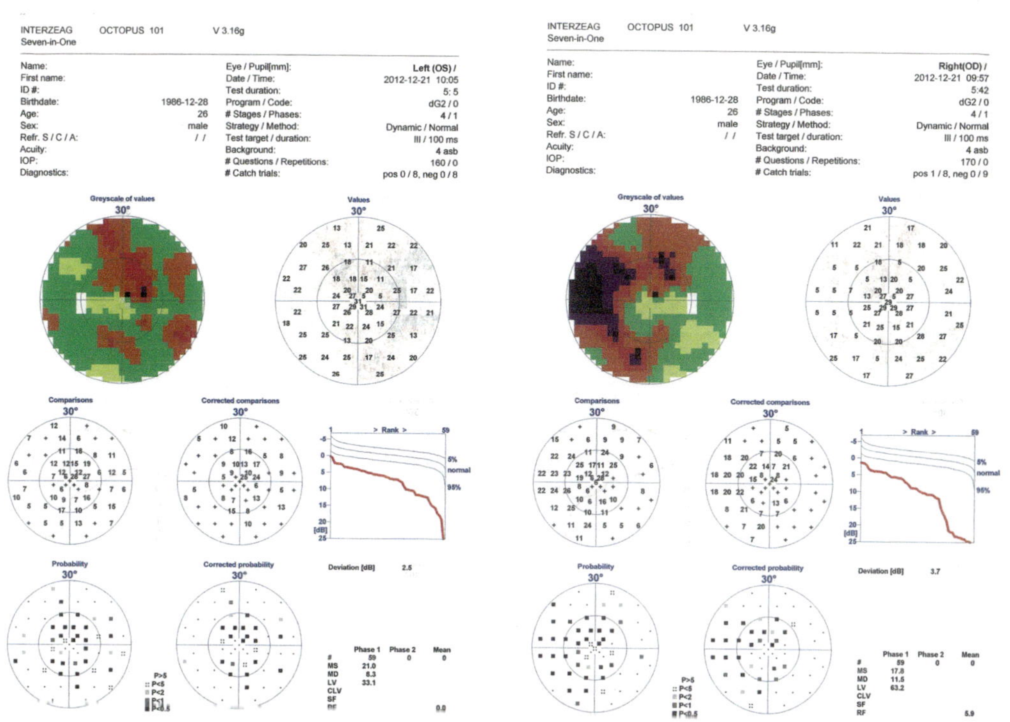

Fig. 4.2 (continued)

The IOP appears to have a dose–response relationship with glaucoma development and progression. Data from a prospective collaborative glaucoma study conducted in five centers during a 13-year period indicated the relative risk (RR) for developing glaucoma rises in a dose–response fashion with a baseline IOP. For example, the RR was 10.5 times greater in patients who had a baseline IOP of 24 mmHg or higher than in patients who had an IOP of less than 16 mmHg [55]. Furthermore, lowering the IOP has been proven to delay the progression of glaucoma [2, 41].

However, some patients continue to lose visual function even though the follow-up IOP is adequately controlled. In this situation, IOP fluctuation may be considered first, regardless of whether the cause is glaucoma itself or non-adherence to eye drops. Intraocular pressure fluctuation has been demonstrated to be a risk factor for VF progression in studies such as the Advanced Glaucoma Intervention Study (AGIS), which revealed that each 1 mmHg increase in IOP fluctuation increased the risk of VF progression by 30% [43, 56–58]. However, this effect has not been consistently repeated in other studies [59, 60]. The significance of IOP fluctuation and VF progression has yet to be fully established in the current literature. In addition, IOP-independent factors such as ocular blood flow and corneal hysteresis may play a role. These factors are still being researched and not clearly understood.

4.5 Drug Delivery Methods

4.5.1 Barriers for Ocular Drug Delivery

4.5.1.1 Drug Loss from Ocular Surface

When eye drops instilled into the sac of conjunctiva, the flow of lacrimal fluid would wash instilled drug out of the ocular surface to the nasolacrimal duct or elsewhere in few minutes. Systemic absorption of instilled drug may also

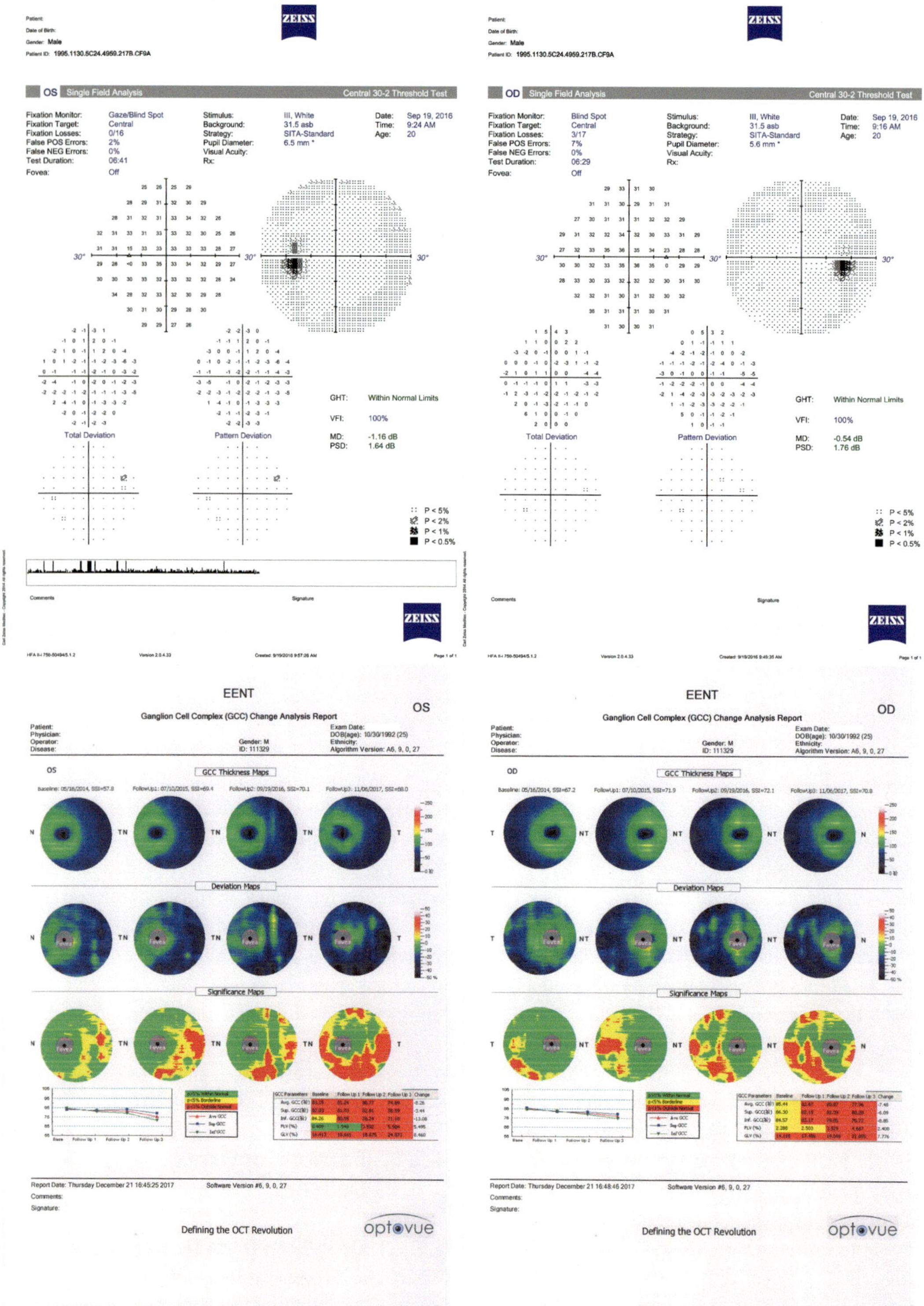

Fig. 4.3 An example of progression detected by OCT. The upper left and upper right boxes display the Humphrey VFs of the left and right eyes, respectively, of a young POAG patient examined in 2016. The VFs were within normal limits for both eyes at the year of 2016. The lower left and lower right boxes provide OCT examination change analysis reports for the same patient comparing ganglion cell complex (GCC) thickness from 2014 to 2017. The alignment comparison shows significant thinning of GCC thickness over 4 years

take place either directly from the conjunctival sac via local blood capillaries or after the solution flow to the nasal cavity. Generally most of applied dose is absorbed into systemic circulation, leading to eye drops the low ocular bioavailability of <5% [61], and this proportion would be even smaller when the wrong administration method occurred (Fig. 4.4).

4.5.1.2 Lacrimal Fluid-Eye Barriers

Corneal epithelium is the main barrier which limits topically applied drug absorption from the lacrimal fluid into the eye. Due to the particular structure of cornea, hydrophobic drugs have typically at least an order of magnitude higher permeability in the cornea than the hydrophilic drugs.

The conjunctiva is a more leaky tissue than the cornea, of which surface area is about 20 times more than that of the cornea. Drug transport across the conjunctiva has aroused increasing interests for conjunctiva fairly permeable to the hydrophilic and large molecules, such as peptides and proteins [62].

Drugs in clinic are generally small and lipophilic. Thus, the corneal route is currently dominating. In both cornea and conjunctiva, principles of passive diffusion have been extensively investigated, but the role of active transporters is only sparsely studied.

4.5.1.3 Blood–Ocular Barriers

Blood–ocular barriers dominate in keeping the eye from the toxicants in systemic circulation. These barriers could be classified as blood–aqueous barrier and blood–retina barrier.

The anterior blood–aqueous barrier, which is composed of the endothelial cells in the uvea, hinders the access of plasma albumin into the aqueous humor and simultaneously limits the hydrophilic drugs from plasma into the aqueous humor. In some conditions such as inflammation, the integrity of this barrier might be disrupted and unlimited drug might distribute into the anterior chamber.

The blood–retina barrier between bloodstream and eye is composed of retinal pigment epithelium (RPE) and the tight junctions of retinal capillaries. Systemic administered drugs easily gain access to the choroidal extravascular space, but further distribution into the retina is restricted by the RPE and retinal endothelia.

These barriers are specific depending on different administration routes (topical instillation, local injection, and systemic). As a result, various factors need to be considered when to develop a suitable formulation for ocular use, aiming to improve the resulting drug concentration and the duration on targeting tissue.

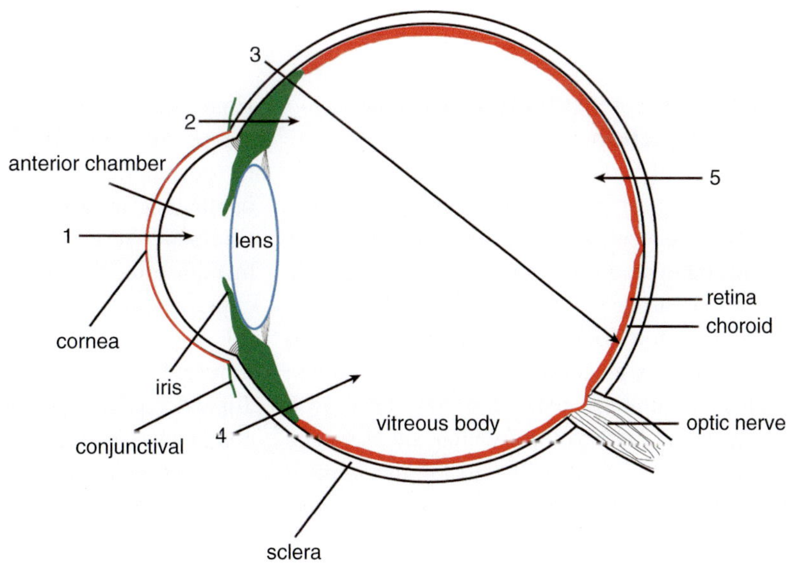

Fig. 4.4 Anatomical structure of human eye and administration routes for ocular drug delivery. The numbers refer to some major administration routes as following: (1) topical instillation via corneal pathway, (2) topical instillation via noncorneal pathway, (3) subretinal injection, (4) intravitreal injection, and (5) systemic administration via blood–retinal barrier

4.5.2 Corneal and Noncorneal Pathway

The corneal and noncorneal pathways are the main absorption routes for the topical instilled drug intraocular delivery. As mentioned above, drug permeation into the eye via corneal pathway is extremely inefficient, especially for hydrophilic and large molecules. Although noncorneal pathway might be more permeable, it should be noted that drug delivery across the conjunctiva and sclera into the intraocular tissues is also limited due to the presence of the local capillary beds that eliminates the drug from target sites. Despite such puzzles, for intraocular delivery of numerous drugs (e.g., timolol maleate, gentamicin, and prostaglandin PGF 2α) with poor corneal permeability, the noncorneal pathway may be the better choice with the help of improved drug delivery systems such as gels, ointments, and subconjunctival implants.

4.5.3 Topical Delivery

Topical delivery of anti-glaucoma drugs is widely used in clinic for the convenience and good patient compliance. There are about six classes of drug to low IOP, and most of them applied by eye drops. In this section, characteristic of topical instillation and local injection, recent development of drug delivery systems, and common drugs in clinical use will be discussed.

4.5.3.1 Topical Instillation and Local Injection

Topical instillation is the most popular administration route for ocular drug delivery. It is noninvasive, convenient to use, and without a need for hospitalization. However, when instilled on the ocular surface, conventional eye drops tend to have a short contact time (usually 1–3 min) led by various precorneal factors (e.g. solution drainage, blinking, tear film, tear turn over, and induced lacrimation), which are the main reasons for only a small part of the applied dose reaching the intraocular tissues by topical instillation (usually <5%). The duration of drug residence on ocular surface can extend by formulation design (e.g., gels, emulsions). Some defects also exist when eye drops used for chronic ocular diseases such as glaucoma. Noncompliance and therapeutic failure with eye drops would increase related to the incorrect drop instillation, especially for the elder or the youth, also high dosing frequency leading to forgetfulness. Moreover, long-term use of eye drops containing preservatives or permeation enhancers might lead to ocular surface injury or even systemic side effects caused by nasolacrimal duct elimination of eye drops [63].

Local injection (e.g., intravitreal, intracameral, subconjunctival) could induce a higher intraocular drug concentration than topical instillation, for avoiding several anterior ocular barriers by a physical method. Although with high bioavailability, such invasive administration routes are with low patient compliance, and have a need for professional medical staff and equipment. For therapy of chronic ocular diseases, multiple injections would sometimes cause severe side effects such as endophthalmitis and retinal detachment [64]. With the development of sustained drug delivery systems, less injection frequency would benefit glaucoma therapy.

For medical therapy of glaucoma in clinic, topical instillation of anti-glaucoma drug remains the first-line treatment. Local injection can also be used in rare cases.

4.5.3.2 Drug Delivery Vehicles for Topical Instillation

High ocular permeation and long drug-ocular contact time are crucial for efficient intraocular drug delivery via eye drops. About 90% of ophthalmic products in the market are in a conventional eye drop form [65], for their easy to manufacture, high patient compliance, and cost effectiveness.

Solution

Topical aqueous solution is with most patient compliance among various ophthalmic preparations. An instilled drug solution provides a pulse drug permeation, followed by rapidly decreasing profile. Another common noninvasive ophthalmic preparation is suspension, which is the dispersion of insoluble drug in an aqueous solvent containing one or more suitable suspending and dispersing agents. Instilled poor soluble particles have a retention in precorneal pocket, leading to an extended drug–ocular contact time. Duration of drug action for suspension is particle size dependent. Smaller size particles promote the drug absorption into ocular tissues, while larger particles have a longer retention time. Thus, an optimal particle size is expected to result in optimum drug efficiency [66].

To improve bioavailability of eye drops, various additives are essential especially permeation enhancers and viscosity enhancers. Permeation enhancers could improve corneal permeability by modifying the corneal integrity, including polyoxyethylene glycol ethers (lauryl, stearyl, and oleyl), sodium taurocholate, cremophor EL, and so on. Viscosity enhancers could promote drug retain on ocular surface by enhancing formulation viscosity, including various cellulose derivatives, polyalcohol, and so on. Other additives such as preservatives and osmotic pressure regulators are sometimes also necessary. Notably, care should be taken in the selection of additives due to high sensitivity of ocular tissues [67].

Emulsions

An emulsion-based formulation could improve ocular bioavailability of drugs mainly for increasing solubility and ocular residence time. Two types of emulsions exploited as vehicles for active substances: oil in water (o/w) and water in oil (w/o) emulsion systems. For ocular drug delivery, o/w emulsion is more widely preferred for better ocular tolerance.

Ointments

Ophthalmic ointments are the formulations, in which drug is embedded in the matrix composing of semisolid and a solid hydrocarbon (paraffin) with a melting point at physiological ocular surface temperature (34 °C). Ointments have a long resistance time on ocular surface, which improves ocular bioavailability, and promote sustained release of the drug, but with relative low compliance.

Gels

Polymeric gels could be classified into two distinct groups as preformed gels and in situ forming gels, both of which could decrease topically applied drugs systemic absorption, eventually improving drug bioavailability and decreasing the side effects [68, 69].

The high efficacy of ophthalmic preformed gels could ascribe to the increase of ocular residence time, related to enhanced viscosity and mucoadhesive properties. The mucoadhesives for performed gels include water-soluble polymers that are linear chains, and water-insoluble polymers that are swellable networks joined by cross-linking agents. Typically, these polymers have high molecular weight (5000–10,000 Da) and cannot cross biological membranes, for example, sodium carboxymethylcellulose (CMC-Na), polyacrylic acid (PAA), and sodium hyaluronate. Besides viscosity and rheological behavior, mucoadhesive and wetting properties are crucial parameters which should be considered in formulation design.

In situ forming gels are the polymeric solutions undergoing sol–gel phase transition to form viscoelastic gels responding to environmental stimuli, including changes in temperature, pH, ions, or others. For ocular delivery, thermosensitive gels are more focused and various thermosensitive polymers have been reported such as poloxamers, polycaprolactone, poly(lactide), poly(N-isopropylacrylamide), and so on. These polymers are firstly mixed with drugs at low temperature in the solution state, which can be concisely administered and forms an in situ gel depot at physiological temperature, leading to an extended ocular residence time.

4.5.3.3 Typical Drugs

1. Prostaglandin analogues

   Prostaglandin analogues, the most effective to lower IOP in open-angle glaucoma by topical instillation, could increase uveoscleral aqueous humor outflow and are the preferred first-line therapy. Moreover, prostaglandin analogues are lack of systemic side effects. There are also limited local reactions such as conjunctival hyperemia, lengthening and darkening of eyelashes, brown discoloration of the iris, and so on (Table 4.2).

2. β-blockers

   The β-blockers might be the most widely used eye drops for IOP controlling, which decrease aqueous humor production through blocking β-receptor on ciliary body non-pigmented epithelium cells, and apply to both primary angle-closure and open-angle glaucoma. Combined application of two or more different β-blockers should be avoided. Ocular irritation and dry eyes are the occasional local reactions. Systemic side effects are often in cardiovascular and respiratory system, as a result, patients with severe diseases in those systems should use β-blockers with caution.

3. β-agonists

   The β-agonists increase aqueous humor outflow by trabecular meshwork and uveoscleral pathway to lower IOP.

4. α-agonists

   The α-agonists could decrease aqueous humor production and increase aqueous humor uveoscleral outflow at the same time.

5. Carbonic anhydrase inhibitors

   Carbonic anhydrase inhibitors suppress carbonic anhydrase in ciliary body non-pigmented epithelium cells to decrease aqueous humor production. Systemic side effects could reduce to some extent by topical instillation.

6. Cholinergic agents

   Cholinergic agents lower IOP through increasing aqueous humor outflow.

4.5.4 Systemic Delivery

Systemic delivery of drug to lower IOP is the supplementary strategy for low efficacy of topical instillation or as the medication prior to surgery. Systemically administered compounds could penetrate the leaky vessels of the ciliary body and diffuse through the iris into aqueous humor, which is the major transport pathway for many lipophilic compounds such as acetazolamide and tetracycline.

Drug penetrates into the vitreous body after systemic administration by one of the three accesses [61]:

1. Penetrating into the posterior chamber and diffusing into the vitreous.
2. Penetrating across the blood–retinal barrier.
3. Penetrating into the vitreous body from the posterior chamber or across the vitreous.

Drug must diffuse from the posterior chamber into the deeper segments of the vitreous body while competing with the parallel elimination of the posterior aqueous humor through the anterior chamber and the normal aqueous humor egress pathways. Extremely lipophilic compounds may gain entry into the vitreous via penetration of the blood–retinal barriers. Notably, there might be some systemic reactions after high-dose or long-term treatment.

Two main classes of drug are used in clinic.

4.5.4.1 Carbonic Anhydrase Inhibitors

Acetazolamide: Inhibit carbonic anhydrase in ciliary body to decrease aqueous humor production. The tablets are taken orally 1–3 times per day, 125–250 mg every time. Sulfanilamide allergies are disabled, and patients with severe hepatic and renal dysfunction or respiratory acidosis are better to refuse. Common adverse effects are numbness of lips, face, and fingers, gastrointestinal irritation, and longer taken would induce lithangiuria, renal colic, metabolic acidosis, and hypokalemia. Potassium chloride and sodium bicarbonate are often combined to reduce adverse effects.

Methazolamide: Similar to acetazolamide in mechanism of action, but with better ocular permeability than acetazolamide. The main side effect is on blood picture.

4.5.4.2 Hypertonic Dehydrant

Mannitol: The usual dose is 1.0–1.5 g/(kg/day). Rapid intravenous drip could lower IOP quickly for about 6 h. The elder, children, and patients with hypertension, cardiac insufficiency, or renal insufficiency should use with caution.

Sorbitol: The usual dose is 1.0–2.0 g/(kg/day). Similar to mannitol in mechanism of action and notes.

Table 4.2 Typical drugs via topical delivery for glaucoma in the market

Class	Generic name/trade name	%w/v	Preparation	Usage
Prostaglandin analogues	Latanoprost/Xalatan	0.005	Aqueous solution	1 drop/night
	Latanoprost/Vyzulta	0.024	Aqueous solution	1 drop/day
	Travoprost/Travatan Z	0.004	Aqueous solution	1 drop/night
	Bimatoprost/Lumigan	0.03	Aqueous solution	1 drop/day
	Tafluprost/Zioptan	0.0015	Aqueous solution	1 drop/night
	Unoprostone/Rescula	0.15	Aqueous solution	1 drop/12 h
β-blockers	Timolol/Timoptic	0.25	Aqueous solution/gel	1 drop/12 h
	Timolol/Timoptic	0.5	Aqueous solution/gel	1 drop/12 h
	Betaxolol/Betoptic S	0.25	Aqueous solution	1 drop/12 h
	Levobunolol/Betagan	0.5	Aqueous solution	1–2 drops/day
	Levobunolol/Betagan	0.25	Aqueous solution	1–2 drops/12 h
	Metipranolol/Optipranolol	0.3	Aqueous solution	1–2 drops/12 h
β-Agonists	Dipivefrin/Propine	0.1	Aqueous solution	1 drop/12 h
α-Agonists	Brimonidine/Alphagan P	0.1	Aqueous solution	1 drop/8 h
	Brimonidine/Alphagan P	0.15	Aqueous solution	1 drop/8 h
	Brimonidine/Mirvaso	0.33	Gel	Once daily
	Apraclonidine/Iopidine	0.5	Aqueous solution	1–2 drops/8 h
Carbonic anhydrase inhibitors	Dorzolamide/Trusopt	2	Aqueous solution	1 drop/8 h
	Dorzolamide+Timolol/Cosopt	2 + 0.5	Aqueous solution	1 drop/12 h
	Brinzolamide/Azopt	1	Suspension	1 drop/8 h
	Brinzolamide/Simbrinza	0.2	Suspension	1 drop/8 h
Cholinergic agents	Pilocarpine/Isopto Carpine	1	Aqueous solution	1 drop/6 h, from lower to higher concentration
	Pilocarpine/Isopto Carpine	2	Aqueous solution	
	Pilocarpine/Isopto Carpine	4	Aqueous solution	
	Carbachol/Miostat	0.01	Aqueous solution	1.5 mL/injection

4.6 Drug Delivery Systems

Eye drops (sterile solutions, emulsions, or suspensions) are most widely used formulations for topical administration, which take up of over 90% of total ophthalmic dosage forms in the market. However, there are still some limitations.

1. Rapid clearance from ocular surface

   The instilled drugs can be rapidly eliminated through the nasolacrimal duct. Tear clearance and dilutive effect lead to reduced residence time in the tear film (only 2–3 min), causing a low bioavailability (<5%). Moreover, most of the applied high dose droplet into the nasolacrimal duct can be absorbed into systemic circulation, which might induce systemic side effects.

2. Noncompliance

The correct instillation of eye drops was not an easily achieved work for the youth or geriatric population. Wrong administration of the drops and high dosing frequency usually cause forgetfulness, which is the main cause for therapeutic failure. Some studies aiming to explore patient compliance to topical drug regimens reveal the improvement of the adherence with less administration times.

A suitable ocular drug delivery system should promote the drug overcome the protective barriers of the eye without causing permanent tissue damages. There are three major objectives of drug delivery for glaucoma: reduced frequency of administration, increasing drug absorption on target site, and less drug transporting into systemic circulation.

4.6.1 Sustained Release Drug Delivery Systems

Traditional eye drops usually have low bioavailability and patient compliance, unsatisfying efficacy, and systemic side effects. Sustained release drug delivery systems could extend drug duration of action, resulting in less treating times and improved bioavailability, eventually to improve patient compliance. Several strategies for sustained drug release are discussed in this section.

4.6.1.1 Sustained Eye Drops

Thickeners into eye drops could increase viscosity of the preparation. As a result, residence time of the drug on the ocular surface extends, which promotes drug efficacy. Some cellulose derivatives, sodium hyaluronate and chitosan, are the typically used thickeners.

4.6.1.2 Polymeric Gels

Performed Gels

The polymeric materials in performed gels could adhere to mucoprotein on ocular surface to extend drug residence time. Although it could improve drug bioavailability and decrease systemic side effects, there are still some disadvantages such as inaccurate dose. It is reported that corneal permeability of 0.4% acetazolamide hydrogel was better than drops, and had similar IOP controlling efficacy but longer action time than the solution [70]. There are also publications revealing that 0.1% brimonidine hydrogel and 0.5% timolol hydrogel using bioadhesive PAMAM–PEG acrylate conjugate as framework are both better than their solutions in solubilization and bioavailability [71].

In Situ Forming Gels

The in situ forming gels, which are liquid in vitro, would transform into semisolid status on ocular surface. They are more rational preparation than bioadhesive performed gels for more concise dose. The in situ forming gels in research could be classified into temperature sensitive gels, pH-sensitive gels, ion-activated gels, and composite gels (Figs. 4.5, 4.6, and 4.7).

4.6.1.3 Colloidal Systems

There are many challenges in developing ocular drug delivery systems such as poor solubility of drug, difficulties in delivery of macromolecules, in vivo instability, intestinal absorption, sustained and targeted delivery to lesion, therapeutic effectiveness, generalized side effects, and plasma fluctuations of drugs. Among various novel drug delivery systems, colloidal systems based on nanotechnology arouse wide concern to solve those questions.

Benefits of colloidal systems for ocular drug delivery: Increase drug solubility in disperse systems, improve drug absorption, protect drug from degradation, sustained and controlled drug release, reduce frequency of administration, and targeting drug delivery.

Nowadays, colloidal systems are widely applied for the treatment of ocular diseases. There are a large number of systems in present researches such as microemulsions, nanoemulsions, nanosuspension, nanoparticles, liposomes, niosomes, micelles, and so on.

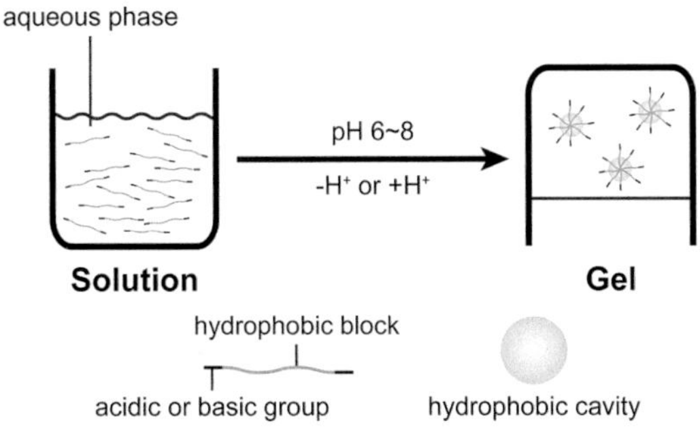

Fig. 4.5 Mechanism of pH-sensitive in situ forming gels

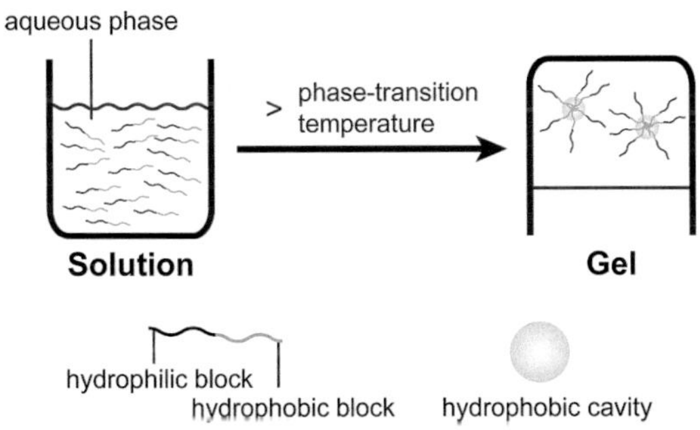

Fig. 4.6 Mechanism of temperature sensitive in situ forming gels

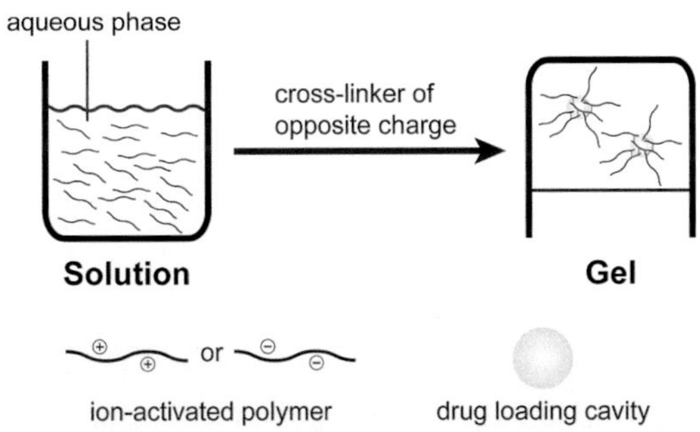

Fig. 4.7 Mechanism of ion-activated in situ forming gels

Microemulsions and Nanoemulsions

Microemulsions are disperse systems composed of water phase and oil phase that require surfactant and co-surfactant agents to stabilize the interface between two phases [72]. They have a transparent appearance, thermodynamic stability, and a small droplet size in the dispersed phase. Microemulsions are promising ocular drug delivery systems for their long-term stability, easy to prepare and sterilize, low toxicity and irritancy, and considerable drug-loading capacity. Microemulsions could deliver lipophilic and hydrophilic drug through their respective medium (aqueous medium or lipoid medium), and surfactant and co-surfactant in them could play a role as permeation enhancers to increase drug intraocular transport, hence improve the bioavailability. Sustained release of drug in microemulsions can also decrease the frequency of application, which benefits patients suffering from chronic diseases. Apart from the advantages of microemulsions mentioned above, nanoemulsions have smaller size, indeed with stronger corneal permeation ability, resulting in an increased bioavailability [73].

Nanosuspension

Nanosuspension is the system of nanosized water-insoluble drug particles suspended in an appropriate medium, which is stabilized by other excipients, such as surfactants and viscosity enhancers [74]. Such a dosage form could be prepared by pearl milling, high-pressure homogenization, and precipitation techniques. Besides sustained drug release and improved bioavailability, it is free from irritation to ocular tissues, and could be an inert carrier for ocular delivery.

Nanoparticles (NPs)

The polymeric nanoparticulate system comprises particles in the range of 1–1000 nm with drug adsorbed, entrapped, conjugated, or encapsulated in it. Depending on the methods of preparation, it can be classified as nanospheres or nanocapsules, having different drug release profile [75]. Nanospheres are small solid spheres constituting of dense solid polymeric network with large surface area. Drugs are incorporated in the matrix or adsorbed on the surface. Nanocapsules have small central cavity (oily droplet) surrounded by a polymeric membrane. After binding to these particles, the drug absorption in the eye is enhanced significantly in comparison to eye drop solutions owing to the much slower ocular elimination rate of particles. Besides, smaller particles are better tolerated than larger particles. Numerous polymers can be used to construct NPs such as biodegradable polymers like polylactides (PLA), poly(lactic-co-glycolic acid) (PLGA), polyacrylamide, poly(methyl methacrylate), and natural polymers like chitosan, gelatin, and albumin.

Lipid nanoparticles applied for ocular drug delivery has satisfying ability to increase drug solubility and improve drug release profile [76]. Solid lipid nanoparticles (SLNs), usually with a solid lipid core and stabilized by surfactants in aqueous dispersion, are able to carry both hydrophobic and hydrophilic molecules. Generally, SLNs could decrease degradation of loading drugs and show good biocompatibility. However, there are some defects restricting their further application, such as low drug-loading capacity and high drug leaking during storage due to polymorphic transition of lipid molecules. When it comes to the methods for more stable lipid nanoparticles, compared with surface modification to SLN, nanostructure lipid carriers (NLS) are more acceptable. NLS containing solid lipid and liquid lipid show improved drug incorporation and release properties for their special nanostructures.

Liposomes

Liposomes are bilayered lipid vesicles composed of altering aqueous compartments enclosed by lipid bilayers (mainly phospholipids and cholesterol), with the diameter ranged from 10 to 1000 nm or greater. Liposomes could encapsulate hydrophobic (in lipid bilayers), hydrophilic (in aqueous compartments), and amphiphilic drugs. For ocular use, liposomes could improve bioavailability of ophthalmic drugs after topical instillation and have no toxicity and low antigenicity [77]. Besides, positively charged liposomes have prolonged precorneal residence time than the negative or neutral charged, due to electrostatic interaction with the negatively charged corneal epithelium.

Niosomes

Niosomes are bilayered vesicular systems formed by self-assembly of hydrated non-ionic surfactants [78]. Like liposomes, niosomes could deliver drug in controlled manner to enhance bioavailability, while niosomes have longer shelf life and lower cost than liposomes. Niosomes usually suspend in water-based medium with higher patient compliance than oily dosage forms. Due to hydrophilic, amphiphilic, and lipophilic moieties together contained structure, niosomes can entrap both hydrophilic and lipophilic drug with various solubility.

Nanomicelles

Nanomicelles are ultramicroscopic globular structures consisting of exterior hydrophilic polar heads and an interior hydrophobic fatty acyl chain, which are able to deliver poorly soluble drugs as well as protect them from degradation. Nanomicelles are the most frequently utilized approach to formulate therapeutic agents into a clear aqueous solution, but disadvantages such as limited drug-loading capacity and poor physical stability restrict their further application [79].

Dendrimers

Dendrimers are repetitively branched molecules which are available in different molecular weights with amine, hydroxyl, or carboxyl functional group as terminals. The highly branched structure of dendrimers allows for incorporation of wide range of drugs, hydrophobic or hydrophilic. And terminal groups can be used to be conjugated to other functional chemical groups. In ocular drug delivery, few promising results were reported with these branched polymeric systems, in which poly(amidoamine) (PAMAM) dendrimers are widely employed [80].

Cyclodextrins Inclusion Compound

Cyclodextrins (CDs) are a family of compounds made up of sugar molecules bound together in a ring, with a hydrophilic outer surface made up of six, seven, or eight glucose units, namely, α, β, γ CD, and nowadays various modified CDs have been developed for drug delivery. Soluble CDs have a lipophilic cavity in the center to improve solubility of poorly soluble therapeutic agents, further to increase their bioavailability and stability in solutions and reduced side effects [81]. CDs are novel, chemically stable carriers that could enhance ocular bioavailability of hydrophobic ophthalmic drugs without affecting the barrier function of the eye or increasing the viscosity of the aqueous eye drop formulation.

4.6.2 Contact Lenses

Contact lenses (CLs), which cling to the corneal tear film for vision correction, could be a possible candidate for sustained ocular drug delivery due to their long residence time on ocular surface. They can also minimize drug absorption into the blood stream through the conjunctiva or nasolacrimal duct, leading to improved bioavailability, lower required dosage, and less frequent drug application, thereby improving patient compliance [82]. CLs in the market could be classified into two groups, rigid CLs, mainly made up of poly(methyl methacrylate), and soft CLs (gelatinous), mainly made up of hydroxyethyl methacrylate polymers, also classified as hydrophilic or hydrophobic one by FDA. The hydrophilic CLs have superior ability to hold water and usually used for quite long period (about 1 week). Moreover, addition of silicon in CLs could improve their gaseous permeability and extend the service life to even 1 month without ocular hypoxia.

As rigid CLs are mainly for orthokeratology and expensive, soft CLs which are more comfortable to wear are more studied for therapeutic usage. Drug could be loaded in CLs by various methods, such as soaking CLs in a drug solution, using molecular imprinting technology, importing drug-loading nanoparticles, and so on. Due to concentration gradient between post-lens tear fluid and CLs, also called the sink effects, drug in CLs firstly diffuses into the post-lens tear film and disperses in the tear followed by absorption into the eye (Fig. 4.8).

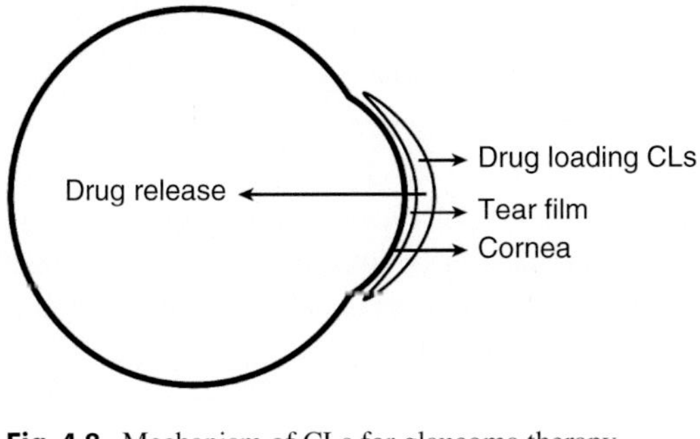

Fig. 4.8 Mechanism of CLs for glaucoma therapy

CLs with ocular adhesion ability and drug release character could increase drug residence time on ocular surface (over 30–2 min for conventional eye drops) and further to improve bioavailability up to 50% (for conventional eye drops, usually no more than 5%), which leads to an increase of therapeutic efficacy and avoids the wastage of drug. Besides, as long-term usage of eye drops sometimes causes ocular irritation for permeation enhancers or perspectives in them, CLs are much safer for free of those ingredients [83].

4.6.2.1 Commercial CLs

Attempts of commercial CLs as sustained drug delivery systems in ophthalmic use are implemented about 50 years ago. The drug incorporates into the CLs and releases through a process named as "soak and release." That means first to soak CLs in drug solutions and the drug could enter into the CLs, and then drug-loading CLs could achieve sustained drug release to the eye. However, low affinity of hydrophilic CLs for most hydrophobic drugs in clinic limits the initial development.

One of the first recorded drug-loading CLs for glaucoma therapy is a 4% pilocarpine solution soaked soft contact lenses [84]. In 1971, it is found that 1% pilocarpine solution soaked CLs were better than 8% pilocarpine solution for IOP control. It is also proved that CLs soaked in 1% pilocarpine for just 2 min were more effective for IOP control than common pilocarpine eye drops in the market [85]. Then in 1974, the effectiveness of the method in glaucoma patients was first proved. Besides, it was showed that increasing exposure time between the lens and the pilocarpine solution may result in a higher equilibrium between them and an extended release time [86]. Vasurfilcon A CLs (CIBA Vision, Duluth, GA) were soaked in timolol maleate (0.65 mg/mL) or brimonidine tartrate (0.2 mg/mL) solution and evaluated their characteristic in vitro and in vivo. In vitro uptake and release experiments showed that both two kinds of CLs uptook or released drug to maximum for approximately 1 h. More importantly, for limited number of patients with glaucoma, when they wore such CLs 30 min per day for 2 weeks, the IOP could be controlled at the level equal to their previous treatments (brimonidine tartrate 2.0% solution using one drop in each eye, twice per day; one drop of 0.25% timolol maleate ophthalmic solution in each eye every 12 h; one drop per day of 0.5% timolol maleate gel-forming solution in each eye). Moreover, quite a lot of drug would be saved as there was vestigial drug in the CLs-soaked solution. After that, the coverage of the CLs above the ophthalmic drops in the eye was recommended to reduce drug wastage.

Despite the positive results related to this harsh method, no research showed a sustained drug release time more than 2 h, which urges the development of modified CLs with longer drug release period.

4.6.2.2 Modified CLs

Vitamin E Imbedding CLs

To achieve longer sustained drug release, an additional barrier in the CL matrix to extend drug diffusion might be useful. However, the establishment of these barriers on the CLs surface is complex owing to the transparency and gaseous permeation demand.

Vitamin E (VE) imbedding CLs have been designed for sustained release of several drugs [87]. Briefly, blank CLs are soaked in a VE ethanolic solution before drug loading, or VE and drug can be loaded simultaneously, then ethanol is extracted with water. This method is preferred to hydrophilic drugs (for example, timolol), for hydrophobic VE acting as a barrier to the release of the drug, thus extending the release time (Fig. 4.9). With various types of CLs tested, VE containing lotrafilcon A CLs showed best ability for sustained release of timolol. The release time was up to 5.5 h when the content of VE was 16%, and with the increase of VE, the release time was 43 h (contained 27% VE) and 192 h (contained 74% VE), respectively [88].

VE imbedding CLs can also be obtained by the "soak and release" method, which induces a lower but homogeneous VE distribution in CLs. Timolol in conventional CLs releases 80% in 30 min, but for VE soaked CLs, timolol releases 75% in 12 h [89].

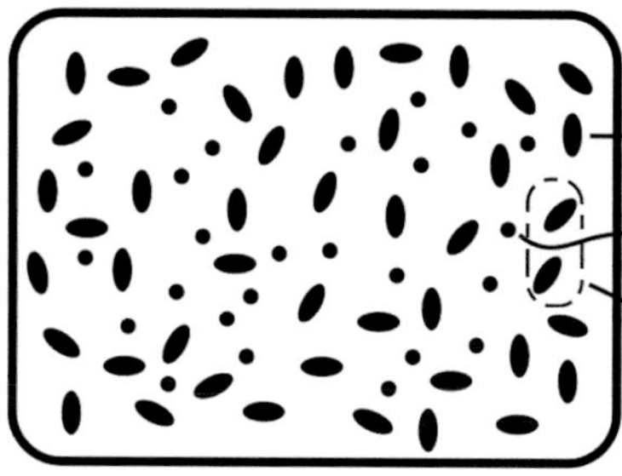

Fig. 4.9 Mechanism of VE imbedding CLs for sustained drug release

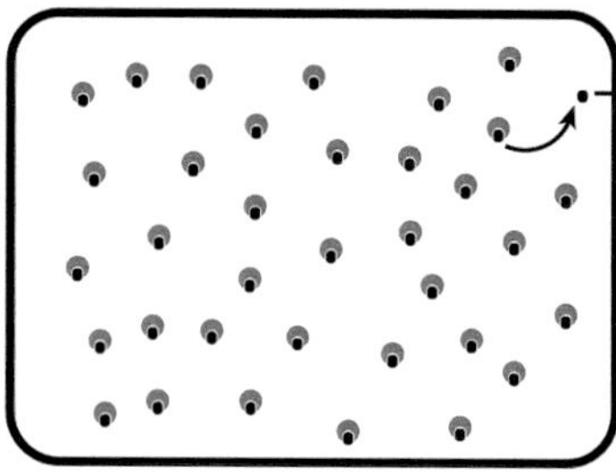

Fig. 4.10 Mechanism of imprinted CLs for sustained drug release

Besides the role as release barrier for hydrophilic drug, VE has been considered as a neuroprotective agent for glaucoma therapy. Imbedding moderate VE in CLs would also have no alteration in the transparency and visual performance of CLs.

Imprinted CLs

Molecular imprinting technology has been a research hotspot for scientists in the field of pharmacy and materials during the last two decades. Through interaction between a template drug and functional monomers during the CLs polymerization process, a memory cavity with a suitable size and chemical groups which could accommodate the drug will appear in CLs (Fig. 4.10) [90]. Monomer composition, diversity, and number of interactions at the recognition position all have effects on the subsequent drug release profile. An appropriate polymer crosslinking degree is crucial in the design of imprinted CLs, for a high crosslinking degree benefit the stability of the imprinted cavities, but lower crosslinker concentrations (<5%) could meet transparency demand and optical performance for CLs.

The first attempt of imprinted soft CLs was applied for timolol. An imprinted CL could load a maximum of 34 μg of timolol, while a conventional CL loads no more than 20 μg. More importantly, imprinted CLs lead to a maximum ocular concentration peak after 5 min followed by a sustained release for 180 min, but for conventional CLs, the sustained release time was 90 min, and timolol in solutions was completely eliminated from the ocular surface in <60 min [91]. Dorzolamide-loaded imprinted CLs also show prolonged release ability than the eye drops [92].

Nanostructures Imbedding CLs

Due to the ability of nanoparticles (either for lipid nanoparticles or polymeric nanoparticles) to increase drug solubility and control their release, nanoparticles imbedding CLs could achieve increased drug-loading capacity and sustained drug release (Fig. 4.11).

As illustrated earlier, lipid nanoparticles or polymeric nanoparticles could increase solubility of both hydrophilic and hydrophobic drugs. Nanoparticles imbedding CLs are usually with high drug-loading capacity, but too much nanoparticles in CLs will hamper their transparency.

Dynamic instability of lipid nanoparticles would cause premature release in storage, as a result, there are limited related researches up to now. Preserving the CLs in a saturated drug solution to prevent premature release would cause wastage of drug. As a result, polymeric nanoparticles imbedding CLs arouse more interest due to their inherent stability.

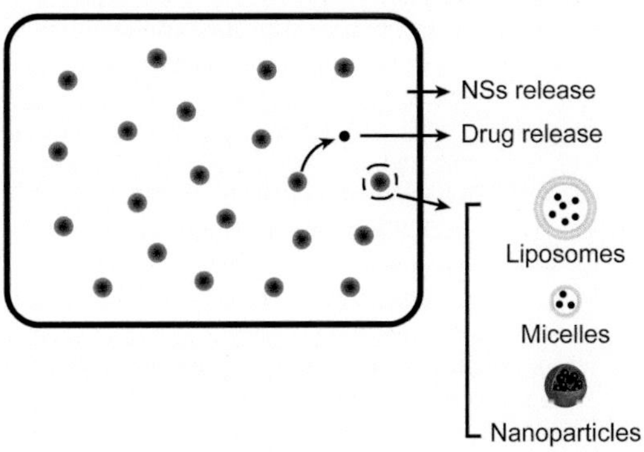

Fig. 4.11 Mechanism of nanostructures imbedding CLs for sustained drug release

The sustained release profile of timolol-loading nanoparticle imbedding CLs has been evaluated [93]. It is found that a continuous release of timolol in therapeutic concentration lasted for 2–4 weeks in a temperature dependent manner (drug releasing at body temperature). This finding is inspiring for storing (lower than body temperature) the drug without premature release. The use of cyclodextrins could also increase the loading capacity of hydrophobic drugs in the hydrophilic polymer matrix of the CLs and prolong their release.

4.6.2.3 Prospects

The usage of CLs can not only improve visual acuity but also provide a more feasible tool for ocular diseases such as glaucoma, for their sustained release profile and high drug-loading capacity. Although there are still some limitations such as ocular compliance problems, CLs might be a promising system for such chronic ocular diseases.

4.6.3 Implantable Reservoirs

One of the advantages of implantable reservoirs is to keep drug release for a quite long time via one administration, especially for those chronic diseases such as glaucoma, which could improve patient compliance. Drug release profile is related to the contact area between eye and the implant, and degradation rate of polymer component.

Implantable reservoirs application could reduce multiple intraocular injections as well as associated complications. For posterior ocular delivery, implants are imported via intravitreal injection through minor surgery. Although with an invasive procedure, implants gain some attention for some merits such as prolonged drug release, local drug release in therapeutic levels, and reduced side effects.

Ophthalmic implants are classified as non-biodegradable and biodegradable one. Polymers such as ethylene vinyl acetate (EVA), polyvinyl alcohol (PVA), and polysulfone capillary fiber (PCF) are common in constructing non-biodegradable implants. One outstanding characteristic of non-biodegradable implants is their near zero order release kinetics [94]. Vitrasert® (ganciclovir, 4.5 mg) and Retisert® (fluocinolone acetonide, 0.59 mg) are representative marketed non-biodegradable implants. Biodegradable implants are more studied for their biocompatible property, as cancellation of extra surgically removed procedure compared to those non-biodegradable implants is a distinctive advantage. Polylactic acid (PLA), poly(lactic-co-glycolic acid) (PLGA), and polyglycolic acid (PGA) are the most common polymers for the construction of biodegradable implants.

For glaucoma therapy, Ocusert® developed and commercialized in the 1970s by ALZA Corporation is an elliptical shaped planar system that is inserted into the cul-de-sac of the eye. The system consists of an inner drug reservoir containing pilocarpine and a polyethylene vinyl acetate (PEVA) membrane to realize sustained release. The system could deliver drug at constant order for up to 1 week.

References

1. European glaucoma society terminology and guidelines for glaucoma, 4th Edition - chapter 3: treatment principles and options supported by the EGS foundation: part 1: foreword; Introduction; glossary; chapter 3 treatment principles and options. Br J Ophthalmol. 2017;101(6):130–95.
2. Heijl A, et al. Reduction of intraocular pressure and glaucoma progression: results from the Early Manifest Glaucoma Trial. Arch Ophthalmol. 2002;120(10):1268–79.
3. Netland PA. Glaucoma medical therapy principles and management. Oxford: Oxford University Press In cooperation with The American Academy of Ophthalmology; 2008.
4. Prum BE Jr, et al. Primary open-angle glaucoma suspect preferred practice pattern (®) guidelines. Ophthalmology. 2016;123(1):P112–51.
5. Prum BE Jr, et al. Primary angle closure preferred practice pattern(®) guidelines. Ophthalmology. 2016;123(1):P1–P40.
6. Sun X, et al. Primary angle closure glaucoma: what we know and what we don't know. Prog Retin Eye Res. 2017;57:26–45.
7. Wilensky JT, et al. Follow-up of angle-closure glaucoma suspects. Am J Ophthalmol. 1993;115(3):338–46.
8. Thomas R, et al. Five year risk of progression of primary angle closure suspects to primary angle closure: a population based study. Br J Ophthalmol. 2003;87(4):450–4.
9. Bain WE. The fellow eye in acute closed-angle glaucoma. Br J Ophthalmol. 1957;41(4):193–9.
10. Lowe RF. Acute angle-closure glaucoma: the second eye: an analysis of 200 cases. Br J Ophthalmol. 1962;46(11):641–50.
11. Saw SM, Gazzard G, Friedman DS. Interventions for angle-closure glaucoma: an evidence-based update. Ophthalmology. 2003;110(10):1869–78. quiz 1878–9, 1930.
12. Ang LP, Aung T, Chew PT. Acute primary angle closure in an Asian population: long-term outcome of the fellow eye after prophylactic laser peripheral iridotomy. Ophthalmology. 2000;107(11):2092–6.
13. European Glaucoma Society Terminology and Guidelines for Glaucoma. 4th edition - chapter 2: classification and terminology supported by the EGS foundation: part 1: foreword; introduction; glossary; chapter 2 classification and terminology. Br J Ophthalmol. 2017;101(5):73–127.
14. Kass MA, et al. The Ocular Hypertension Treatment Study: a randomized trial determines that topical ocular hypotensive medication delays or prevents the onset of primary open-angle glaucoma. Arch Ophthalmol. 2002;120(6):701–13. discussion 829–30.
15. Stewart WC, et al. Cost-effectiveness of treating ocular hypertension. Ophthalmology. 2008;115(1):94–8.
16. Hitchings RA. A practical approach to the management of normal tension glaucoma. In: Essentials in ophthalmology: glaucoma. Berlin: Springer; 2004. p. 147–56.
17. Drance S, Anderson DR, Schulzer M. Risk factors for progression of visual field abnormalities in normal-tension glaucoma. Am J Ophthalmol. 2001;131(6):699–708.
18. Barton K, Hitchings RA. In: Budenz DL, editor. Medical Management of Glaucoma. Manchester: Springer Healthcare; 2013.
19. Hughes E, Spry P, Diamond J. 24-hour monitoring of intraocular pressure in glaucoma management: a retrospective review. J Glaucoma. 2003;12(3):232–6.
20. Wilensky JT, et al. Self-tonometry to manage patients with glaucoma and apparently controlled intraocular pressure. Arch Ophthalmol. 1987;105(8):1072–5.
21. Liu JH, Weinreb RN. Monitoring intraocular pressure for 24 h. Br J Ophthalmol. 2011;95(5):599–600.
22. Mansouri K, Shaarawy T. Continuous intraocular pressure monitoring with a wireless ocular telemetry sensor: initial clinical experience in patients with open angle glaucoma. Br J Ophthalmol. 2011;95(5):627–9.
23. Leske MC, et al. Factors for glaucoma progression and the effect of treatment: the early manifest glaucoma trial. Arch Ophthalmol. 2003;121(1):48–56.

24. Jay JL, Allan D. The benefit of early trabeculectomy versus conventional management in primary open angle glaucoma relative to severity of disease. Eye (Lond). 1989;3(Pt 5):528–35.
25. Migdal C, Gregory W, Hitchings R. Long-term functional outcome after early surgery compared with laser and medicine in open-angle glaucoma. Ophthalmology. 1994;101(10):1651–6. discussion 1657.
26. The Glaucoma Laser Trial (GLT) and glaucoma laser trial follow-up study: 7. Results. Glaucoma Laser Trial Research Group. Am J Ophthalmol. 1995;120(6):718–31.
27. Lichter PR, et al. Interim clinical outcomes in the Collaborative Initial Glaucoma Treatment Study comparing initial treatment randomized to medications or surgery. Ophthalmology. 2001;108(11):1943–53.
28. Hedman K, Larsson LI. The effect of latanoprost compared with timolol in African-American, Asian, Caucasian, and Mexican open-angle glaucoma or ocular hypertensive patients. Surv Ophthalmol. 2002;47(Suppl 1):S77–89.
29. Netland PA, et al. Travoprost compared with latanoprost and timolol in patients with open-angle glaucoma or ocular hypertension. Am J Ophthalmol. 2001;132(4):472–84.
30. Brandt JD, et al. Comparison of once- or twice-daily bimatoprost with twice-daily timolol in patients with elevated IOP: a 3-month clinical trial. Ophthalmology. 2001;108(6):1023–31. discussion 1032.
31. Fechtner RD, Realini T. Fixed combinations of topical glaucoma medications. Curr Opin Ophthalmol. 2004;15(2):132–5.
32. Heijl A, et al. Rates of visual field progression in clinical glaucoma care. Acta Ophthalmol. 2013;91(5):406–12.
33. Heijl A, et al. Natural history of open-angle glaucoma. Ophthalmology. 2009;116(12):2271–6.
34. Leske MC, et al. Predictors of long-term progression in the early manifest glaucoma trial. Ophthalmology. 2007;114(11):1965–72.
35. Jampel HD. Target pressure in glaucoma therapy. J Glaucoma. 1997;6(2):133–8.
36. Heijl A, et al. Measuring visual field progression in the Early Manifest Glaucoma Trial. Acta Ophthalmol Scand. 2003;81(3):286–93.
37. Yu M, et al. Risk of visual field progression in glaucoma patients with progressive retinal nerve fiber layer thinning: a 5-year prospective study. Ophthalmology. 2016;123(6):1201–10.
38. Fitzke FW, et al. Analysis of visual field progression in glaucoma. Br J Ophthalmol. 1996;80(1):40–8.
39. Leung CK, et al. Retinal nerve fiber layer imaging with spectral-domain optical coherence tomography: patterns of retinal nerve fiber layer progression. Ophthalmology. 2012;119(9):1858–66.
40. Sung KR, et al. Progression detection capability of macular thickness in advanced glaucomatous eyes. Ophthalmology. 2012;119(2):308–13.
41. The Advanced Glaucoma Intervention Study (AGIS): 7. The relationship between control of intraocular pressure and visual field deterioration. The AGIS Investigators. Am J Ophthalmol. 2000;130(4):429–40.
42. Musch DC, et al. Visual field progression in the Collaborative Initial Glaucoma Treatment Study the impact of treatment and other baseline factors. Ophthalmology. 2009;116(2):200–7.
43. Nouri-Mahdavi K, et al. Predictive factors for glaucomatous visual field progression in the Advanced Glaucoma Intervention Study. Ophthalmology. 2004;111(9):1627–35.
44. Martus P, et al. Predictive factors for progressive optic nerve damage in various types of chronic open-angle glaucoma. Am J Ophthalmol. 2005;139(6):999–1009.
45. Tezel G, et al. Clinical factors associated with progression of glaucomatous optic disc damage in treated patients. Arch Ophthalmol. 2001;119(6):813–8.
46. Stewart WC, et al. Factors associated with long-term progression or stability in primary open-angle glaucoma. Am J Ophthalmol. 2000;130(3):274–9.
47. Daugeliene L, Yamamoto T, Kitazawa Y. Risk factors for visual field damage progression in normal-tension glaucoma eyes. Graefes Arch Clin Exp Ophthalmol. 1999;237(2):105–8.
48. Suh MH, et al. Glaucoma progression after the first-detected optic disc hemorrhage by optical coherence tomography. J Glaucoma. 2012;21(6):358–66.
49. Medeiros FA, et al. Corneal thickness as a risk factor for visual field loss in patients with preperimetric glaucomatous optic neuropathy. Am J Ophthalmol. 2003;136(5):805–13.
50. Kim JW, Chen PP. Central corneal pachymetry and visual field progression in patients with open-angle glaucoma. Ophthalmology. 2004;111(11):2126–32.
51. Jonas JB, et al. Central corneal thickness correlated with glaucoma damage and rate of progression. Invest Ophthalmol Vis Sci. 2005;46(4):1269–74.
52. Medeiros FA, et al. Corneal hysteresis as a risk factor for glaucoma progression: a prospective longitudinal study. Ophthalmology. 2013;120(8):1533–40.
53. Jonas JB, et al. Predictive factors of the optic nerve head for development or progression of glaucomatous visual field loss. Invest Ophthalmol Vis Sci. 2004;45(8):2613–8.
54. Charlson ME, et al. Nocturnal systemic hypotension increases the risk of glaucoma progression. Ophthalmology. 2014;121(10):2004–12.
55. Armaly MF, et al. Biostatistical analysis of the collaborative glaucoma study. I. Summary report of the risk factors for glaucomatous visual-field defects. Arch Ophthalmol. 1980;98(12):2163–71.
56. Asrani S, et al. Large diurnal fluctuations in intraocular pressure are an independent risk factor in patients with glaucoma. J Glaucoma. 2000;9(2):134–42.
57. Nouri-Mahdavi K, Medeiros FA, Weinreb RN. Fluctuation of intraocular pressure as a predictor of visual field progression. Arch Ophthalmol. 2008;126(8):1168–9. author reply 1169–70.

58. Caprioli J, Coleman AL. Intraocular pressure fluctuation a risk factor for visual field progression at low intraocular pressures in the advanced glaucoma intervention study. Ophthalmology. 2008;115(7):1123–1129.e3.
59. Bengtsson B, et al. Fluctuation of intraocular pressure and glaucoma progression in the early manifest glaucoma trial. Ophthalmology. 2007;114(2):205–9.
60. Gordon MO, et al. Validated prediction model for the development of primary open-angle glaucoma in individuals with ocular hypertension. Ophthalmology. 2007;114(1):10–9.
61. Hughes PM, Olejnik O, Chang-Lin JE, et al. Topical and systemic drug delivery to the posterior segments. Adv Drug Deliv Rev. 2005;57(14):2010–32.
62. Hosoya K, Lee VHL, Kim KJ. Roles of the conjunctiva in ocular drug delivery: a review of conjunctival transport mechanisms and their regulation. Eur J Pharm Biopharm. 2005;60(2):227–40.
63. Baudouin C, Labbé A, Liang H, et al. Preservatives in eyedrops: the good, the bad and the ugly. Prog Retin Eye Res. 2010;29(4):312–34.
64. Jaissle GB, Szurman P, Bartz-Schmidt KU. Ocular side effects and complications of intravitreal triamcinolone acetonide injection. Der Ophthalmologe: Zeitschrift der Deutschen Ophthalmologischen Gesellschaft. 2004;101(2):121–8.
65. Lux A, Maier S, Dinslage S, et al. A comparative bioavailability study of three conventional eye drops versus a single lyophilisate. Br J Ophthalmol. 2003;87(4):436–40.
66. Holló G, Bozkurt B, Irkec M. Brinzolamide/timolol fixed combination: a new ocular suspension for the treatment of open-angle glaucoma and ocular hypertension. Expert Opin Pharmacother. 2009;10(12):2015–24.
67. Prasad D, Chauhan H. Excipients utilized for ophthalmic drug delivery systems. In: Pathak Y, Sutariya V, Hirani AA, editors. Nano-biomaterials for ophthalmic drug delivery. Basel: Springer; 2016. p. 555–82.
68. Vashist A, Vashist A, Gupta YK, et al. Recent advances in hydrogel based drug delivery systems for the human body. J Mater Chem B. 2014;2(2):147–66.
69. Saini R, Saini S, Singh G, et al. In situ gels-a new trends in ophthalmic drug delivery system. Int J Pharm Sci Res. 2015;6:386–90.
70. Tártara LI, Quinteros DA, Saino V, et al. Improvement of acetazolamide ocular permeation using ascorbyl laurate nanostructures as drug delivery system. J Ocul Pharmacol Ther. 2012;28(2):102–9.
71. Holden CA, Tyagi P, Thakur A, et al. Polyamidoamine dendrimer hydrogel for enhanced delivery of antiglaucoma drugs. Nanomedicine. 2012;8(5):776–83.
72. Farid RM, El-Salamouni NS, El-Kamel AH, et al. Lipid-based nanocarriers for ocular drug delivery. In: Andronescu E, Grumezescu AM, editors. Nanostructures for drug delivery; 2017. p. 495–522.
73. Panatieri LF, Brazil NT, Faber K, et al. Nanoemulsions containing a coumarin-rich extract from Pterocaulon balansae (Asteraceae) for the treatment of ocular acanthamoeba keratitis. AAPS PharmSciTech. 2017;18(3):721–8.
74. Kassem MA, Rahman AAA, Ghorab MM, et al. Nanosuspension as an ophthalmic delivery system for certain glucocorticoid drugs. Int J Pharm. 2007;340(1):126–33.
75. Vandervoort J, Ludwig A. Ocular drug delivery: nanomedicine applications. Nanomedicine. 2007;2(1):11–21.
76. Alvarez-Trabado J, Diebold Y, Sanchez A. Designing lipid nanoparticles for topical ocular drug delivery. Int J Pharm. 2017;532(1):204–17.
77. Tsukamoto T, Hironaka K, Fujisawa T, et al. Preparation of bromfenac-loaded liposomes modified with chitosan for ophthalmic drug delivery and evaluation of physicochemical properties and drug release profile. Asian J Pharm Sci. 2013;8(2):104–9.
78. Patidar S, Jain S. Non ionic surfactant based vesicles (niosomes) containing flupirtine maleate as an ocular drug delivery system. J Chem Pharm Res. 2012;4(10):4495–500.
79. Cholkar K, Patel A, Dutt Vadlapudi A, et al. Novel nanomicellar formulation approaches for anterior and posterior segment ocular drug delivery. Recent Pat Nanomed. 2012;2(2):82–95.
80. Kambhampati SP. Dendrimer based nanotherapeutics for ocular drug delivery. Ph.D. dissertation, Wayne State University, Detroit; 2014.
81. Nabih Maria D, Mishra SR, Wang L, et al. Water-soluble complex of curcumin with cyclodextrins: enhanced physical properties for ocular drug delivery. Curr Drug Deliv. 2017;14(6):875–86.
82. Maulvi FA, Soni TG, Shah DO. A review on therapeutic contact lenses for ocular drug delivery. Drug Deliv. 2016;23(8):3017–26.
83. Bengani LC, Hsu KH, Gause S, et al. Contact lenses as a platform for ocular drug delivery. Expert Opin Drug Deliv. 2013;10(11):1483–96.
84. North DP. Treatment of acute glaucoma. Can Med Assoc J. 1971;105(6):561.
85. Kaufman HE, Uotila MH, Gasset AR, et al. The medical uses of soft contact lenses. Trans Am Acad Ophthalmol Otolaryngol. 1971;75(2):361–73.
86. Hillman JS. Management of acute glaucoma with pilocarpine-soaked hydrophilic lens. Br J Ophthalmol. 1974;58(7):674.
87. Peng CC, Kim J, Chauhan A. Extended delivery of hydrophilic drugs from silicone-hydrogel contact lenses containing vitamin E diffusion barriers. Biomaterials. 2010;31(14):4032–47.
88. Fraunfelder FT, Meyer SM. Systemic side effects from ophthalmic timolol and their prevention. J Ocul Pharmacol Ther. 1987;3(2):177–84.

89. Peng CC, Ben-Shlomo A, Mackay EO, et al. Drug delivery by contact lens in spontaneously glaucomatous dogs. Curr Eye Res. 2012;37(3):204–11.
90. González-Chomón C, Concheiro A, Alvarez-Lorenzo C. Soft contact lenses for controlled ocular delivery: 50 years in the making. Ther Deliv. 2013;4(9):1141–61.
91. Alvarez-Lorenzo C, Hiratani H, Gómez-Amoza JL, et al. Soft contact lenses capable of sustained delivery of timolol. J Pharm Sci. 2002;91(10):2182–92.
92. Nikouei BM, Vahabzadeh SA, Mohajeri SA. Preparation of a molecularly imprinted soft contact lens as a new ocular drug delivery system for dorzolamide. Curr Drug Deliv. 2013;10(3):279–85.
93. Jung HJ, Chauhan A. Temperature sensitive contact lenses for triggered ophthalmic drug delivery. Biomaterials. 2012;33(7):2289–300.
94. Lee SS, Hughes P, Ross AD, et al. Biodegradable implants for sustained drug release in the eye. Pharm Res. 2010;27(10):2043–53.

Medical Therapy for Glaucoma-IOP Lowering Agents

5

Anna C. Momont and Paul L. Kaufman

Abstract

Pharmacologic agents that lower intraocular pressure (IOP) are the first line of treatment for the majority of glaucoma patients. Classically these medications can be split into two groups: those that suppress aqueous production, and those that enhance aqueous outflow. Multiple formulations and combinations now exist in order to limit side effects and improve adherence. This chapter will review glaucoma medications that are currently available, those that will be available in the near future, and some "farther-down-the-road" technologies.

Keywords

Glaucoma · Glaucoma medical treatment Glaucoma pharmacology · Intraocular pressure · Gene therapy · Stem cell therapy

5.1 Introduction

The use of medication to lower intraocular pressure dates back to the 1870s when pilocarpine and physostigmine were described in the treatment of glaucoma [1]. Since that time multiple medications have been used with varying success to lower eye pressure in an attempt to slow glaucoma progression. Although multiple factors have been implicated in the development and progression of glaucoma, IOP remains the only clinically modifiable target. Lowering intraocular pressure has been shown to slow or halt the progression of primary open angle glaucoma [2, 3], ocular hypertension [4], and normal tension glaucoma [5].

Intraocular pressure can be lowered with laser treatment to the trabecular meshwork, incisional surgery, and oral therapy, but topical therapy remains the mainstay of treatment. The search for the ideal medication would lead to an agent that produces uniformly low intraocular pressure around the clock in essentially all patients, and has limited side effects promoting good adherence, and physical and chemical compatibility with other agents to allow fixed combinations with other medications in one drop.

IOP-lowering medications fall into two main categories: suppressors of aqueous humor formation and enhancers of aqueous humor outflow (Fig. 5.1). Those that cause suppression of aqueous humor production include β-adrenergic antagonists, α2-adrenergic agonists, and carbonic anhydrase inhibitors. Agents that improve aqueous outflow through the trabecular meshwork/Schlemm's canal/distal conventional outflow pathways include cholinergic agents and,

A. C. Momont · P. L. Kaufman (✉)
University of Wisconsin, Department of Ophthalmology and Visual Sciences, Madison, WI, USA
e-mail: Paul.Kaufman@wisc.edu

X. Sun, Y. Dai (eds.), *Medical Treatment of Glaucoma*,
https://doi.org/10.1007/978-981-13-2733-9_5

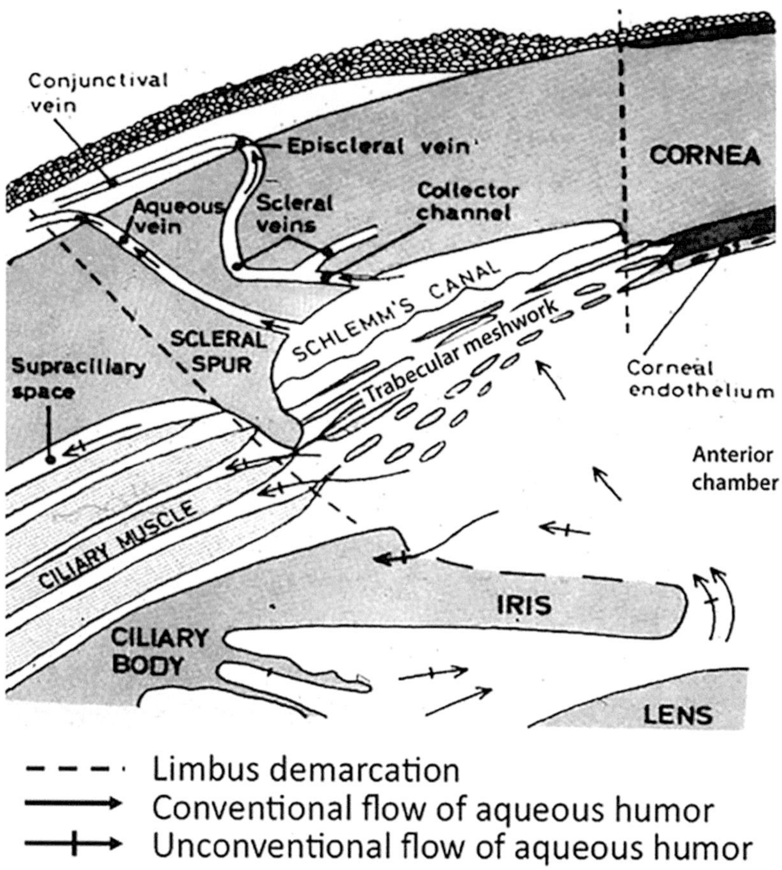

Fig. 5.1 Aqueous humor outflow pathways (figure courtesy of Björn Svedbergh). Aqueous humor, produced by the ciliary body, exits the eye through the trabecular meshwork/Schlemm's canal, also known as the conventional pathway (plain arrows), and the uveoscleral pathway, also known as the unconventional pathway (crossed arrows). Resistance in the trabecular meshwork, Schlemm's canal, and downstream collector channels results in elevation in intraocular pressure

most recently, rho kinase inhibitors and nitric oxide-donating moieties. Prostaglandin analogs improve aqueous outflow through the uveoscleral pathway (Table 5.1).

Throughout the text, efficacy of IOP control is reported in terms of percent reduction in IOP. Of course, comparing percent reductions in IOP is only useful if starting IOPs are similar, as a larger percent reduction will be seen with a higher starting IOP for the same physiological effect on any given parameter of aqueous dynamics. It can generally be assumed that starting IOP in all studies was between 21 mmHg and 30 mmHg, typically averaging in the mid-20s, although in some older studies the range of baseline IOP was not given, and patients were only described as having ocular hypertension. Very few efficacy studies exist that specifically address patients with baseline IOP below 21 mmHg or carry a diagnosis of normal tension glaucoma.

5.2 Adrenergic Antagonists

β-adrenergic receptor antagonists (β-blockers) are sympatholytics that prevent transmission of impulses from adrenergic post-ganglionic fibers. Propranolol, the first available systemic β-blocker, was noted to have IOP effects with intravenous administration [6]. Topical timolol became available in 1978 and continues to be the most widely used β-blocker. β-blockers are divided into two classes: (1) non-selective, inhibiting both β1- and β2-adrenoceptors, and (2) selective for β1-adrenoceptor inhibition (cardioselective; e.g., betaxolol). β-blockers reduce IOP by binding to and occupying β_2-adrenergic receptor sites on the ciliary epithelia such that neither the neurotransmitter (norepinephrine) released from sympathetic neurons *nor* circulating or humoral catechlolamines (epinephrine) can stimulate the epithelia to produce aqueous humor.

Table 5.1 Summary of topical IOP lowering medications

Medication class	Available agents	Dosing	Mechanism of action	Adverse effects	Special considerations
Prostaglandin analogs	Latanoprost Travoprost Bimatoprost Tafluprost	Every evening	Increased aqueous humor outflow through the uveoscleral pathway	Hyperemia, hypertrichosis, iris darkening, increase in pigmentation of periocular skin, and orbital fat atrophy. Less common: Uveitis, cystoid macular edema, iris cysts, and reactivation of herpes simplex keratitis	First-line treatment in majority of patients due to duration of action throughout 24 h period and low incidence of side effects
Beta blockers	Timolol Carteolol Levobunolol Betaxolol	Every morning or twice daily	Decreased aqueous humor production	Hyperemia, dry eye, and ocular discomfort. Systemic side effects include bradycardia, arrhythmia, bronchospasm, impotence, and fatigue. These are lessened with selective beta1-blockers or nasolacrimal occlusion	First- or second-line treatment, use is limited by systemic side effects affecting the cardiovascular and pulmonary systems
Alpha adrenergic (α2) agonists	Brimonidine Apraclonidine	Three times daily	Decreased aqueous humor production	Local side effects are common: Blepharoconjunctivitis and follicular conjunctivitis. Systemic: Dry mouth, headache, and fatigue	Absolute contraindication in children due to cardiorespiratory depression
Carbonic anhydrase inhibitors	Dorzolamide Brinzolamide	Three times daily	Decreased aqueous humor production	Stinging and burning and possible worsening of endothelial dysfunction. A bad taste is the only frequently reported systemic side effect	Avoid in patients with sulfa allergy. More serious side effects reported with systemic sulfonamides include myelosuppression and aplastic anemia
Muscarinic cholinergic agonists	Pilocarpine Carbachol Echothiophate	Four times [carbachol only 3x/ day] daily	Decreased aqueous outflow resistance through the trabecular meshwork and Schlemm's canal	Brow ache, blurred vision, myopia, miosis, narrowing of the angle, uveitis, and retinal detachment. Systemic side effects: Nausea, diarrhea, sweating, and cardiovascular instability. Respiratory paralysis from succinylcholine	Useful prior to laser iridotomy and may be used to break angle closure attack
Rho kinase inhibitors	Ripasudil Netarsudil	Ripasudil twice daily; netarsudil once daily	Decreased aqueous humor outflow resistance through the trabecular meshwork and Schlemm's canal	Hyperemia, subconjunctival hemorrhage, and blurred vision	Netarsudil also decreases aqueous humor production by inhibiting the norepinephrine transporter and may reduce episcleral venous pressure

(continued)

Table 5.1 (continued)

Medication class	Available agents	Dosing	Mechanism of action	Adverse effects	Special considerations
Nitric oxide agents	Latanoprostene bunod	Every evening	Decreased aqueous outflow resistance through the trabecular meshwork and Schlemm's canal and increased outflow through the uveoscleral pathway	Hyperemia, hypertrichosis, irritation, and punctate keratitis	Hybrid molecule of latanoprost and NO-donating moiety

5.2.1 Non-Selective β-Blockers

5.2.1.1 Timolol

Timolol is a non-selective β-blocker that lowers IOP by inhibiting aqueous production [7]. Multiple studies have shown the efficacy of timolol in the treatment of glaucoma [8–12]. In a meta-analysis of 11 randomized, controlled trials comparing timolol to latanoprost, the percent reductions in IOP were 26.9(±2.3) and 30.2(±3.4), respectively [13]. The overnight IOP-lowering ability of timolol has been shown to be blunted in healthy individuals [14] and when compared to latanoprost, timolol has less effect on IOP during night-time hours [15] despite similar IOP-lowering during waking hours. Normal aqueous production is reduced by approximately 50% at night when total catecholaminergic tone is low and the ciliary epithelia are in essence "asleep." Blocking β_2-adrenergic receptors on the ciliary epithelia has no additional effect on aqueous production during this time. Timolol generally causes a marked decrease in IOP at the onset of treatment which then stabilizes to a slightly higher level over time [16].

Timolol is available in 0.25% and 0.5% concentrations and is generally dosed twice daily. Once-daily administration may be sufficient to effectively control daytime IOP when the majority of effect is seen [17], and simplifying the dosing regimen may lead to improved adherence. A gel-forming solution is marketed for a longer duration of effect as well as decreased systemic absorption. A preservative-free formulation is also available for those with a benzalkonium chloride (BAK) allergy or preservative sensitivity. Timolol is available in fixed combination formulations with brimonidine (US Combigan) and dorzolamide (US Cosopt) as well as with prostaglandin analogs such as travoprost (Europe Xalacom).

Local side effects of timolol include conjunctival hyperemia, ocular discomfort, superficial punctate keratitis, and reduction in tear flow with resultant dry eye syndrome [18–20]. The use of timolol is limited by systemic side effects related to β1-blockade on the adrenoceptors of the heart. This includes bradycardia, heart block, and arrhythmia, as well as congestive heart failure [18, 19, 21]. In addition, by blocking β2-adrenoceptors of the bronchioles, timolol can cause bronchospasm in patients with asthma or chronic obstructive pulmonary disease (COPD) [18, 19, 21, 22]. Timolol is contraindicated in patients with myasthenia gravis as it may worsen symptoms [23], and in patients with diabetes at risk for hypoglycemia as it may blunt early warning signs of low blood sugar [24]. Additional reported systemic side effects include anxiety, depression, impotence, fatigue, and alterations in cholesterol profiles [18, 19]. Nasolacrimal occlusion following topical timolol instillation can reduce plasma levels and decrease systemic side effects while improving the dose-response and duration of effect [25].

5.2.1.2 Other Non-selective β-Blockers

Other topical non-selective β-blockers include levobunolol, metipranolol, and carteolol. Levobunolol is metabolized to dihydrolevobunolol in the eye and shows similar IOP-lowering and adverse effects when compared to timolol [26]. Studies have shown that once-daily levobunolol is effective in IOP-lowering in the majority of patients [17, 27]. Metipranolol has similar IOP reduction when compared to timolol, with slightly more stinging and burning [28, 29]. An association with granulomatous anterior uveitis has led to discontinuation of metipranolol in multiple countries [30]. Carteolol is a non-selective β-blocker with similar IOP-lowering to timolol [31, 32] but with slight sympathomimetic activity [33]. In theory, this sympathomimetic activity may balance the sympatholytic activity and allow the use of carteolol in patients with cardiac compromise. However, in reality, carteolol demonstrates β-blocking effects on heart rate and blood pressure and should be avoided in patients with cardiopulmonary insufficiency, similar to the other compounds in this class [31]. The sympathomimetic effects are likely responsible for a beneficial effect on cholesterol [34].

5.2.2 Selective β-Blockers

5.2.2.1 Betaxolol

Betaxolol is a relatively selective β1-blocker that exerts its effects by inhibiting aqueous production [35] possibly through weak β2 antagonism on the ciliary body. The IOP-lowering effect of betaxolol is 18–26% [36–38], less than that of timolol.

The ocular side effects of betaxolol are similar to those of other β-blockers and include burning and stinging with instillation, as well as hyperemia and dry eye. Betaxolol has fewer systemic side effects when compared to timolol and other non-selective β-blockers. The relative β1-selective blockade leads to less effect on forced expiratory volume in patients with asthma [39, 40]. However, there is evidence of an effect on lung function in some patients with asthma, and so care should be taken when treating these patients with any β-blocking agent [41, 42]. There is also evidence that betaxolol has fewer cardiovascular side effects including bradycardia and arrhythmias, possibly due to high binding to plasma proteins and a low free plasma concentration [43]. Changing from timolol to betaxolol may also improve or resolve side effects of the central nervous system including depression, emotional lability, and impotence in some patients [44].

5.2.3 Summary

Topical β-blockers transformed the landscape of glaucoma management, offering patients a well-tolerated topical therapy that is effective in lowering IOP. In most treatment algorithms β-blockers are considered second-line treatment after prostaglandin analogs. However, due to lower cost and greater availability, as well as fast onset of action, β-blocking agents may be used as first-line treatment in many circumstances. Their use is primarily limited by systemic side effects affecting the cardiovascular and pulmonary systems, which can be lessened by choosing a selective β1-blockers or by discussing nasolacrimal occlusion with the patient.

5.3 Adrenergic Agonists

Adrenergic agonists may also be called sympathomimetic agents, and mimic the effects of stimulation of adrenergic sympathetic nerves and receptors.

5.3.1 Epinephrine

Epinephrine or adrenalin is a direct-acting sympathomimetic amine, and has been used to treat glaucoma dating back to the 1920s. Epinephrine stimulates β2-, α1-, and α2-adrenoceptors in the eye, which leads to an increase in aqueous outflow through the trabecular meshwork [45] and uveoscleral pathways [46]. Epinephrine also increases aqueous humor production in the first hours after instillation due to adrenergic stimulation at the ciliary epithelia. Twice-daily application of a 2% epinephrine solution leads to a 15–25% IOP lowering [47, 48], but its use is limited by significant ocular and systemic side effects. The α1-adrenergic stimulation causes transient mydriasis which can blur the vision and can lead to angle closure attacks in patients with narrow anterior chamber angles. Epinephrine has also been linked with the development of cystoid macular edema in aphakic and pseudophakic eyes, adrenochrome deposits in the conjunctiva and cornea, as well as significant systemic side effects including tachycardia, arrhythmia, and elevated blood pressure [49].

5.3.2 Dipivalyl Epinephrine

Dipivalyl epinephrine (DFE) is a prodrug of epinephrine which is converted to epinephrine by hydrolysis within the eye. By adding two ester groups to the epinephrine molecule the lipophilic character of the molecule is improved, allowing it to cross the cornea more readily, leading to similar IOP-lowering at much lower concentrations [50]. IOP reduction and ocular side effects with DFE are similar to epinephrine but with fewer systemic side effects.

5.3.3 Selective α2-Adrenergic Agents

Selective α_2-adrenergic agonists were developed in order to minimize the sympatheticomimetic side effects related to β- and α_1-adrenergic response. Selective α_2-adrenergic agonists reduce sympathetic neuronal tone at the ciliary processes, leading to a decrease in aqueous humor production. Clonidine, the first available selective agonist, lowers intraocular pressure but also easily crosses the blood-brain barrier. Clonidine is no longer in use clinically as use may result in systemic hypotension through stimulation of vasomotor centers in the brainstem. Topical clonidine eye drops 0.25% and 0.5% have also been shown to lower the ophthalmic artery pressure [51].

5.3.3.1 Apraclonidine

A second-generation α_2-agonist, apraclonidine, contains a para-amino group making it more hydrophilic and decreasing transport through the blood–brain barrier. Apraclonidine reduces IOP by 20–30%, mainly by decreasing aqueous humor production [52, 53]. Although apraclonidine has an improved side effect profile when compared to clonidine, it still may reduce heart rate and blood pressure and causes dry nose and dry mouth in 20% of patients [54]. Unfortunately, dermatitis, follicular conjunctivitis, and blepharoconjunctivitis are common [55] and may occur in up to 48% of users [56]. Due to this high rate of ocular side effects, as well as tachyphylaxis, apraclonidine is marketed primarily for short term pressure spikes with recommended use before and after laser procedures or after phacoemulsification.

5.3.3.2 Brimonidine

Brimonidine is a third-generation, highly-selective α_2-agonist and is the only adrenergic agonist in wide use today. The addition of a quinoxaline ring and bromine side group, rather than chlorine, differentiates it from the first- and second-generation drugs in this class. This formulation was found to have a significantly higher affinity for α_2-adrenoceptors [57]. Brimonidine lowers intraocular pressure both by reducing aqueous production and increasing outflow via the uveoscleral pathway [58]. The peak effect of brimonidine occurs at 2–3 h after installation and lowers pressure by 20–30% [59]. In a randomized, double-masked, multicenter trial brimonidine 0.2% was compared to timolol 0.5%. Brimonidine subjects achieved a significantly lower IOP 2 h after instillation (peak effect), but brimonidine was not as effective as timolol 12 h after instillation (trough effect) [60]. When compared to latanoprost 0.005%, brimonidine 0.2% had less effect on IOP in a large meta-analysis of 14 trials [61]. Brimonidine has also been studied as an adjunctive therapy, with an additional lowering of intraocular pressure when used in addition to either a β-blocker or latanoprost [62]. It is also available in a fixed combination therapy both with timolol (US Combigan) and brinzolamide (US Simbrinza).

Limited evidence for neuroprotection independent of IOP-lowering has also been published. This may be related to an upregulation of basic fibroblast growth factor in photoreceptors [63]. In a rat model of elevated IOP, systemic brimonidine was associated with a statistically significant reduction in retinal ganglion cell loss [64]. In the Low-Pressure Glaucoma Treatment Study, less visual field progression was seen in patients treated with brimonidine 0.2% compared to those treated with timolol 0.5%, despite similar reduction in IOP [65].

The most commonly reported systemic side effects from brimonidine include dry mouth, fatigue, and headache [66, 67]. Unlike less selective α-adrenergic agonists or β-blocker treatment, there has been no association with significant effects on heart rate, blood pressure, or lung function in adults [66, 67]. However, brimonidine and iopidine are absolutely contraindicated in children due to systemic side effects. This can include CNS depression leading to poor arousability and extreme fatigue [68, 69], as well as cardiorespiratory depression [70, 71].

The incidence of ocular side effects, although less than with apraclonidine, is common, including blepharoconjunctivitis and follicular conjunctivitis in 7.8–12.7% of patients with 1 year of follow-up [60, 72]. The rates of allergic conjunctivitis may be much higher long-term, reported at 32.3% in a survey of 26 years of data in one teaching hospital [73]. There are also concerns that brimonidine may increase the likelihood of allergy to subsequent eye drops [74]. Brimonidine 0.1% and 0.15% are available as Alphagan P with Purite® rather than benzalkonium chloride (BAK) as a preservative. This may improve tolerability in those with BAK allergy or sensitivity to preservative.

Another less common, but oft-overlooked side effect of brimonidine treatment is granulomatous anterior uveitis. Sporadic case reports have emerged since 2000; the largest published series was 19 eyes of 12 patients that occurred between 7 days and 5 years after treatment initiation [75]. The uveitis resolved following cessation of brimonidine, without recurrence and frequently without the use of topical corticosteroids. In other case reports a rechallenge with brimonidine caused a recurrence [76, 77]. Elevated IOP has been reported in patients with follicular conjunctivitis related to brimonidine [78], and in this study as well as in the author's own experience (AM), discontinuation of brimonidine leads to improvement in IOP frequently without additional therapy.

5.3.4 Summary

Adrenergic agonists include epinephrine, dipivalyl epinephrine, and clonidine, which are of historical significance, and the selective α_2-agonists include apraclonidine and brimonidine, which are still in widespread clinical use today. Brimonidine remains an important tool in IOP reduction, generally as an adjunctive therapy rather than first-line treatment. Apraclonidine is used for short-term pressure control peri-operatively or after laser procedures. The use of both brimonidine and apraclonidine is limited by a high rate of ocular side effects, and they are absolutely contraindicated in children due to serious systemic side effects.

5.4 Cholinergic Agents

Parasympathomimetics or cholinergic agents were the first class of ocular hypotensive medications used to treat glaucoma, dating back at least to 1876 with the introduction of eserine (physostigmine), followed a year later by pilocarpine. The parasympathomimetics are divided into either direct or indirect action on the muscarinic receptors of the eye. Muscarinic activation leads to contraction of the ciliary muscle and increased tension on the scleral spur, with expansion of the trabecular meshwork and dilation of Schlemm's canal leading to decreased resistance to aqueous outflow through the trabecular meshwork and consequent reduction in IOP. This class of medications is also known collectively as "miotics" due to constrictive effects on the pupil. The miosis is not causative in the reduction in outflow resistance and complete removal of the iris in a monkey model had no effect on either the outflow resistance or IOP response to pilocarpine [79]. However, disinsertion of the ciliary muscle from the scleral spur eliminates the response, indicating that the effect depends completely on the ciliary muscle altering the configuration of the meshwork and Schlemm's canal [80]. The m3 muscarinic receptor subtype is responsible for trabecular outflow, miosis, and accommodation, all three of the anterior segment responses to the cholinergic agents. There is a high rate of ocular side effects related to the miosis and accommodation, and it has not been possible to separate these responses in favor of outflow as they all occur in a similar dose range.

5.4.1 Pilocarpine

Pilocarpine is a direct-acting muscarinic agonist and is the most commonly used cholinergic agent. It is available in concentrations of 1, 2, and 4%, and IOP response is estimated at a 20–30% reduction [81]. The effect of pilocarpine lasts approximately 6 h; thus, frequent dosing—4 to 6 times daily—is required for a sustained effect. Higher concentrations are generally necessary for heavily pigmented eyes. Pilocarpine gel and ocular delivery devices have been developed to reduce dosing frequency and improve adherence. In addition to the primary indication of IOP-lowering, pilocarpine is used for its miotic effects, including flattening of the peripheral iris prior to laser iridotomy and in helping to break an acute attack of primary angle closure.

The ocular side effects of pilocarpine are primarily related to the drug effects on the ciliary muscle and iris sphincter muscle. Blurred vision results from the accommodation and myopia induced by ciliary muscle contraction and consequent lens rounding, thickening, and forward translation [82]. Vision may also become dimmed from induced miosis, especially in patients with incipient cataracts. Patients frequently complain of brow ache secondary to ciliary spasm, although this may improve with longer duration of treatment. Lens opacities and cataract formation [83], retinal detachments [84], and narrowing of the iridocorneal angle with resultant angle closure [85] have all been reported with miotic agents. Systemic side effects with pilocarpine include nausea, vomiting, diarrhea, sweating, and bronchospasm [85]. Paradoxical effects on the cardiovascular system have been observed with both bradycardia and tachycardia, as well as episodes of hypotension followed by hypertension [49].

5.4.2 Carbachol

Carbachol is a synthetic cholinergic and works both as a direct agonist at muscarinic receptors and as an indirect parasympathomimetic through inhibition of cholinesterase [86]. Concentrations of 0.75, 1.5, and 3% used three times daily have been used. Carbachol is hydrophilic and requires benzalkonium chloride to promote penetration through the cornea. Ocular and systemic side effects are similar to those seen with pilocarpine but are generally more severe [87].

5.4.3 Other Cholinergic Agents

Ecothiopate, demecarium bromide, and diisopropyl fluorophosphates are indirect-acting parasympathomimetics that lead to increased levels of the muscarinic neurotransmitter acetylcholine via cholinesterase inhibition. They are potent and long-acting medications with limited usefulness due to the high rate and severity of ocular and systemic side effects in line with other cholinergics. Anticholinesterase eye drops have been associated with a prolonged response to succinylcholine, a muscle relaxant used during general anesthesia, and should be discontinued several weeks prior to any surgery where succinylcholine may be used [88, 89].

5.4.4 Summary

Although cholinergic agents have fallen out of usage with preference for newer classes of agents with fewer side effects and less frequent dosing, pilocarpine remains a useful medication in some clinical situations. Increased aqueous outflow through the trabecular meshwork may be beneficial in patients with pigmentary glaucoma and pseudoexfoliation. In addition, patients who prefer to avoid surgery or are poor surgical candidates are more likely to tolerate the frequent dosing and ocular side effects if pilocarpine is necessary to control IOP.

5.5 Carbonic Anhydrase Inhibitors

Carbonic anhydrase is a zinc-containing enzyme with 14 isoenzymes found in humans, all with different subcellular localization and tissue distribution [90]. The enzyme catalyzes the hydration of carbon dioxide to bicarbonate. Isoforms II and IV are present in the non-pigmented epithelial cells of the ciliary processes and are involved in active secretion of aqueous humor through the production of bicarbonate. Carbonic anhydrase inhibitors (CAIs) decrease aqueous production by up to 50% by inhibition of this enzyme. There is a need for essentially complete inhibition of carbonic anhydrase activity in the ciliary epithelium (>99%) in order to inhibit aqueous production and probably near total (>99.9%) inhibition to maximally inhibit aqueous humor formation. In addition to direct inhibition of aqueous secretion, induced metabolic acidosis at high systemic doses of CAI further decreases secretion.

5.5.1 Systemic Carbonic Anhydrase Inhibitors

In the 1950s acetazolamide, a sulfonamide-derived compound and carbonic anhydrase inhibitor (CAI), was discovered to lower IOP by 20–30% [91, 92]. Standard dosing of acetazolamide is 250 mg tablets four times daily or 500 mg sustained release capsules twice daily, and it is also available as an intravenous injection that is useful for patients who are unable to tolerate oral formulations due to nausea and vomiting brought on by acutely high IOP. The use of acetazolamide has also been approved for altitude sickness, congestive heart failure, idiopathic intracranial hypertension, and seizures.

Methazolamide is an alternative systemic CAI available as a 25 mg, 50 mg, or 100 mg tablet to be taken three times daily. It has slightly less IOP-lowering effect when compared to acetazolamide [93] and for some patients may lead to fewer or less severe side effects [94]. Methazolamide is metabolized in part by the liver, whereas acetazolamide is excreted unchanged through the kidney.

Oral CAIs have significant systemic side effects which limit their usefulness in chronic glaucoma management. Paresthesias, fatigue, and gastrointestinal effects, including loss of appetite, nausea, and diarrhea, are all common. More serious side effects related to the action of CAI on the kidneys include renal stones, metabolic acidosis, and hypokalemia. As a sulfonamide derivative both acetazolamide and methazolamide may induce aplastic anemia and agranulocytosis [95] and use is contraindicated in patients with a history of allergy to sulfa medications. In addition, sulfonamide-induced angle closure associated with acute myopia and ciliary body effusion has been reported with both acetazolamide and methazolamide [96], as have several cases of Stevens–Johnson syndrome [97–99]. Both of these conditions must be recognized by the treating eye doctor with immediate discontinuation of the causative medication and initiation of supportive treatment.

5.5.2 Topical Carbonic Anhydrase Inhibitors

Topical formulations of CAIs, first dorzolamide and then brinzolamide, were introduced in the 1990s, 40 years after oral formulations were introduced. The delay was related to difficulty in finding a topical formulation that could lead to near-100% inhibition of carbonic anhydrase, which is necessary to lower IOP.

5.5.3 Dorzolamide

Dorzolamide is an inhibitor of carbonic anhydrase isoenzyme II and a weak inhibitor of isoenzyme

IV, leading to aqueous suppression [100]. In a rabbit model, dorzolamide inhibited 100% of carbonic anhydrase activity in the iris and ciliary body [101]. Optimal dosing is 2% at least three times daily [102]. In one comparative study dorzolamide 2% solution administered three times daily lowered IOP 23%, which was similar to betaxolol (21%) and timolol (25%) [103]. Dorzolamide is an effective adjunctive therapy when added to either timolol or latanoprost, although it may have less IOP-lowering effect than addition of brimonidine [104]. However, there is evidence of improved nocturnal IOP control when compared to timolol and brimonidine [15, 105] as well as an advantageous effect on ocular perfusion pressure [15] and retinal blood flow [106].

Dorzolamide lacks the systemic side effects of the systemic CAIs [101, 103]. However, as a sulfonamide derivative the potential for idiosyncratic aplastic anemia and myelosuppression does exist. The ocular side effects include stinging, burning, itching, and tearing [103]. Carbonic anhydrase is involved in corneal endothelial function, and in patients with guttae an increase in corneal thickness has been observed [107]. Although rarely clinically relevant, CAIs should be considered as a cause of worsening endothelial function. A bad taste in the mouth is the most commonly reported systemic side effect, reported by 25% of subjects in one study, but is an uncommon cause for discontinuation of therapy [101]. Dorzolamide should be avoided in patients with a history of sulfa allergy.

5.5.4 Brinzolamide

Brinzolamide is a selective inhibitor of carbonic anhydrase isoenzyme II and is similar in action to dorzolamide. Brinzolamide 1% offers similar effectiveness in IOP-lowering when compared to dorzolamide 2% and is less effective than timolol 0.5% [108]. Brinzolamide 1% twice daily had similar IOP-lowering when compared to three times daily dosing (19.1% vs. 20.3% reduction) [108].

Significantly less stinging, burning, and irritation are seen with topical brinzolamide when compared to dorzolamide [109]. The most common non-ocular side effect is bad taste in the mouth, and similar to dorzolamide no severe systemic side effects have been reported.

5.5.5 Summary

CAIs provide a powerful tool for IOP-lowering. Systemic CAIs have limited application for most patients due to their side effect profile. However, they are very useful with acute IOP spikes such as those seen post-operatively or with acute angle closure. They may also be used in chronic application for patients who are not surgical candidates. Topical CAIs provide a well-tolerated adjunctive therapy in IOP-lowering and may have a better effect on 24-h IOP-lowering when compared to timolol. For this reason, they have been popular in fixed combination formulations with timolol (US Cosopt) and brimonidine (US Simbrinza).

5.6 Prostaglandin Analogs

Prostaglandins are autacoids, that is, hormones that are synthesized, released, and act locally. They mediate a wide variety of physiological functions throughout the body, including smooth muscle and vascular relaxation, blood flow regulation, vascular permeability, and some aspects of inflammatory responses. In low doses some prostaglandins, especially PGF_{2a}, lower IOP primarily by increasing uveoscleral outflow of aqueous, likely through stimulation of matrix metalloproteinase synthesis and release, with consequent remodeling of the extracellular matrix between the ciliary muscle bundles [110]. PGF_{2a} has only a minor effect on trabecular meshwork outflow facility [111], while EP_2 and EP_4 agonists have larger facility-increasing effects.

5.6.1 Latanoprost

Unoprostone was the first PGA available, reaching the Japanese market in 1994, with modest

IOP-lowering effect. Two years later latanoprost was introduced and revolutionized glaucoma medical management. Latanoprost is a prostaglandin $F_{2\alpha}$ prodrug analog, with the acid residue replaced by an isopropyl ester side chain. The inactive isopropyl ester prodrug is hydrolyzed by esterases to the active acid form within the cornea and anterior chamber. IOP reduction with latanoprost 0.005% is 30–35% from baseline, and when applied in the evening it had greater IOP lowering (35%) than either timolol applied twice daily (27%) or latanoprost applied in the morning (31% reduction) [112]. Latanoprost provides excellent 24-h IOP reduction with some effect persisting to 48 h [113]. Peak efficacy occurs between 8 and 24 h after administration, and evening administration is generally recommended as it appears to best flatten the diurnal pressure curve. Long-term treatment has proven safe and effective, with little to no IOP upward drift over time [114, 115]. Many studies have documented the existence of non-responders, reportedly between 5 and 16% of patients [114, 116, 117]. Latanoprost remains by far the most frequently prescribed PGA worldwide.

5.6.2 Travoprost

Travoprost is also a prostaglandin $F_{2\alpha}$ analog, and is also an isopropyl ester prodrug which is hydrolyzed by corneal esterases into the biologically active form. Travoprost 0.004% lowers IOP similarly to latanoprost [118, 119], and is safe and well tolerated. The brand name Travatan Z replaces standard BAK with an ionic buffered preservative (SofZia®) that may benefit patients with a history of BAK allergy.

5.6.3 Bimatoprost

Bimatoprost has been described as a prostamide, a synthetic structural analog of prostaglandin $F_{2\alpha}$ with a unique amide group. It has been suggested that this compound does not require hydrolysis by corneal esterases and may activate a novel prostaglandin receptor (named as a "prostamide" receptor to distinguish it from the prostaglandin family). This is highly controversial, especially because of the patent and proprietary considerations. To add still further complexity, some research suggests that a prostamide metabolite is in fact a $PGF_{2\alpha}$ agonist [119]. Bimatoprost 0.03% is similar to latanoprost 0.005% in IOP-lowering magnitude [120]. The current commercially available form of bimatoprost is a 0.01% solution, and a 12-month randomized controlled trial showed no difference in IOP-lowering compared to the 0.03% solution, but significantly less hyperemia and improved tolerability with the lower concentration [121].

5.6.4 Tafluprost

Tafluprost is a prostaglandin analog with similar IOP-lowering effect to other PGAs [122]. It is available in a preservative-free formulation, and thus is useful in patients with a known BAK allergy or sensitivity to preservatives.

5.6.5 Comparison of Prostaglandin Analogs and Side Effects

Some studies have suggested that switching between classes of PGAs may offer additional IOP-lowering, especially for those patients classified as non-responders [123–125]. Although some have argued that this results from variation in corneal esterases or PGA receptors, it may also be due to lack of proper controls in these studies with resultant regression to the mean or to improved adherence with a change in therapy [119]. Additionally, differences in medication concentration may be more significant with PGAs than with other classes of medication, as PGAs are known to elevate IOP at higher concentrations. Thus, differing responses to different PGAs may reflect medication concentration rather than inherent differences in efficacy between compounds.

Side effects of all PGAs include conjunctival hyperemia, hypertrichosis, darkening of the iris (except for very dark and very blue irides), and periocular skin pigmentation. Enophthalmos and orbital fat atrophy have also been reported with chronic use [126]. Less common but more serious ocular side effects include iris cysts, cystoid macular edema (CME), anterior uveitis, and reactivation of herpes simplex keratitis (HSK) [127]. The risk of CME is extremely low in patients with no history of previous intraocular surgery or uveitis and is relatively low in patients at high risk (i.e., a history of aphakia, ruptured capsule, uveitis, or retinal vascular disease) [128, 129]. Prostaglandins are known mediators of ocular inflammation, and so it is not surprising that an association between PGA therapy and de novo anterior uveitis has been reported [128, 130]. The uveitis is readily reversible with discontinuation of the PGA with or without topical steroids. Reactivation of HSK with PGA therapy has been reported [131, 132]. However, in a large review of claims records the rate of diagnosis of HSK or pharmacy claims for antiviral medications was not associated with any glaucoma therapies [133].

5.6.6 Summary

PGAs provide excellent IOP reduction throughout a 24-hour period as well as a low incidence of local side effects and no systemic side effects. This profile has made them the first line for medical management of glaucoma in the majority of patients. The evidence supports that the medications in this class all have a similar mechanism of action and are similarly effective in lowering IOP. However, some patients may benefit more from one PGA vs. another for a variety of reasons, including individual differences in response, available preservative and preservative-free formulations leading to differences in tolerance, and cost.

5.7 Nitric Oxide Agents

Latanoprostene bunod became available in early 2018 in the USA. It is a hybrid molecule of latanoprost and butanediol mononitrate, a nitric oxide (NO)-donating moiety. NO inhibits actomyosin contractility and degrades the actin microfilament network and cell–extracellular matrix (ECM) adhesion in the trabecular meshwork, at least in part by inhibiting the rho-signaling cascade, leading to relaxation of the meshwork and dilation of Schlemm's canal, and thereby decreasing resistance to aqueous humor outflow [134].

In the phase II VOYAGER study latanoprostene bunod 0.024% showed greater lowering of mean diurnal IOP at 28 days (9 mmHg) when compared to latanoprost (7.8 mmHg) [134]. A phase 3 study of latanoprostene bunod 0.024% showed mean diurnal IOP significantly lower compared to timolol 0.5% with IOP reduction of 34.9% in the LBN group and 19.5% in the timolol group [135]. IOP-lowering appears to be maintained through 1 year of follow-up [136].

Ocular side effects are similar to prostaglandin analogs including conjunctival hyperemia, hypertrichosis, ocular irritation, and punctate keratitis. Stinging on instillation seems to be increased with latanoprost bunod when compared to latanoprost [134]. No significant systemic side effects have been identified to date.

5.8 Rho Kinase Inhibitors

Rho kinase inhibitors also decrease IOP by improving aqueous outflow through the trabecular meshwork. Rho kinase (ROCK) expression has been found in the trabecular meshwork, Schlemm's canal, ciliary muscle, and in the optic nerve [137]. ROCK is involved in smooth muscle and trabecular meshwork cell contraction through the interaction of actin and myosin, and inhibition of this action leads to relaxation of the trabecular meshwork and inner wall of Schlemm's canal, and weakening of cell-ECM focal adhesions in the meshwork and dilation of the canal, all combining to decrease resistance to aqueous outflow. There is additional interest in rho kinase inhibitors related to neuroprotection. Animal studies have shown benefit in optic nerve head blood flow in rabbits [138] and axonal regeneration in a nerve crush model in cats [139].

5.8.1 Ripasudil

Ripasudil is a fluorinated derivative of fasudil, a ROCK inhibitor marketed for cerebral vasospasm, and first became available for use in Japan in 2014. At peak, IOP is decreased by 4.5 mmHg in patients with ocular hypertension or primary open angle glaucoma with 0.4% ripasudil [140]. Significant additional lowering of IOP was noted in a phase 3 study in patients already on latanoprost 0.005% or timolol 0.5% [141]. Conjunctival hyperemia is not uncommon, and conjunctival follicles have been reported [142]. No significant systemic effects have been reported.

5.8.2 Netarsudil

Netarsudil is a rho kinase inhibitor that also inhibits the norepinephrine transporter. Via the former it increases trabecular meshwork outflow facility, and via the latter it decreases production of aqueous humor [143]. Preliminary evidence suggests that it may also decrease episcleral venous pressure. Netarsudil was approved for use in the USA in 2018. A large phase 3 study showed non-inferiority to timolol with both daily and twice-daily dosing of netarsudil 0.02% [143]. Conjunctival hyperemia was the most common side effect, reported in 50–59% of subjects; blurred vision was also commonly reported at 7.2% with once-daily dosing and 16.2% with twice-daily dosing. With twice-daily dosing discontinuation from the study due to adverse events was 30%.

5.9 Fixed Combination Agents

Fixed combination agents are available for several medications and have the benefit of simplifying treatment and improving adherence. In addition, there is less exposure to preservatives when one drop is needed in place of two.

Combination of dorzolamide 2% and timolol 0.5% is available in both brand name and generic formulations. Both compounds suppress aqueous humor production, through different pathways, and studies have shown that use of dorzolamide and timolol is superior to monotherapy with either drug alone [144]. Preservative-free fixed combination dorzolamide/timolol is available as Cosopt PF for patients with BAK allergy or preservative hypersensitivity. Brimonidine 0.2% and timolol 0.5% are also available as a fixed combination as Combigan (US) and show improved IOP control compared to the components alone [145]. Simbrinza (US), a fixed combination of brinzolamide 1% and brimonidine 0.2%, has also shown significantly lower IOP when compared to monotherapy with either component alone and is non-inferior to using the two medications separately [146]. This is the only fixed combination currently available without timolol, and so may benefit those patients who cannot tolerate a β-blocker due to the systemic side effects. A fixed combination of latanoprost 0.005% and netarsudil 0.02% has also shown significantly lower IOP than either component alone [147] but is not yet available at the time of this manuscript.

5.10 Hyperosmotic Agents

Systemically administered hyperosmotic agents for the lowering of IOP include oral glycerine and intravenous mannitol. The mechanism of action of this class is related to decreasing vitreous volume through oncotic dehydration. This leads to a rapid, dramatic reduction in IOP. Side effects may be severe and include headache, diuresis, circulatory overload leading to angina, pulmonary edema, and heart failure, and central nervous system effects including seizure and cerebral hemorrhage. Oral glycerine is also associated with nausea and vomiting. Hyperosmotic agents should be used with care and only in cases when significant IOP lowering is needed acutely, such as choroidal hemorrhage, aqueous misdirection, and angle closure glaucoma that is not responding to conservative management.

5.11 Gene Therapy

Topical eye drop therapy is the most common first treatment option for elevated intraocular pressure in the USA. Most patients will be treated with more than one medication over time. Small molecule topical pharmaceuticals have drawbacks: they must be applied frequently, resulting in issues with patient adherence; they may have ocular surface or off-target toxicity or mechanism-based side effects, and some patients are, or become, refractory to small molecule treatment. The chronic nature of glaucoma makes it a good target for novel long-term therapeutic strategies such as stem cell or gene therapy. Gene therapy has achieved a number of successes in retinal applications, where it has been used to improve vision in people with the retinal disease Leber's congenital amaurosis [148–151] and recently choroideremia [152–154], a rare type of inherited eye disease. The first ocular gene therapy, approved in December 2017, was for voretigene neparvovec, sold as Luxturna (Spark Therapeutics Inc), indicated for the treatment of Leber's congenital amaurosis, a biallelic RPE65 mutation-associated retinal dystrophy. These positive results have helped further the field of ocular gene therapy by providing much needed safety and efficacy data for viral vectors (specifically adeno-associated virus or AAV vectors), paving the regulatory way for future therapeutics.

The aim of gene therapy for glaucoma is to up- or down-regulate genes in some of the same pathways targeted by topical drops, with better tissue specificity. Gene therapy could effectively remove the patient from the delivery system and obviate compliance issues, as well as assuring a constant action in the most relevant tissue and pathway [155].

Several classes of compounds, described in detail in the sections above, act on the trabecular meshwork to disrupt the actin cytoskeleton, altering cell shape, contractility, and adhesions and reducing outflow resistance through the relaxation and expansion of the trabecular meshwork and Schlemm's canal [156–159]. These compounds reduce IOP in ocular hypertensive patients in clinical trials [160–162] and both netarsudil, a rho kinase inhibitor, and latanoprostene bunod, a nitric oxide agent, have recently been approved by the FDA. Other compounds of interest that could be used in gene therapy applications for glaucoma include prostanoid EP receptors, adenosine, and Wnt signaling agonists. Lentiviral and self-complementary adeno-associated viral vectors (scAAV) can stably express the green fluorescent protein reporter protein in the trabecular meshwork of live non-human primates for over 2 years [163, 164] and reduce outflow resistance in organ cultured anterior segment models.

Gene therapy delivery techniques, including intracanalicular, intracameral, intravitreal, subretinal, or subconjunctival injection, have been developed and refined to allow targeting different ocular tissues. For glaucoma these include targeting the trabecular meshwork, the inner wall of Schlemm's canal, ciliary body, and optic nerve. The potential for off-target transgene expression in neighboring tissues is a possibility for all delivery methods but may be reduced with more targeted approaches such as medication delivery during canaloplasty or canal-based minimally invasive glaucoma surgery procedures [165]. Elimination of patient-administered topical glaucoma therapy to assure continuous intraocular pressure reduction could optimize therapeutic outcomes in glaucoma.

5.12 Stem Cell and Associated Therapies

As with gene therapy, retinal applications for stem cell therapies are further along in development than those for glaucoma. Some aspects of gene transfer and stem cell applications are similar—there is a relatively small area/number of cells to replace; and visualization of the transplant site and testing of functionality serially and non-invasively are possible. Clinical trials using a variety of cell-based therapies for retinal degenerative diseases include human embryonic stem cell (hES), bone marrow stem cell (BMSC), mesenchymal stem cell (MSC), human neural stem cell (hNSC), and human induced pluripotent stem cells (hiPSC) [166–169].

Advances in mammalian somatic cell reprogramming have facilitated the production of human induced pluripotent stem cells (hiPSCs) [170–173]. hiPSCs have potential for use in transplantation, high throughput drug screening, cell-culture disease modeling, disease gene discovery, and gene therapy testing [169]. In animal and organ culture models, iPSCs have improved function in the outflow pathways, reducing IOP and reducing outflow resistance in animal and organ culture models [174, 175]. One of the biggest allures of hiPSCs is the ability to derive patient-specific material, since allogeneic transplantation may avoid potential complications due to immune rejection. Autologous transplantation of mesenchymal stem cells (MSC) is also a possibility since they can be isolated from bone marrow aspirates from individual patients and expanded in vitro before transplantation [176, 177]. Of particular relevance to glaucoma, MSCs have been programmed/engineered to secrete brain-derived neurotrophic factor and platelet-derived growth factor, both of which play a role in neuroprotection, serve as neurotransmitter modulators, and participate in neuronal plasticity [177–180]. In animal models, these and other constructs have shown some efficacy in retinal ganglion cell neuroprotection [177–181].

Populations of stem cells have been found in glaucoma relevant anterior segment tissues, including the trabecular meshwork [182, 183] and Schwalbe's line [181]. It may be possible to generate a population of cells that are capable of differentiating to a trabecular meshwork and a corneal endothelial lineage to replace both cell types [184]. As trabecular meshwork cellularity declines with age and glaucoma [185], this could be beneficial for many patients.

Potential gene and stem cell therapies for glaucoma will be discussed in more detail in Chap. 7.

References

1. Snell S. On eserine and pilocarpine in glaucoma, and eserine in ocular neuralgia. Br Med J. 1882;1(1118):811–2.
2. Heij A, Leske MC, Bengtsson B, Hyman L, Bengtsson B, Hussein M. Reduction of intraocular pressure and glaucoma progression: results from the early manifest Glaucoma trial. Arch Ophthalmol. 2002;120(10):1268–79.
3. Ederer F, Gaasterland DE, Sullivan EK. The advanced glaucoma intervention study (AGIS): 1. Study design and methods and baseline characteristics of study patients. Control Clin Trials. 1994;15(4):299–325.
4. Kass MA, Heuer DK, Higginbotham EJ, Johnson CA, Keltner JL, Miller JP, et al. The ocular hypertension treatment study: a randomized trial determines that topical ocular hypotensive medication delays or prevents the onset of primary open-angle glaucoma. Arch Ophthalmol. 2002;120(6):701–13. discussion 829–30.
5. Collaborative Normal-Tension Glaucoma Study Group. Comparison of glaucomatous progression between untreated patients with normal-tension glaucoma and patients with therapeutically reduced intraocular pressures. Am J Ophthalmol. 1998;126(4):487–97.
6. Phillips CI, Howitt G, Rowlands DJ. Propranolol as ocular hypotensive agent. Br J Ophthalmol. 1967;51(4):222–6.
7. Coakes RL, Brubaker RF. The mechanism of timolol in lowering intraocular pressure. In the normal eye. Arch Ophthalmol. 1978;96(11):2045–8.
8. Zimmerman TJ. Kaufman HE. Timolol. A beta-adrenergic blocking agent for the treatment of glaucoma. Arch Ophthalmol. 1977;95(4):601–4.
9. Zimmerman TJ, Kaufman HE. Timolol, dose response and duration of action. Arch Ophthalmol. 1977;95(4):605–7.
10. Ritch R, Hargett NA, Podos SM. The effect of 1.5% timolol maleate on intraocular pressure. Acta Ophthalmol. 1978;56(1):6–10.
11. Boger WP 3rd, Steinert RF, Thomas JV. Timolol in the therapy of "ocular hypertension". Surv Ophthalmol. 1980;25(3):195–202.
12. Lin LL, Galin MA, Obstbaum SA, Katz I. Longterm timolol therapy. Surv Ophthalmol. 1979;23(6):377–80.
13. Zhang WY, Po AL, Dua HS, Azuara-Blanco A. Meta-analysis of randomised controlled trials comparing latanoprost with timolol in the treatment of patients with open angle glaucoma or ocular hypertension. Br J Ophthalmol. 2001;85(8):983–90.
14. Topper JE, Brubaker RF. Effects of timolol, epinephrine, and acetazolamide on aqueous flow during sleep. Invest Ophthalmol Vis Sci. 1985;26(10):1315–9.
15. Quaranta L, Gandolfo F, Turano R, Rovida F, Pizzolante T, Musig A, et al. Effects of topical hypotensive drugs on circadian IOP, blood pressure, and calculated diastolic ocular perfusion pressure in patients with glaucoma. Invest Ophthalmol Vis Sci. 2006;47(7):2917–23.
16. Steinert RF, Thomas JV, Boger WP 3rd. Long-term drift and continued efficacy after multiyear timolol therapy. Arch Ophthalmol. 1981;99(1):100–3.
17. Rakofsky SI, Lazar M, Almog Y, LeBlanc RP, Mann C, Orr A, et al. Efficacy and safety of once-daily levobunolol for glaucoma therapy. Can J Ophthalmol. 1989;24(1):2–6.
18. McMahon CD, Shaffer RN, Hoskins HD Jr, Hetherington J Jr. Adverse effects experienced by patients taking timolol. Am J Ophthalmol. 1979;88(4):736–8.
19. Van Buskirk EM. Adverse reactions from timolol administration. Ophthalmology. 1980;87(5):447–50.

20. Bonomi L, Zavarise G, Noya E, Michieletto S. Effects of timolol maleate on tear flow in human eyes. Albrecht Von Graefes Arch Klin Exp Ophthalmol. 1980;213(1):19–22.
21. Nelson WL, Fraunfelder FT, Sills JM, Arrowsmith JB, Kuritsky JN. Adverse respiratory and cardiovascular events attributed to timolol ophthalmic solution, 1978-1985. Am J Ophthalmol. 1986;102(5):606–11.
22. Sadiq SA, Fielding K, Vernon SA. The effect of timolol drops on respiratory function. Eye (Lond). 1998;12(Pt 3a):386–9.
23. Shaivitz SA. Timolol and myasthenia gravis. JAMA. 1979;242(15):1611–2.
24. Velde TM, Kaiser FE. Ophthalmic timolol treatment causing altered hypoglycemic response in a diabetic patient. Arch Intern Med. 1983;143(8):1627.
25. Zimmerman TJ, Sharir M, Nardin GF, Fuqua M. Therapeutic index of pilocarpine, carbachol, and timolol with nasolacrimal occlusion. Am J Ophthalmol. 1992;114(1):1–7.
26. The Levobunolol Study Group (Appended). Levobunolol. A beta-adrenoceptor antagonist effective in the long-term treatment of glaucoma. Ophthalmology. 1985;92(9):1271–6.
27. Wandel T, Charap AD, Lewis RA, Partamian L, Cobb S, Lue JC, et al. Glaucoma treatment with once-daily levobunolol. Am J Ophthalmol. 1986;101(3):298–304.
28. Muller O, Knobel HR. Effectiveness and tolerance of metipranolol--results of a multi-center long-term study in Switzerland. Klin Monbl Augenheilkd. 1986;188(1):62–3.
29. Bleckmann H, Duy TP, Grajewski O. Therapeutic efficacy of metipranolol eye drops 0.3% versus timolol eye drops 0.25%. In: Merté HJ, editor. Metipranolol. Vienna: Springer; 1984.
30. Akingbehin T, Villada JR. Metipranolol-associated granulomatous anterior uveitis. Br J Ophthalmol. 1991;75(9):519–23.
31. Schnarr KD. Comparative multicenter study of carteolol eyedrops with other beta blockers in 768 patients under normal conditions. Klin Monbl Augenheilkd. 1988;192(2):167–72.
32. Stewart WC, Shields MB, Allen RC, Lewis RA, Cohen JS, Hoskins HD, et al. A 3-month comparison of 1% and 2% carteolol and 0.5% timolol in open-angle glaucoma. Graefes Arch Clin Exp Ophthalmol. 1991;229(3):258–61.
33. Frishman WH, Covey S. Penbutolol and carteolol: two new beta-adrenergic blockers with partial agonism. J Clin Pharmacol. 1990;30(5):412–21.
34. van Brummelen P. The relevance of intrinsic sympathomimetic activity for beta-blocker-induced changes in plasma lipids. J Cardiovasc Pharmacol. 1983;5(Suppl 1):S51–5.
35. Reiss GR, Brubaker RF. The mechanism of betaxolol, a new ocular hypotensive agent. Ophthalmology. 1983;90(11):1369–72.
36. Caldwell DR, Salisbury CR, Guzek JP. Effects of topical betaxolol in ocular hypertensive patients. Arch Ophthalmol. 1984;102(4):539–40.
37. Feghali JG, Kaufman PL. Decreased intraocular pressure in the hypertensive human eye with betaxolol, a beta 1-adrenergic antagonist. Am J Ophthalmol. 1985;100(6):777–82.
38. Stewart RH, Kimbrough RL, Ward RL. Betaxolol vs timolol. A six-month double-blind comparison. Arch Ophthalmol. 1986;104(1):46–8.
39. Dunn TL, Gerber MJ, Shen AS, Fernandez E, Iseman MD, Cherniack RM. The effect of topical ophthalmic instillation of timolol and betaxolol on lung function in asthmatic subjects. Am Rev Respir Dis. 1986;133(2):264–8.
40. Schoene RB, Abuan T, Ward RL, Beasley CH. Effects of topical betaxolol, timolol, and placebo on pulmonary function in asthmatic bronchitis. Am J Ophthalmol. 1984;97(1):86–92.
41. Harris LS, Greenstein SH, Bloom AF. Respiratory difficulties with betaxolol. Am J Ophthalmol. 1986;102(2):274–5.
42. Roholt PC. Betaxolol and restrictive airway disease. Case report. Arch Ophthalmol. 1987;105(9):1172.
43. Vuori ML, Ali-Melkkila T, Kaila T, Iisalo E, Saari KM. Beta 1- and beta 2-antagonist activity of topically applied betaxolol and timolol in the systemic circulation. Acta Ophthalmol. 1993;71(5):682–5.
44. Lynch MG, Whitson JT, Brown RH, Nguyen H, Drake MM. Topical beta-blocker therapy and central nervous system side effects. A preliminary study comparing betaxolol and timolol. Arch Ophthalmol. 1988;106(7):908–11.
45. Wang YL, Hayashi M, Yablonski ME, Toris CB. Effects of multiple dosing of epinephrine on aqueous humor dynamics in human eyes. J Ocul Pharmacol Ther. 2002;18(1):53–63.
46. Schenker HI, Yablonski ME, Podos SM. Linder L. Fluorophotometric study of epinephrine and timolol in human subjects. Arch Ophthalmol. 1981;99(7):1212–6.
47. Garner LL, Johnstone WW, Ballintine EJ, Carroll ME. Effect of 2% levo-rotary epinephrine on the intraocular pressure of the glaucomatous eye. AMA Arch Ophthalmol. 1959;62(2):230–8.
48. Becker B, Pettit TH, Gay AJ. Topical epinephrine therapy of open-angle glaucoma. Arch Ophthalmol. 1961;66:219–25.
49. Costagliola C, dell'Omo R, Romano MR, Rinaldi M, Zeppa L, Parmeggiani F. Pharmacotherapy of intraocular pressure: part I. Parasympathomimetic, sympathomimetic and sympatholytics. Expert Opin Pharmacother. 2009;10(16):2663–77.
50. Mandell AI, Stentz F, Kitabchi AE. Dipivalyl epinephrine: a new pro-drug in the treatment of glaucoma. Ophthalmology. 1978;85(3):268–75.
51. Krieglstein GK, Gramer E. The response of ophthalmic arterial pressure to topically applied clonidine. Albrecht Von Graefes Arch Klin Exp Ophthalmol. 1978;207(1):1–5.
52. Gharagozloo NZ, Relf SJ, Brubaker RF. Aqueous flow is reduced by the alpha-adrenergic agonist, apraclonidine hydrochloride (ALO 2145). Ophthalmology. 1988;95(9):1217–20.

53. Abrams DA, Robin AL, Pollack IP, de Faller JM, DeSantis L. The safety and efficacy of topical 1% ALO 2145 (p-aminoclonidine hydrochloride) in normal volunteers. Arch Ophthalmol. 1987;105(9):1205–7.
54. Stewart WC, Ritch R, Shin DH, Lehmann RP, Shrader CE, van Buskirk EM. The efficacy of apraclonidine as an adjunct to timolol therapy. Apraclonidine adjunctive therapy study group. Arch Ophthalmol. 1995;113(3):287–92.
55. Stewart WC. Effect and side effects of apraclonidine. Klin Monbl Augenheilkd. 1996;209(1):A7–13.
56. Butler P, Mannschreck M, Lin S, Hwang I, Alvarado J. Clinical experience with the long-term use of 1% apraclonidine. Incidence of allergic reactions. Arch Ophthalmol. 1995;113(3):293–6.
57. Burke J, Schwartz M. Preclinical evaluation of brimonidine. Surv Ophthalmol. 1996;41(Suppl 1):S9–18.
58. Toris CB, Gleason ML, Camras CB, Yablonski ME. Effects of brimonidine on aqueous humor dynamics in human eyes. Arch Ophthalmol. 1995;113(12):1514–7.
59. Walters TR. Development and use of brimonidine in treating acute and chronic elevations of intraocular pressure: a review of safety, efficacy, dose response, and dosing studies. Surv Ophthalmol. 1996;41(Suppl 1):S19–26.
60. Katz LJ. Brimonidine tartrate 0.2% twice daily vs timolol 0.5% twice daily: 1-year results in glaucoma patients. Brimonidine study group. Am J Ophthalmol. 1999;127(1):20–6.
61. Fung AT, Reid SE, Jones MP, Healey PR, McCluskey PJ, Craig JC. Meta-analysis of randomised controlled trials comparing latanoprost with brimonidine in the treatment of open-angle glaucoma, ocular hypertension or normal-tension glaucoma. Br J Ophthalmol. 2007;91(1):62–8.
62. Lee DA, Gornbein JA. Effectiveness and safety of brimonidine as adjunctive therapy for patients with elevated intraocular pressure in a large, open-label community trial. J Glaucoma. 2001;10(3):220–6.
63. Wen R, Cheng T, Li Y, Cao W, Steinberg RH. Alpha 2-adrenergic agonists induce basic fibroblast growth factor expression in photoreceptors in vivo and ameliorate light damage. J Neurosci. 1996;16(19):5986–92.
64. WoldeMussie E, Ruiz G, Wijono M, Wheeler LA. Neuroprotection of retinal ganglion cells by brimonidine in rats with laser-induced chronic ocular hypertension. Invest Ophthalmol Vis Sci. 2001;42(12):2849–55.
65. Krupin T, Liebmann JM, Greenfield DS, Ritch R, Gardiner S. A randomized trial of brimonidine versus timolol in preserving visual function: results from the low-pressure Glaucoma treatment study. Am J Ophthalmol. 2011;151(4):671–81.
66. RP LB. Twelve-month results of an ongoing randomized trial comparing brimonidine tartrate 0.2% and timolol 0.5% given twice daily in patients with glaucoma or ocular hypertension. Brimonidine study group 2. Ophthalmology. 1998;105(10):1960–7.
67. Melamed S, David R. Ongoing clinical assessment of the safety profile and efficacy of brimonidine compared with timolol: year-three results. Brimonidine study group II. Clin Ther. 2000;22(1):103–11.
68. Enyedi LB, Freedman SF. Safety and efficacy of brimonidine in children with glaucoma. J AAPOS. 2001;5(5):281–4.
69. Carlsen JO, Zabriskie NA, Kwon YH, Barbe ME, Scott WE. Apparent central nervous system depression in infants after the use of topical brimonidine. Am J Ophthalmol. 1999;128(2):255–6.
70. Soto-Perez-de-Celis E, Skvirsky DO, Cisneros BG. Unintentional ingestion of brimonidine antiglaucoma drops: a case report and review of the literature. Pediatr Emerg Care. 2007;23(9):657–8.
71. Vanhaesebrouck S, Cossey V, Cosaert K, Allegaert K, Naulaers G. Cardiorespiratory depression and hyperglycemia after unintentional ingestion of brimonidine in a neonate. Eur J Ophthalmol. 2009;19(4):694–5.
72. Schuman JS, Horwitz B, Choplin NT, David R, Albracht D, Chen K. A 1-year study of brimonidine twice daily in glaucoma and ocular hypertension. A controlled, randomized, multicenter clinical trial. Chronic Brimonidine study group. Arch Ophthalmol. 1997;115(7):847–52.
73. Rahman MQ, Montgomery DM, Lazaridou MN. Surveillance of glaucoma medical therapy in a Glasgow teaching hospital: 26 years' experience. Br J Ophthalmol. 2009;93(12):1572–5.
74. Osborne SA, Montgomery DM, Morris D, McKay IC. Alphagan allergy may increase the propensity for multiple eye-drop allergy. Eye (Lond). 2005;19(2):129–37.
75. Beltz J, Zamir E. Brimonidine induced anterior uveitis. Ocul Immunol Inflamm. 2016;24(2):128–33.
76. Byles DB, Frith P, Salmon JF. Anterior uveitis as a side effect of topical brimonidine. Am J Ophthalmol. 2000;130(3):287–91.
77. Cates CA, Jeffrey MN. Granulomatous anterior uveitis associated with 0.2% topical brimonidine. Eye (Lond). 2003;17(5):670–1.
78. Watts P, Hawksworth N. Delayed hypersensitivity to brimonidine tartrate 0.2% associated with high intraocular pressure. Eye (Lond). 2002;16(2):132–5.
79. Kaufman PL. Aqueous humor dynamics following total iridectomy in the cynomolgus monkey. Invest Ophthalmol Vis Sci. 1979;18(8):870–4.
80. Kaufman PL, Barany EH. Loss of acute pilocarpine effect on outflow facility following surgical disinsertion and retrodisplacement of the ciliary muscle from the scleral spur in the cynomolgus monkey. Investig Ophthalmol. 1976;15(10):793–807.
81. Drance SM, Nash PA. The dose response of human intraocular pressure to pilocarpine. Can J Ophthalmol. 1971;6(1):9–13.
82. Poinoosawmy D, Nagasubramanian S, Brown NA. Effect of pilocarpine on visual acuity and on the dimensions of the cornea and anterior chamber. Br J Ophthalmol. 1976;60(10):676–9.
83. Levene RZ. Uniocular miotic therapy. Trans Sect Ophthalmol Am Acad Ophthalmol Otolaryngol. 1975;79(2):Op376–80.

84. Pape LG, Forbes M. Retinal detachment and miotic therapy. Am J Ophthalmol. 1978;85(4):558–66.
85. Zimmerman TJ, Wheeler TM. Miotics: side effects and ways to avoid them. Ophthalmology. 1982;89(1):76–80.
86. Duncan G, Collison DJ. Role of the non-neuronal cholinergic system in the eye: a review. Life Sci. 2003;72(18–19):2013–9.
87. Reichert RW, Shields MB, Stewart WC. Intraocular pressure response to replacing pilocarpine with carbachol. Am J Ophthalmol. 1988;106(6):747–8.
88. Pantuck EJ. Ecothiopate iodide eye drops and prolonged response to suxamethonium. Br J Anaesth. 1966;38(5):406–7.
89. Gesztes T. Prolonged apnoea after suxamethonium injection associated with eye drops containing an anticholinesterase agent. Br J Anaesth. 1966;38(5):408–9.
90. Supuran CT, Scozzafava A, Casini A. Carbonic anhydrase inhibitors. Med Res Rev. 2003;23(2):146–89.
91. Becker B. Decrease in intraocular pressure in man by a carbonic anhydrase inhibitor, diamox; a preliminary report. Am J Ophthalmol. 1954;37(1):13–5.
92. Grant WM, Trotter RR. Diamox (acetazolamide) in treatment of glaucoma. AMA Arch Ophthalmol. 1954;51(6):735–9.
93. Dahlen K, Epstein DL, Grant WM, Hutchinson BT, Prien EL Jr, Krall JMA. Repeated dose-response study of methazolamide in glaucoma. Arch Ophthalmol. 1978;96(12):2214–8.
94. Lichter PR. Reducing side effects of carbonic anhydrase inhibitors. Ophthalmology. 1981;88(3):266–9.
95. Fraunfelder FT, Meyer SM, Bagby GC Jr, Dreis MW. Hematologic reactions to carbonic anhydrase inhibitors. Am J Ophthalmol. 1985;100(1):79–81.
96. Murphy RM, Bakir B, O'Brien C, Wiggs JL, Pasquale LR. Drug-induced bilateral secondary angle-closure Glaucoma: a literature synthesis. J Glaucoma. 2016;25(2):e99–105.
97. Her Y, Kil MS, Park JH, Kim CW, Kim SS. Stevens-Johnson syndrome induced by acetazolamide. J Dermatol. 2011;38(3):272–5.
98. Shirato S, Kagaya F, Suzuki Y, Joukou S. Stevens-Johnson syndrome induced by methazolamide treatment. Arch Ophthalmol. 1997;115(4):550–3.
99. Sud RN, Grewal SS. Stevens Johnson syndrome due to Diamox. Indian J Ophthalmol. 1981;29(2):101–3.
100. Hoyng PF, van Beek LM. Pharmacological therapy for glaucoma: a review. Drugs. 2000;59(3):411–34.
101. Sugrue MF, Mallorga P, Schwam H, Baldwin JJ, Ponticello GS. A comparison of L-671,152 and MK-927, two topically effective ocular hypotensive carbonic anhydrase inhibitors, in experimental animals. Curr Eye Res. 1990;9(6):607–15.
102. Pfeiffer N. Dorzolamide: development and clinical application of a topical carbonic anhydrase inhibitor. Surv Ophthalmol. 1997;42(2):137–51.
103. Strahlman E, Tipping R, Vogel R. A double-masked, randomized 1-year study comparing dorzolamide (Trusopt), timolol, and betaxolol. International Dorzolamide Study Group. Arch Ophthalmol. 1995;113(8):1009–16.
104. Cheng JW, Cheng SW, Yu DY, Wei RL, Lu GC. Meta-analysis of alpha2-adrenergic agonists versus carbonic anhydrase inhibitors as adjunctive therapy. Curr Med Res Opin. 2012;28(4):543–50.
105. Orzalesi N, Rossetti L, Invernizzi T, Bottoli A, Autelitano A. Effect of timolol, latanoprost, and dorzolamide on circadian IOP in glaucoma or ocular hypertension. Invest Ophthalmol Vis Sci. 2000;41(9):2566–73.
106. Costagliola C, Campa C, Parmeggiani F, Incorvaia C, Perri P, D'Angelo S, et al. Effect of 2% dorzolamide on retinal blood flow: a study on juvenile primary open-angle glaucoma patients already receiving 0.5% timolol. Br J Clin Pharmacol. 2007;63(3):376–9.
107. Wirtitsch MG, Findl O, Heinzl H, Drexler W. Effect of dorzolamide hydrochloride on central corneal thickness in humans with cornea guttata. Arch Ophthalmol. 2007;125(10):1345–50.
108. Silver LH. Clinical efficacy and safety of brinzolamide (Azopt), a new topical carbonic anhydrase inhibitor for primary open-angle glaucoma and ocular hypertension. Brinzolamide primary therapy study group. Am J Ophthalmol. 1998;126(3):400–8.
109. Silver LH. Ocular comfort of brinzolamide 1.0% ophthalmic suspension compared with dorzolamide 2.0% ophthalmic solution: results from two multicenter comfort studies. Brinzolamide comfort study group. Surv Ophthalmol. 2000;44(Suppl 2):S141–5.
110. Toris CB, Gabelt BT, Kaufman PL. Update on the mechanism of action of topical prostaglandins for intraocular pressure reduction. Surv Ophthalmol. 2008;53(Suppl1):S107–20.
111. Toris CB, Camras CB, Yablonski ME, Brubaker RF. Effects of exogenous prostaglandins on aqueous humor dynamics and blood-aqueous barrier function. Surv Ophthalmol. 1997;41(Suppl 2):S69–75.
112. Alm A, Camras CB, Watson PG. Phase III latanoprost studies in Scandinavia, the United Kingdom and the United States. Surv Ophthalmol. 1997;41(Suppl 2):S105–10.
113. Larsson LI, Mishima HK, Takamatsu M, Orzalesi N, Rossetti L. The effect of latanoprost on circadian intraocular pressure. Surv Ophthalmol. 2002;47(Suppl 1):S90–6.
114. Costagliola C, Del Prete A, Verolino M, Antinozzi P, Fusco R, Parmeggiani F, et al. Effect of 0.005% latanoprost once daily on intraocular pressure in glaucomatous patients not adequately controlled by beta-blockers twice daily: a 3-year follow-up. Experience and incidence of side effects in a prospective study on 76 patients. Graefes Arch Clin Exp Ophthalmol. 2002;240(5):379–86.
115. Perry CM, McGavin JK, Culy CR, Ibbotson T. Latanoprost: an update of its use in glaucoma and ocular hypertension. Drugs Aging. 2003;20(8):597–630.

116. Susanna R Jr, Chew P, Kitazawa Y. Current status of prostaglandin therapy: latanoprost and unoprostone. Surv Ophthalmol. 2002;47(Suppl 1):S97–104.
117. Goldberg I, Li XY, Selaru P, Paggiarino D. A 5-year, randomized, open-label safety study of latanoprost and usual care in patients with open-angle glaucoma or ocular hypertension. Eur J Ophthalmol. 2008;18(3):408–16.
118. Netland PA, Landry T, Sullivan EK, Andrew R, Silver L, Weiner A, et al. Travoprost compared with latanoprost and timolol in patients with open-angle glaucoma or ocular hypertension. Am J Ophthalmol. 2001;132(4):472–84.
119. Bean GW, Camras CB. Commercially available prostaglandin analogs for the reduction of intraocular pressure: similarities and differences. Surv Ophthalmol. 2008;53(Suppl1):S69–84.
120. Gandolfi S, Simmons ST, Sturm R, Chen K, Van Denburgh AM. Three-month comparison of bimatoprost and latanoprost in patients with glaucoma and ocular hypertension. Adv Ther. 2001;18(3):110–21.
121. Katz LJ, Cohen JS, Batoosingh AL, Felix C, Shu V, Schiffman RM. Twelve-month, randomized, controlled trial of bimatoprost 0.01%, 0.0125%, and 0.03% in patients with glaucoma or ocular hypertension. Am J Ophthalmol. 2010;149(4):661–71.e1.
122. Swymer C, Neville MW. Tafluprost: the first preservative-free prostaglandin to treat open-angle glaucoma and ocular hypertension. Ann Pharmacother. 2012;46(11):1506–10.
123. Gandolfi SA, Cimino L. Effect of bimatoprost on patients with primary open-angle glaucoma or ocular hypertension who are nonresponders to latanoprost. Ophthalmology. 2003;110(3):609–14.
124. Kaback M, Geanon J, Katz G, Ripkin D, Przydryga J. Ocular hypotensive efficacy of travoprost in patients unsuccessfully treated with latanoprost. Curr Med Res Opin. 2004;20(9):1341–5.
125. Williams RD. Efficacy of bimatoprost in glaucoma and ocular hypertension unresponsive to latanoprost. Adv Ther. 2002;19(6):275–81.
126. Costagliola C, dell'Omo R, Romano MR, Rinaldi M, Zeppa L, Parmeggiani F. Pharmacotherapy of intraocular pressure - part II. Carbonic anhydrase inhibitors, prostaglandin analogues and prostamides. Expert Opin Pharmacother. 2009;10(17):2859–70.
127. Alm A, Grierson I, Shields MB. Side effects associated with prostaglandin analog therapy. Surv Ophthalmol. 2008;53(Suppl1):S93–105.
128. Warwar RE, Bullock JD, Ballal D. Cystoid macular edema and anterior uveitis associated with latanoprost use. Experience and incidence in a retrospective review of 94 patients. Ophthalmology. 1998;105(2):263–8.
129. Lima MC, Paranhos A Jr, Salim S, Honkanen R, Devgan L, Wand M, et al. Visually significant cystoid macular edema in pseudophakic and aphakic patients with glaucoma receiving latanoprost. J Glaucoma. 2000;9(4):317–21.
130. Fechtner RD, Khouri AS, Zimmerman TJ, Bullock J, Feldman R, Kulkarni P, et al. Anterior uveitis associated with latanoprost. Am J Ophthalmol. 1998;126(1):37–41.
131. Wand M, Gilbert CM, Liesegang TJ. Latanoprost and herpes simplex keratitis. Am J Ophthalmol. 1999;127(5):602–4.
132. Kroll DM, Schuman JS. Reactivation of herpes simplex virus keratitis after initiating bimatoprost treatment for glaucoma. Am J Ophthalmol. 2002;133(3):401–3.
133. Bean G, Reardon G, Zimmerman TJ. Association between ocular herpes simplex virus and topical ocular hypotensive therapy. J Glaucoma. 2004;13(5):361–4.
134. Weinreb RN, Ong T, Scassellati Sforzolini B, Vittitow JL, Singh K, Kaufman PL. A randomised, controlled comparison of latanoprostene bunod and latanoprost 0.005% in the treatment of ocular hypertension and open angle glaucoma: the VOYAGER study. Br J Ophthalmol. 2015;99(6):738–45.
135. Weinreb RN, Scassellati Sforzolini B, Vittitow J, Liebmann J. Latanoprostene bunod 0.024% versus timolol maleate 0.5% in subjects with open-angle glaucoma or ocular hypertension: the APOLLO study. Ophthalmology. 2016;123(5):965–73.
136. Kawase K, Vittitow JL, Weinreb RN, Araie M. Long-term safety and efficacy of latanoprostene bunod 0.024% in Japanese subjects with open-angle glaucoma or ocular hypertension: the JUPITER study. Adv Ther. 2016;33(9):1612–27.
137. Wang SK, Chang RT. An emerging treatment option for glaucoma: rho kinase inhibitors. Clin Ophthalmol. 2014;8:883–90.
138. Sugiyama T, Shibata M, Kajiura S, Okuno T, Tonari M, Oku H, et al. Effects of fasudil, a rho-associated protein kinase inhibitor, on optic nerve head blood flow in rabbits. Invest Ophthalmol Vis Sci. 2011;52(1):64–9.
139. Sagawa H, Terasaki H, Nakamura M, Ichikawa M, Yata T, Tokita Y, et al. A novel ROCK inhibitor, Y-39983, promotes regeneration of crushed axons of retinal ganglion cells into the optic nerve of adult cats. Exp Neurol. 2007;205(1):230–40.
140. Tanihara H, Inoue T, Yamamoto T, Kuwayama Y, Abe H, Araie M. Phase 2 randomized clinical study of a rho kinase inhibitor, K-115, in primary open-angle glaucoma and ocular hypertension. Am J Ophthalmol. 2013;156(4):731–6.
141. Tanihara H, Inoue T, Yamamoto T, Kuwayama Y, Abe H, Suganami H, et al. Additive intraocular pressure-lowering effects of the rho kinase inhibitor ripasudil (K-115) combined with timolol or latanoprost: a report of 2 randomized clinical trials. JAMA Ophthalmol. 2015;133(7):755–61.
142. Tanihara H, Inoue T, Yamamoto T, Kuwayama Y, Abe H, Araie M. Phase 1 clinical trials of a selective rho kinase inhibitor, K-115. JAMA Ophthalmol. 2013;131(10):1288–95.
143. Serle JB, Katz LJ, McLaurin E, Heah T, Ramirez-Davis N, Usner DW, et al. Two phase 3 clinical trials comparing the safety and efficacy of netarsudil

to timolol in patients with elevated intraocular pressure: rho kinase elevated IOP treatment trial 1 and 2 (ROCKET-1 and ROCKET-2). Am J Ophthalmol. 2018;186:116–27.

144. Ormrod D, McClellan K. Topical dorzolamide 2%/timolol 0.5%: a review of its use in the treatment of open-angle glaucoma. Drugs Aging. 2000;17(6):477–96.
145. Craven ER, Walters TR, Williams R, Chou C, Cheetham JK, Schiffman R. Brimonidine and timolol fixed-combination therapy versus monotherapy: a 3-month randomized trial in patients with glaucoma or ocular hypertension. J Ocul Pharmacol Ther. 2005;21(4):337–48.
146. Sharma S, Trikha S, Perera SA, Aung T. Clinical effectiveness of brinzolamide 1%-brimonidine 0.2% fixed combination for primary open-angle glaucoma and ocular hypertension. Clin Ophthalmol. 2015;9:2201–7.
147. Lewis RA, Levy B, Ramirez N, Kopczynski CC, Usner DW, Novack GD. Fixed-dose combination of AR-13324 and latanoprost: a double-masked, 28-day, randomised, controlled study in patients with open-angle glaucoma or ocular hypertension. Br J Ophthalmol. 2016;100(3):339–44.
148. Vignal C, Uretsky S, Fitoussi S, Galy A, Blouin L, Girmens JF, Bidot S, Thomasson N, Bouquet C, Valero S, Meunier S, Combal JP, Gilly B, Katz B, Sahel JA. Safety of rAAV2/2-ND4 gene therapy for Leber hereditary optic neuropathy. Ophthalmology. 2018;125(6):945–7. pii: S0161-6420(17)33673-4.
149. Kumaran N, Michaelides M, Smith AJ, Ali RR, Bainbridge JWB. Retinal gene therapy. Br Med Bull. 2018;126(1):13–25.
150. Guy J, Feuer WJ, Davis JL, Porciatti V, Gonzalez PJ, Koilkonda RD, Yuan H, Hauswirth WW, Lam BL. Gene therapy for leber hereditary optic neuropathy: low- and medium-dose visual results. Ophthalmology. 2017;124(11):1621–34.
151. Ashtari M, Nikonova ES, Marshall KA, Young GJ, Aravand P, Pan W, Ying GS, Willett AE, Mahmoudian M, Maguire AM, Bennett J. The role of the human visual cortex in assessment of the long-term durability of retinal gene therapy in follow-on RPE65 clinical trial patients. Ophthalmology. 2017;124(6):873–83.
152. Duong TT, Vasireddy V, Ramachandran P, Herrera PS, Leo L, Merkel C, Bennett J, Mills JA. Use of induced pluripotent stem cell models to probe the pathogenesis of Choroideremia and to develop a potential treatment. Stem Cell Res. 2018;27:140–50.
153. Patrício MI, MacLaren RE. Retinal gene therapy for choroideremia: in vitro testing for gene augmentation using an adeno-associated viral (aav) vector. Methods Mol Biol. 2018;1715:89–97.
154. MacLaren RE, Groppe M, Barnard AR, Cottriall CL, Tolmachova T, Seymour L, Clark KR, During MJ, Cremers FP, Black GC, Lotery AJ, Downes SM, Webster AR, Seabra MC. Retinal gene therapy in patients with choroideremia: initial findings from a phase 1/2 clinical trial. Lancet. 2014;383(9923):1129–37.
155. Kaufman PL. Enhancing trabecular outflow by disrupting the actin cytoskeleton, increasing uveoscleral outflow with prostaglandins, and understanding the pathophysiology of presbyopia interrogating mother nature: asking why, asking how, recognizing the signs, following the trail. Exp Eye Res. 2008;86:3–17.
156. Rasmussen CA, Kaufman PL. Novel therapeutic approaches for glaucoma. Drugs Fut. 2011;36(4):287.
157. Kaufman PL, Rasmussen CA. Advances in glaucoma treatment and management: outflow drugs. Invest Ophthalmol Vis Sci. 2012;53(5):2495–500.
158. Tian B, Gabelt BT, Geiger B, Kaufman PL. The role of the actomyosin system in regulating trabecular fluid outflow. Exp Eye Res. 2009;88(4):713–7.
159. Tian B, Kaufman PL. Comparisons of actin filament disruptors and rho kinase inhibitors as potential antiglaucoma medications. Expert Rev Ophthalmol. 2012;7(2):177–87.
160. Kazemi A, McLaren JW, Kopczynski CC, Heah TG, Novack GD, Sit AJ. The effects of netarsudil ophthalmic solution on aqueous humor dynamics in a randomized study in humans. J Ocul Pharmacol Ther. 2018;34(5):380–6.
161. Serle JB, Katz LJ, McLaurin E, Heah T, Ramirez-Davis N, Usner DW, Novack GD, Kopczynski CC, ROCKET-1 and ROCKET-2 Study Groups. Two phase 3 clinical trials comparing the safety and efficacy of Netarsudil to Timolol in patients with elevated intraocular pressure: rho kinase elevated IOP treatment trial 1 and 2 (ROCKET-1 and ROCKET-2). Am J Ophthalmol. 2018;186:116–27.
162. Weinreb RN, Liebmann JM, Martin KR, Kaufman PL, Vittitow JL. Latanoprostene bunod 0.024% in subjects with open-angle glaucoma or ocular hypertension: pooled phase 3 study findings. J Glaucoma. 2018;27(1):7–15.
163. Barraza RA, Rasmussen CA, Loewen N, Cameron JD, Gabelt BT, Teo WL, Kaufman PL, Poeschla EM. Prolonged transgene expression with lentiviral vectors in the aqueous humor outflow pathway of nonhuman primates. Hum Gene Ther. 2009;20(3):191–200.
164. Buie LK, Rasmussen CA, Porterfield EC, Ramgolam VS, Choi VW, Markovic-Plese S, Samulski RJ, Kaufman PL, Borrás T. Self-complementary AAV virus (scAAV) safe and long-term gene transfer in the trabecular meshwork of living rats and monkeys. Invest Ophthalmol Vis Sci. 2010;51(1):236–48.
165. Aktas Z, Tian B, McDonald J, Yamamato R, Larsen C, Kiland J, Kaufman PL, Rasmussen CA. Application of canaloplasty in glaucoma gene therapy: where are we? J Ocul Pharmacol Ther. 2014;30(2–3):277–82.
166. Lewallen M, Xie T. Cell-based therapies for retinal degenerative diseases: a thousand strategies. J Glaucoma. 2013;22(Suppl 5):S42–5.

167. Eveleth DD. Cell-based therapies for ocular disease. J Ocul Pharmacol Ther. 2013;29(10):844–54.
168. Cyranoski D. Stem cells cruise to clinic. Nature. 2013;494(7438):413.
169. Wright LS, Phillips MJ, Pinilla I, Hei D, Gamm DM. Induced pluripotent stem cells as custom therapeutics for retinal repair: Progress and rationale. Exp Eye Res. 2014;123:161–72. pii: S0014-4835(13)00345-X.
170. Phillips MJ, Capowski EE, Petersen A, Jansen AD, Barlow K, Edwards KL, Gamm DM. Generation of a rod-specific NRL reporter line in human pluripotent stem cells. Sci Rep. 2018;8(1):2370.
171. Leach LL, Croze RH, Hu Q, Nadar VP, Clevenger TN, Pennington BO, Gamm DM, Clegg DO. Induced pluripotent stem cell-derived retinal pigmented epithelium: a comparative study between cell lines and differentiation methods. J Ocul Pharmacol Ther. 2016;32(5):317–30.
172. Singh R, Phillips MJ, Kuai D, Meyer J, Martin JM, Smith MA, Perez ET, Shen W, Wallace KA, Capowski EE, Wright LS, Gamm DM. Functional analysis of serially expanded human iPS cell-derived RPE cultures. Invest Ophthalmol Vis Sci. 2013;54(10):6767–78.
173. Langer KB, Ohlemacher SK, Phillips MJ, Fligor CM, Jiang P, Gamm DM, Meyer JS. Retinal ganglion cell diversity and subtype specification from human pluripotent stem cells. Stem Cell Reports. 2018;10(4):1282–93.
174. Zhu W, Jain A, Gramlich OW, Tucker BA, Sheffield VC, Kuehn MH. Restoration of aqueous humor outflow following transplantation of iPSC-derived trabecular meshwork cells in a transgenic mouse model of glaucoma. Invest Ophthalmol Vis Sci. 2017;58(4):2054–62.
175. Abu-Hassan DW, Li X, Ryan EI, Acott TS, Kelley MJ. Induced pluripotent stem cells restore function in a human cell loss model of open-angle glaucoma. Stem Cells. 2015;33(3):751–61. https://doi.org/10.1002/stem.1885.
176. Johnson TV, DeKorver NW, Levasseur VA, Osborne A, Tassoni A, Lorber B, Heller JP, Villasmil R, Bull ND, Martin KR, Tomarev SI. Identification of retinal ganglion cell neuroprotection conferred by platelet-derived growth factor through analysis of the mesenchymal stem cell secretome. Brain. 2014;137:503–19.
177. Levkovitch-Verbin H, Sadan O, Vander S, Rosner M, Barhum Y, Melamed E, Offen D, Melamed S. Intravitreal injections of neurotrophic factors secreting mesenchymal stem cells are neuroprotective in rat eyes following optic nerve transection. Invest Ophthalmol Vis Sci. 2010;51:6394–400.
178. Harper MM, Grozdanic SD, Blits B, Kuehn MH, Zamzow D, Buss JE, Kardon RH, Sakaguchi DS. Transplantation of bdnf secreting mesenchymal stem cells provides neuroprotection in chronically hypertensive rat eyes. Invest Ophthalmol Vis Sci. 2011;52:4506–15.
179. Johnson TV, Bull ND, Hunt DP, Marina N, Tomarev SI, Martin KR. Neuroprotective effects of intravitreal mesenchymal stem cell transplantation in experimental glaucoma. Invest Ophthalmol Vis Sci. 2010;51(4):2051–9.
180. Osborne A, Sanderson J, Martin KR. Neuroprotective effects of human mesenchymal stem cells and platelet-derived growth factor on human retinal ganglion cells. Stem Cells. 2018;36(1):65–78. https://doi.org/10.1002/stem.2722.
181. Divya MS, Rasheed VA, Schmidt T, Lalitha S, Hattar S, James J. Intraocular injection of ES cell-derived neural progenitors improve visual function in retinal ganglion cell-depleted mouse models. Front Cell Neurosci. 2017;11:295. https://doi.org/10.3389/fncel.2017.00295. eCollection 2017.
182. Braunger BM, Ademoglu B, Koschade SE, Fuchshofer R, Gabelt BT, Kiland JA, Hennes-Beann EA, Brunner KG, Kaufman PL, Tamm ER. Identification of adult stem cells in Schwalbe's line region of the primate eye. Invest Ophthalmol Vis Sci. 2014;55(11):7499–507.
183. Yun H, Zhou Y, Wills A, Du Y. Stem cells in the trabecular meshwork for regulating intraocular pressure. J Ocul Pharmacol Ther. 2016;32(5):253–60. https://doi.org/10.1089/jop.2016.0005.
184. Zhang Y, Cai S, Tseng SCG, Zhu YT. Isolation and expansion of multipotent progenitors from human trabecular meshwork. Sci Rep. 2018;8(1):2814.
185. Alvarado J, Murphy C, Juster R. Trabecular meshwork cellularity in primary open-angle glaucoma and nonglaucomatous normals. Ophthalmology. 1984;91(6):564–79.

6 Combined Use of Pharmaceutical Agents

Junyi Chen and Xinghuai Sun

Abstract

A combination of anti-glaucoma drugs is often required to achieve the target intraocular pressure when treating glaucoma. The efficacy and safety of combining these drugs are discussed in the first part of this chapter. Since patients with glaucoma also often suffer from systemic illnesses, such as hypertension, cardiovascular disease, and respiratory diseases, we also discuss the potential problems associated with glaucoma medications and systemic therapies for these conditions in this chapter. Elevated intraocular pressure or glaucoma can occur following many ophthalmic therapeutic procedures. How to identify and treat this type of glaucoma is discussed. Finally, combined uses of systemic and topical agents to control higher IOP are briefly discussed at the end of the chapter.

Keywords

Anti-glaucoma drugs · Combined use
Systemic disease · Triamcinolone acetonide
Dexamethasone intravitreal implant
Systemic agents

Glaucoma is the most common cause of irreversible blindness, for which the only effective treatment is to reduce the intraocular pressure (IOP) to within a target range. Typical treatment for glaucoma is initiated with topical medical therapy, and pharmaceutical agents comprising five categories of anti-glaucoma medications are currently commonly used to reduce IOP: (1) beta-blockers;

J. Chen
Department of Ophthalmology & Visual Science, Eye & ENT Hospital, Shanghai Medical College, Fudan University, Shanghai, China

NHC Key Laboratory of Myopia (Fudan University), Key Laboratory of Myopia, Chinese Academy of Medical Sciences, Shanghai, China

Shanghai Key Laboratory of Visual Impairment and Restoration (Fudan University), Shanghai, China

X. Sun (✉)
Department of Ophthalmology & Visual Science, Eye & ENT Hospital, Shanghai Medical College, Fudan University, Shanghai, China

NHC Key Laboratory of Myopia (Fudan University), Key Laboratory of Myopia, Chinese Academy of Medical Sciences, Shanghai, China

Shanghai Key Laboratory of Visual Impairment and Restoration (Fudan University), Shanghai, China

State Key Laboratory of Medical Neurobiology, Institutes of Brain Science and Collaborative Innovation Center for Brain Science, Fudan University, Shanghai, China
e-mail: xhsun@shmu.edu.cn

X. Sun, Y. Dai (eds.), *Medical Treatment of Glaucoma*,
https://doi.org/10.1007/978-981-13-2733-9_6

(2) alpha-adrenergic agonists; (3) carbonic anhydrase inhibitors (CAIs); (4) prostaglandin analogues (PGAs); and (5) cholinergics (miotics). The use of a single therapeutic to treat glaucoma (monotherapy) is beneficial to both the clinician and patient. However, in actual clinical practice, glaucoma patients often require combination therapy to achieve the target IOP and may also have a variety of concurrent conditions that require systemic medications [1, 2]. Many glaucoma medications also have associated side effects and can interact with other prescribed therapies. Therefore, the safe and effective combination of drugs is an issue that clinicians must consider carefully when treating patients with glaucoma.

6.1 Combinations of Anti-glaucoma Agents

Historically, beta-blockers were the preferred agent for treating glaucoma. However, the use of prostaglandin analogues (PGAs) as a monotherapy has emerged as a first-line treatment for patients with primary open-angle glaucoma (POAG) or ocular hypertension. PGSs are beneficial due to the high IOP-reduction efficacy (decreasing the IOP by approximately 30%), diurnal and circadian IOP regulation, and control of IOP fluctuations.

For the combined use of anti-glaucoma agents, there are some principles we should keep in mind (Fig. 6.1). Firstly, the aim of combined use is to complement each medication to strengthen their effect of lowering IOP. There are combinations of IOP-lowering agents each with different mechanisms, including: (1) enhancing the aqueous humor outflow in combination with decreasing aqueous humor formation; (2) increasing aqueous humor outflow by trabecular meshwork (pressure-sensitive outflow, traditional pathway) in combination with uveoscleral outflow (pressure-insensitive outflow, non-traditional pathway); or (3) suppressing aqueous humor formation through inhibiting carbonic anhydrase combined with a β_2-receptor blockade. Secondly, these situations should be avoided for the combined use of anti-glaucoma agents (e.g., one β-blocker in combination with another β-blocker, or one PGA in combination with another PGA). In these cases, control of IOP will not be enhanced and there will be increased adverse reactions.

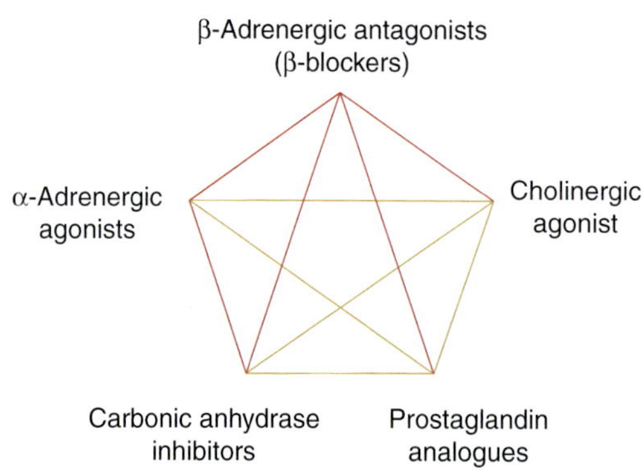

Fig. 6.1 Combined use of five categories of anti-glaucoma medications. Red line: available fixed combinations

Recently, fixed combinations of anti-glaucoma agents have been commonly prescribed for glaucoma patients who require two or more eyedrops to control IOP. Fixed combinations are medications (i.e., two drugs, occasionally three drugs) combined in a single bottle. They have the potential benefits of improved convenience, patient adherence, and psychological effects, as well as reduced drug wash-out, adverse effects due to preservatives, and cost. In general, the efficacy of fixed combination formulations is similar to that of the components instilled separately. However, the adverse effects and contraindications are the same as each drug given individually. It is an interesting clinical phenomenon that fewer ocular adverse effects may occur when using the fixed combinations than when both drugs individually administered.

6.1.1 Requirement for Adjunctive Glaucoma Therapies

In this section, we mainly discuss the efficacy of adjunct therapies for patients who have been previously treated with PGA as a first-line therapeutic, but the target IOP has not been reached. In both published reports and clinical settings, there are many patients who must be treated with adjunctive agents to sufficiently reduce the IOP, despite prior PGA treatment. The Ocular Hypertension Treatment Study (OHTS) [1] investigated the treatment efficacy of various medications for patients with glaucoma exhibiting an increased IOP. The results revealed that more than 40% of the enrolled patients required at least two medications to reduce the target IOP by ≥20% of the baseline level. In addition, the recent Collaborative Initial Glaucoma Treatment Study (CIGTS) [2] is assessing the efficacy of a trabeculectomy as a potential first-line therapy for patients who have been newly diagnosed with glaucoma. It has been found that the majority of the patients included in the treatment group of the CIGTS require a minimum of two medications to achieve an aggressive reduction of about 35% from baseline.

Selecting an appropriate adjunctive therapy for the treatment of glaucoma is challenging. Thus, several criteria have been established to aid in the selection of an agent that can be used in conjunction with a PGA, including: (1) whether the agent is safe and well-tolerated are the most important factors to be considered; (2) the agent's efficacy. For patients who are being treated with a monotherapy, an additional reduction of 15% is expected following treatment with a second medication; (3) the second agent's mechanism of action. For example, the enhanced aqueous outflow induced by a PGA can be complimented by selecting an adjunctive therapy that reduces the IOP through decreasing aqueous humor production; and (4) the convenience of the regimen, which should be straight-forward to ensure patient compliance.

6.1.2 β-Adrenergic Antagonists

Combining topical β-adrenergic antagonists, or a β-blocker (an aqueous inflow suppressant that reduces the production of cyclic adenosine monophosphate [cAMP] in the ciliary epithelium), with the aqueous-outflow-enhancing properties of a PGA, (increases outflow via the uveoscleral pathway and decreases outflow resistance to a variable extent), makes sense clinically because the mechanisms of action of these drugs are complementary. Several clinical studies have reported that such combinations did indeed achieve an additional reduction in IOP and were equally effective at lowering IOPs with a PGA and β-blocker in either fixed or unfixed combinations. However, some studies have not been encouraging regarding this combination. Bucci et al. found a similar reduction in the mean diurnal IOP with latanoprost and timolol compared with that achieved with latanoprost alone (6.1 ± 0.3 mmHg vs 5.5 ± 0.3 mmHg, respectively) [3]. Moreover, Manni et al. recently observed no significant difference in the mean diurnal IOP between patients treated with 0.03% bimatoprost or latanoprost and timolol combination therapy after 6 months of treatment [4]. In addition, Higginbotham et al. compared treatment with latanoprost alone with that of fixed latanoprost and timolol combination therapy, and found that the fixed combination produced a final mean diurnal IOP < 1 mmHg lower than that of latanoprost monotherapy (19.9 ± 3.4 vs 20.8 ± 4.6 mmHg, respectively) after 6 months of treatment [5]. Since β-blockers do not contribute additional IOP-lowering efficacy, no combined PGA/β-blocker agents have been formally approved for clinical use by the US Food and Drug Administration.

6.1.3 α-Adrenergic Agonists

Brimonidine is a α_2-selective agent that is currently the most commonly used α-adrenergic agonist for the treatment of glaucoma. While it is recommended that brimonidine be administered three times daily, clinicians typically prescribe two doses per day when used as an adjunctive therapy. In a large, open-label, phase IV community trial conducted in 2001, when brimonidine was combined with latanoprost, the IOP was reduced by an additional 32% (5.9 mmHg; $p < 0.001$) [6]. Other post-marketing studies have shown that both 0.2% brimonidine and 0.15% brimonidine-P as adjunctive therapies can effectively reduce the IOP by an additional 2.0–5.1 mmHg when used with a PGA [7, 8].

6.1.4 Topical Carbonic Anhydrase Inhibitors

Topical carbonic anhydrase inhibitors (CAIs), which include brinzolamide and dorzolamide, decrease IOP via suppressing the production of aqueous humors. Studies evaluating the efficacy of dorzolamide as an adjunctive therapy to latanoprost have shown additional IOP reductions of as high as 3 mmHg and overall IOP reductions of approximately 40% from baseline [9, 10]. It has also been found that brinzolamide can act additively with a PGA, by reducing the IOP by an additional 4.2 mmHg (18.4%) when administered to patients with POAG or ocular hypertension undergoing treatment with travoprost, and an additional IOP reduction of 5.2 mmHg (24.6%) when used as an adjunct agent with latanoprost [11, 12]. In addition, topical CAI combined with a PGA has been found to effectively and continuously control IOP for 24 h. Nakamoto and Yasuda demonstrated a significant reduction in both the diurnal and nocturnal mean IOP in 22 patients with normal-tension glaucoma treated for 8 weeks with brinzolamide and latanoprost combination therapy compared to latanoprost treatment alone [13].

6.2 Interactions Between Glaucoma Agents and Other Systemic Therapies

The prevalence of both glaucoma and various other systemic diseases gradually increases with age. Therefore, glaucoma patients may have a variety of concurrent conditions that require systemic medication. Many glaucoma medications potentially cause systemic side effects and/or interact with other prescription agents.

6.2.1 Hypertension and Cardiovascular Risk

Several risk factors associated with POAG have been established, such as age, ethnicity, family history, myopia, ocular hypertension, and vascular conditions (e.g., systemic hypertension, systemic hypotension, low diastolic perfusion pressure, and impaired ocular blood flow). Moreover, since treatments for systemic hypertension can impact the incidence or progression of POAG, they are also considered to be risk factors.

Diastolic ocular perfusion pressure (DOPP) is the driving force responsible for the movement of blood into the eye and is calculated as the diastolic blood pressure (DBP) minus the IOP. In the Baltimore Eye Survey, systemic hypotension and low DOPP increased the prevalence of POAG. While a reduction in the IOP will improve DOPP, a decreased DBP will exacerbate DOPP. Therefore, medication that alters either the IOP or blood pressure can affect the perfusion pressure. There are evidences that have shown that nocturnal hypotension is involved in glaucoma pathogenesis. Moreover, in patients with nocturnal hypotension, visual field defect progression has been associated with systemic antihypertensives. While angiotensin-converting enzyme (ACE) inhibitors and calcium channel blockers (CCBs) have been shown to exacerbate normal nocturnal hypotension, treatment with β-blockers and angiotensin receptor blockers have not. Langman et al. [14] showed that oral β-blockers exert significant protection against glaucoma (OR: 0.77), whereas oral CCBs and ACE inhibitors significantly increased the risk of developing glaucoma (OR 1.34 and 1.16, respectively). Moreover, in the same study, the use of diuretics did not exhibit any significant effect [14]. In the Rotterdam Study, patients using CCBs were found to have a significantly increased (1.8-fold) risk of developing glaucoma [15]. In addition, treatment with β-blockers was not associated with a significantly reduced risk of developing glaucoma (OR: 0.60), and other antihypertensive therapies did not have an impact on open-angle glaucoma incidence [15]. Thus, β-blockers appear to be extremely well-tolerated antihypertensive agents in patients with glaucoma, and there is evidence to suggest that they may also exert a protective effect. In contrast, other medications (e.g., diuretics, CCBs, and ACE blockers) have been linked to a higher risk of developing glaucoma [16–18].

In addition to the impact of systemic hypertensive drugs on the progression of glaucoma, anti-glaucoma agents (especially β-blockers) can also interact with hypertensive drugs. Systemic β-blockers can exacerbate hypotension or bradycardia when combined with a topical β-blocker. Therefore, it is important to monitor the blood pressure and heart rate of glaucoma patients. ACE inhibitors are used to treat hypertension and can potentially cause hypotension. CCBs may interact with topical β-blockers and can cause an irregular heartbeat. Cardiac glycosides combined with CCBs and β-blockers can also slow the heart rate [19].

Bradycardia and hypotension are potential responses to the administration of topical apraclonidine. A significant decrease in the changes in the heart rate and blood pressure was found to be associated with these factors compared to the effect exhibited by ophthalmic timolol. Brimonidine was found to have a minimal effect on both heart rate and blood pressure.

6.2.2 Asthma and Obstructive Lung Disease

An inhibition of lung bronchodilating β_2-receptors has been shown to exaggerate and induce bronchospasms in patients with asthma or obstructive lung disease with a significant reactive component. Therefore, a β-adrenergic blocker should not be prescribed to patients with asthma unless other treatment options are exhausted and the patient's diseases are stable and mild to moderate in severity; in such situations, betaxolol, a β_1-selective β-adrenergic blocker, is the recommended treatment. Since patients with chronic obstructive pulmonary disease (COPD) have a differential degree of reactive airway disease compared to patients with asthma, ophthalmic β-adrenergic blockers may be potential treatment options if they suffer concomitant glaucoma [20]. One meta-analysis found that systemic β_1-selective blockers were safe for patients with COPD of mild to moderate severity [21].

6.2.3 Depression

Historically, it was widely believed that β-blockers were a category of drugs linked to depression, cognitive dysfunction, insomnia, memory loss, and other neuropsychiatric disturbances. Since the first case report in 1967, several case reports and series have been published to support these associations. The majority of these reports were associated with propranolol, a highly lipophilic early-generation β-blocker. However, over time, randomized clinical trials and meta-analyses have presented data that argues against a causal association between β-blockers and depression. A population-based cohort study by Kaiserman et al. investigated whether there was a relationship between ophthalmic β-blockers and depression, and found no difference between the subjects using β-blockers and those who were not, even after adjusting for age [22]. These findings add to the existing evidence from clinical trials and population-based studies that support a lack of a relationship between β-blockers and depression.

6.3 Medical Management for Elevated IOP After Ophthalmic Procedures

Elevated IOP and secondary glaucoma may occur following ophthalmic procedures. Since the risk factors differ between each ophthalmic procedure, follow-up monitoring is of particular importance for patients who are at an increased risk of developing IOP. The pathophysiology can be attributed to both open- and closed-angle mechanisms and can strongly influence the management of secondary elevated IOP. Regardless of the reasons for elevated IOP, treatment with cartelolol, one of non-selective β-blockers but with intrinsic sympathomimetic action (ISA), is seemingly adequate for those cases after ophthalmic procedures because it also has significant inhibitory effect on the inflammatory response caused by surgery.

6.3.1 Increased IOP/Glaucoma After Pars Plana Vitrectomy

A common complication associated with pars plana vitrectomy (PPV) is elevated IOP. Han et al. conducted a prospective study that found an acute increase in IOP of 5–22 mmHg within 48 h of PPV and an acute increase in IOP of >30 mmHg in 60% and 36% of patients, respectively. The majority of post-vitrectomy glaucoma is secondary open-angle glaucoma (OAG), with approximately 20% of cases attributed to angle closure mechanisms. OAG can be caused by gas expansion without angle closure, inflammation, the use of silicone oil without a pupillary block, responses to corticosteroids, or blood-mediated mechanisms. A pupillary block mediated by intraocular gas, silicone oil, fibrin, or an intraocular lens, and ciliary body edema and irido-corneal apposition comprise angle closure mechanisms [23].

It is important to monitor IOP during the early postoperative period when a long-acting gas is used, and the associated tonometer should be noted. The IOP was found to be underestimated by pneumatic tonometry performed on gas-filled eyes from a human autopsy. It was found that the pressure readings from the Tono-Pen (Reichert Technologies, NY, USA) were similar to that of Goldmann applanation tonometry, whereas the IOP was underestimated by pneumatic tonometry in a clinical study involving 84 gas-filled eyes [24].

Management may consist of using topical therapies used as a monotherapy or in combination with surgery and/or laser treatment. Topical therapies (e.g., cycloplegics, corticosteroids, β-blockers, and PGAs) have been found to successfully control IOP in 30–78% of patients. Whether PGAs can be used to treat patients who have undergone a vitrectomy remains controversial due to the potential reactivation of inflammation and detrimental effects on the blood–aqueous barrier. However, studies involving human subjects have shown that there are no changes in the blood–aqueous barrier following treatment with latanoprost. Furthermore, experimental studies have found that neither latanoprost nor other PGAs induce chemotaxis, a marker of inflammation [25]. Therefore, PGAs are no longer prohibited for the treatment of postoperative intraocular hypertension. Finally, it is important to note that the use of PGAs in eyes after a vitrectomy is associated with a potential risk of cystoid macular edema (i.e., eyes with aphakia or pseudophakia) [26].

6.3.2 Glaucoma Associated with Penetrating Keratoplasty

Penetrating keratoplasty (PKP) can be complicated during both early and late postoperative periods by a significant elevation in IOP. The incidence of glaucoma following PKP is associated with the following factors: recipients older than 60 years; aphakia, preexisting glaucoma; bullous keratopathy; herpetic keratitis; trauma; keratoconus; anterior segment reconstruction; vitrectomy; and a preoperative diagnosis of adherent leukoma [27].

In some cases, postoperative glaucoma after PKP is associated with elevated pressure caused by mechanisms common to other intraocular methods (e.g., uveitis, hemorrhage, pupillary block, and steroid-induced glaucoma). There are two other mechanisms associated with postoperative glaucoma that are exclusive to the eyes following PKP: (1) trabecular meshwork collapse may occur due to a loss of anterior support following an incision of the Descemet membrane, which can be further complicated in eyes with aphakia due to reduced posterior support resulting from a loss in zonular tension. The anterior chamber angle may be compressed by PKP techniques, which may cause an early increase in postoperative IOP promoting the development of chronic glaucoma arising from peripheral anterior synechiae; and (2) graft rejection may also increase the IOP, which will likely require long-term treatment with steroids and anti-glaucoma medications [28–32].

While medicinal therapies should be administered first, most attempts to treat early postoperative elevations in IOP typically fail. The β-blockers, especially cartelolol, are recommended to control elevated IOP [33]. Although CAIs are not significantly effective, they can be used to treat chronic glaucoma. It is important to note that eyes exhibiting compromised endothelial cell functionality may be more susceptible to corneal decompensation following treatment with topical CAIs. Generally, a miotic agent should not be used. If the optic nerve head or graft survival is threatened by chronic IOP elevation, surgery is recommended.

6.3.3 IOP Elevation After Glaucoma Laser Treatment (Laser Iridotomy or Laser Trabeculoplasty)

Few complications are associated with laser treatment for glaucoma. However, up to 50% of patients experience a transient spike in IOP due to laser induced inflammation. The elevated IOP that occurs post-laser treatment is more frequent and severe in eyes with a darker iris. Elevated IOP is usually observed and occurs 1–4 h following a laser iridotomy or trabeculoplasty and is typically self-limiting. Anti-inflammatory drops and IOP-lowering agents, such as an α-adrenergic agonist, β-blocker, CAIs, or osmotic agent, are suggested treatment options. Most physicians recommend one drop of topical apraclonidine or topical brimonidine prior to treatment to prevent increased IOP post-laser surgery, and some also recommend one drop after treatment because these drugs are effective and lack adverse effects with short-term use. It is common for the IOP to return to pretreatment levels or lower within 24 h naturally; however, elevated IOP can be severe and sustained in glaucoma caused by combination mechanisms, which exhibit an abnormal outflow prior to surgery (e.g., exfoliative syndrome or pigment dispersion). Therefore, these patients should be informed before undergoing laser surgery that filtering surgery may be needed should there be an uncontrollable increase in IOP.

6.3.4 Elevated IOP After an Intravitreal Injection of Triamcinolone Acetonide or Dexamethasone Implant

An intravitreal injection of corticosteroids (e.g., triamcinolone acetonide or dexamethasone implant) has become a popular treatment for diabetic macular edema, macular edema associated with retinal vein occlusion, and several posterior-pole inflammatory conditions. Approximately one-third of eyes undergoing these treatments will exhibit a short-lived increase in IOP [34, 35]. In some patients, a persistent elevation in IOP may require topical medication, laser trabeculoplasty, or even a trabeculectomy to reduce the pressure and prevent the onset or progression of damage to the optic nerve. Risk factors for elevated IOP during the post-injection period include preexisting glaucoma, younger age, high doses of triamcinolone, high baseline IOP, uveitis, or repeated injections [36, 37].

The mechanism associated with how glucocorticoids increase IOP by reducing outflow facility remains poorly understood. One common explanation is that an accumulation of glycosaminoglycans in the trabecular meshwork caused by glucocorticoids stabilizes lysosomal membranes and inhibits the release of catabolic enzymes [38]. The first step in managing this clinical condition is the administration of an anti-glaucoma medication to control IOP. All IOP-lowering agents, especially PGAs, are safe and effective in patients with steroid-induced glaucoma [39]. It is necessary to stop or remove glucocorticoids to control the elevated IOP. Substituting therapies for those with a decreased risk of inducing IOP elevation is preferred in cases requiring glucocorticoid treatment. Filtering surgery or laser trabeculoplasty should be recommended when the prescribed treatments cannot successfully control the IOP and there is risk that the optic nerve could be damaged.

6.4 Systemic and Topical Agents for Highly Elevated IOP

There is another combination use of systemic agents if topical drugs cannot control a highly increased IOP. Systemic therapy for a higher IOP may be administered orally (e.g., CAI, diuretics, and hypertonic agents) or intravenously (e.g., CAI, diuretics, and hypertonic agents). The most common oral CAIs are sustained-release acetazolamide and methazolamide, which begin to lower IOP within 1 h of treatment, exhibiting a maximal response within 2–4 h and is maintained for 6–8 h. No advantage has been found for patients receiving an oral administration of CAI.

Hyperosmotic agents, including oral glycerol and intravenous mannitol, are used to control acute episodes of elevated IOP or a very high IOP in chronic cases, commonly as combined usage with topical eye drops. The IOP begins to decline within 15 min of the administration of intravenous mannitol, its maximal effect is observed within 30–60 min, and the effect is maintained for 3–8 h.

Systemic agents are not intended for prolonged use and only recommended for emergency situation, since their IOP-lowering effects are transient and are associated with more adverse effects. It should be kept in the mind that topical drugs are basic agents used for glaucoma control, whereas systemic agents are prescribed to meet emergency conditions.

References

1. Kass MA, Heuer DK, Higginbotham EJ, et al. The ocular hypertension treatment study: a randomized trial determines that topical ocular hypotensive medication delays or prevents the onset of primary open angle glaucoma. Arch Ophthalmol. 2002;120(6):701–13.
2. Lichter PR, Musch DC, Gillespie BW, et al. Interim clinical outcomes in the collaborative initial glaucoma treatment study comparing initial treatment randomized to medications or surgery. Ophthalmology. 2001;108(11):1943–53.
3. Bucci MG. Intraocular pressure-lowering effects of latanoprost monotherapy versus latanoprost or pilocarpine in combination with timolol: a randomized, observer-masked multicenter study in patients with open-angle glaucoma. Italian Latanoprost Study Group. J Glaucoma. 1999;8(1):24–30.
4. Manni G, Centofanti M, Parravano M, et al. A 6-month randomized clinical trial of bimatoprost 0.03% versus the association of timolol 0.5% and latanoprost 0.005% in glaucomatous patients. Graefes Arch Clin Exp Ophthalmol. 2004;242(9):767–70.
5. Higginbotham EJ, Feldman R, Stiles M, et al. Latanoprost and timolol combination therapy vs. monotherapy: one-year randomized trial. Arch Ophthalmol. 2002;120(7):915–22.
6. Lee DA, Gornbein JA. Effectiveness and safety of brimonidine as adjunctive therapy for patients with elevated intraocular pressure in a large, open-label community trial. J Glaucoma. 2001;10(3):220–6.
7. Erdogan H, Toker I, Arici MK, et al. A short-term study of the additive effect of latanoprost 0.005% and brimonidine 0.2%. Jpn J Ophthalmol. 2003;47(5):473–8.
8. Mundorf T, Noecker RJ, Earl M. Ocular hypotensive efficacy of brimonidine 0.15% as adjunctive therapy with latanoprost 0.005% in patients with open-angle glaucoma or ocular hypertension. Adv Ther. 2007;24:302–9.
9. Arici MK, Topalkara A, Guler C. Additive effect of latanoprost and dorzolamide in patients with elevated intraocular pressure. Int Ophthalmol. 1998;22(1):37–42.
10. Chiselita D, Apatachioae I, Poiata I. The ocular hypotensive effect of the combination of latanoprost with dorzolamide. Oftalmologia. 1999;46(4):39–45.
11. Franks W, Brinzolamide Study Group. Ocular hypotensive efficacy and safety of brinzolamide ophthalmic suspension 1% added to travoprost ophthalmic solution 0.004% therapy in patients with open-angle glaucoma or ocular hypertension. Curr Med Res Opin. 2006;22(9):1643–9.
12. Shoji N, Ogata H, Suyama H, et al. Intraocular pressure lowering effect of brinzolamide 1.0% as adjunctive therapy to latanoprost 0.005% in patients with open-angle glaucoma or ocular hypertension: an uncontrolled, open-label study. Curr Med Res Opin. 2005;21(4):503–8.
13. Nakamoto K, Yasuda N. Effect of concomitant use of latanoprost and brinzolamide on 24-hour variation of IOP in normal-tension glaucoma. J Glaucoma. 2007;16(4):352–7.
14. Langman MJ, Lancashire RJ, Cheng KK, et al. Systemic hypertension and glaucoma: mechanisms in common and co-occurrence. Br J Ophthalmol. 2005;89(8):960–3.
15. Khawaja AP, Chan MP, Broadway DC, et al. Systemic medication and intraocular pressure in a British population: the EPIC-Norfolk Eye Study. Ophthalmology. 2014;121(8):1501–7.
16. Deokule S, Weinreb RN. Relationships among systemic blood pressure, intraocular pressure, and open-angle glaucoma. Can J Ophthalmol. 2008;43(3):302–7.
17. Tielsch JM, Katz J, Sommer A, et al. Hypertension, perfusion pressure, and primary open-angle glaucoma. A population-based assessment. Arch Ophthalmol. 1995;113(2):216–21.
18. Hayreh SS, Zimmerman MB, Podhajsky P, et al. Nocturnal arterial hypotension and its role in optic nerve head and ocular ischemic disorders. Am J Ophthalmol. 1994;117(5):603–24.
19. Muskens RP, de Voogd S, Wolfs RC, et al. Systemic antihypertensive medication and incident open-angle glaucoma. Ophthalmology. 2007;114(12):2221–6.
20. Salpeter SR, Ormiston TM, Salpeter EE, et al. Cardioselective beta-blockers for chronic obstructive pulmonary disease: a meta-analysis. Respir Med. 2003;97(10):1094–101.
21. Salpeter SR, Ormiston TM, Salpeter EE. Cardioselective beta-blockers in patients with reactive airway disease: a meta-analysis. Ann Intern Med. 2002;137(9):715–25.

22. Kaiserman I, Kaiserman N, Elhayany A, et al. Topical beta-blockers are not associated with an increased risk of treatment for depression. Ophthalmology. 2006;113(7):1077–80.
23. Honavar SG, Goyal M, Majji AB, et al. Glaucoma after pars plana vitrectomy and silicone oil injection for complicated retinal detachments. Ophthalmology. 1999;106(1):169–76. discussion 177.
24. Hines MW, Jost BF, Fogelman KL. Oculab Tono-Pen, Goldmann applanation tonometry, and pneumatic tonometry for intraocular pressure assessment in gas-filled eyes. Am J Ophthalmol. 1988;106(2):174–9.
25. Stjernschantz JW. From PGF(2alpha)-isopropyl ester to latanoprost: a review of the development of xalatan: the Proctor Lecture. Invest Ophthalmol Vis Sci. 2001;42(6):1134–45.
26. Schumer RA, Camras CB, Mandahl AK. Latanoprost and cystoid macular edema: is there a causal relation? Curr Opin Ophthalmol. 2000;11(2):94–100.
27. Karesh JW, Nirankari VS. Factors associated with glaucoma after penetrating keratoplasty. Am J Ophthalmol. 1983;96(2):160–4.
28. Foulks GN. Glaucoma associated with penetrating keratoplasty. Ophthalmology. 1987;94(7):871–4.
29. Goldberg DB, Schanzlin DJ, Brown SI. Incidence of increased intraocular pressure after keratoplasty. Am J Ophthalmol. 1981;92(3):372–7.
30. Zimmerman TJ, Krupin T, Grodzki W, et al. The effect of suture depth on outflow facility in penetrating keratoplasty. Arch Ophthalmol. 1978;96(3):505–6.
31. Olson RJ, Kaufman HE. A mathematical description of causative factors and prevention of elevated intraocular pressure after keratoplasty. Invest Ophthalmol Vis Sci. 1977;16(12):1085–92.
32. Polack FM. Graft rejection and glaucoma. Am J Ophthalmol. 1986;101(3):294–7.
33. Olson RJ, Kaufman HE, Zimmerman TJ. Effects of timolol and Daranide on elevated intraocular pressure after aphakic keratoplasty. Ann Ophthalmol. 1979;11(12):1833–6.
34. Vasconcelos-Santos DV, Nehemy PG, Schachat AP, et al. Secondary ocular hypertension after intravitreal injection of 4 mg of triamcinolone acetonide: incidence and risk factors. Retina. 2008;28(4):573–80.
35. Boyer DS, Yoon YH, Belfort R Jr, et al. Three-year, randomized, sham-controlled trial of dexamethasone intravitreal implant in patients with diabetic macular edema. Ophthalmology. 2014;121(10):1904–14.
36. Inatani M, Iwao K, Kawaji T, et al. Intraocular pressure elevation after injection of triamcinolone acetonide: a multicenter retrospective case-control study. Am J Ophthalmol. 2008;145(4):676–81.
37. Galor A, Margolis R, Brasil OM, et al. Adverse events after intravitreal triamcinolone in patients with and without uveitis. Ophthalmology. 2007;114(10):1912–8.
38. Francois J. The importance of the mucopolysaccharides in intraocular pressure regulation. Investig Ophthalmol. 1975;14(3):173–6.
39. Scherer WJ, Hauber FA. Effect of latanoprost on intraocular pressure in steroid-induced glaucoma. J Glaucoma. 2000;9(2):179–82.

Novel Therapeutic Targets for Glaucoma: Disease Modification Treatment, Neuroprotection, and Neuroregeneration

7

Jacky Man Kwong Kwong and Iok-Hou Pang

Abstract

Current treatments for primary open-angle glaucoma, be they medication or surgery, only manage the symptom of ocular hypertension. They do not address the underlying mechanisms of pathogenesis or pathophysiology of the disease. Therefore, they do not alter the progression of the glaucomatous pathological changes. In contrast, this chapter explores potential therapeutic targets that aim to correct and/or reverse the pathological changes based on our understanding of the molecular and cellular mechanisms involved in the disorder. Therapies based on these targets, which are related to the trabecular meshwork, retina, or optic nerve, if proven successful, will revolutionize the treatment of this devastating blinding disease.

J. M. K. Kwong
Stein Eye Institute, Glaucoma Division, Department of Ophthalmology, David Geffen School of Medicine, University of California Los Angeles, Los Angeles, CA, USA
e-mail: kwong@jsei.ucla.edu

I.-H. Pang (✉)
Pharmaceutical Sciences, North Texas Eye Research Institute, University of North Texas Health Science Center, Fort Worth, TX, USA
e-mail: iok-hou.pang@unthsc.edu

X. Sun, Y. Dai (eds.), *Medical Treatment of Glaucoma*,
https://doi.org/10.1007/978-981-13-2733-9_7

Keywords

Glaucoma · Therapy · Therapeutic target
Disease modification · Neuroprotection
Neurorescue · Neuroregeneration

Abbreviations

4-PBA	4-Phenylbutyrate
ACE	Angiotensin-converting enzyme
ACh	Acetylcholine
ADSC	Adipose tissue-derived mesenchymal stromal cell
AGIS	Advanced Glaucoma Intervention Study
APC	Adenomatosis polyposis coli
AT1-R	Angiotensin II type 1 receptor
Aβ	Amyloid-β
BAMBI	BMP and activin membrane-bound inhibitor
BBB	Blood–brain barrier
BDNF	Brain-derived neurotrophic factor
BMP	Bone morphogenic protein
BMSC	Bone marrow-derived mesenchymal stromal cell
Brn	Brain-specific homeobox/POU domain protein
CIGT	Collaborative Initial Glaucoma Treatment Study Trial
CK1α	Casein kinase 1α
CNS	Central nervous system
CNTF	Ciliary neurotrophic factor

CNTG	Collaborative Normal Tension Glaucoma Study
DPSC	Dental pulp-derived mesenchymal-like cell
Dsh	Dishevelled
EAAT1	Excitotoxic amino acid transporter 1
ECM	Extracellular matrix
EGCG	Epigallocatechin-3-gallate
EMGT	Early Manifest Glaucoma Trial
EPO	Erythropoietin
ERG	Electroretinograph(y)
ERK	Extracellular signal-regulated kinase
ET	Endothelin
ETA	Endothelin A receptor
ETB	Endothelin B receptor
FasL	Fas ligand
Fz	Frizzled family receptors
GAP-43	Growth-associated protein-43
GGA	Geranylgeranylacetone/Teprenone
GLAST	Glutamate/aspartate transporters
GSK	Glycogen synthase kinase
HSF	Heat shock factor
HSP	Heat shock protein
IL	Interleukin
IOP	Intraocular pressure
JNK	c-Jun N-terminal kinase
LBP	L. barbarum polysaccharide
LRP	Lipoprotein receptor-related protein
MMP	Matrix metalloproteinase
MSC	Mesenchymal stromal cell
nAChR	Nicotinic acetylcholine receptor
NGF	Nerve growth factor
NMDA	*N*-methyl-D-aspartate
NMNAT1	Nicotinamide/nicotinic acid mononucleotide adenylyltransferase 1
NO	Nitric oxide
NOS	Nitric oxide synthase
OEC	Olfactory ensheathing cell
ONH	Optic nerve head
OXPHOS	Oxidative phosphorylation
p75NTR	p75 neurotrophin receptor
PERG	Pattern electroretinograph(y)
POAG	Primary open-angle glaucoma
PP2A	Protein phosphatase 2A
PPS	Peripapillary sclera
RAS	Renin–angiotensin system
RGC	Retinal ganglion cell
ROCK	Rho-associated coiled-coil protein kinase
ROS	Reactive oxygen species
SAA	Serum amyloid A
sFRP-1	Secreted frizzled-related protein-1
TCF/LEF	T-cell factor/lymphoid enhancing factor
Tfam	Mitochondrial transcription factor A
TGF	Transforming growth factor
TM	Trabecular meshwork
TNF	Tumor necrosis factor
TPGS	D-α-Tocopherol polyethylene glycol 1000 succinate
TRK	Tropomyosin-related kinase
Txn	Thioredoxin
Txnip	Thioredoxin-interacting protein

7.1 Introduction

7.1.1 Current Glaucoma Medications: Only Symptomatic Relief

As discussed in previous chapters, currently available medical treatments for primary open-angle glaucoma (POAG) aim simply to lower intraocular pressure (IOP) without managing or ameliorating the underlying disease process in the trabecular meshwork (TM). Because of that, the pathological changes continue to progress and deteriorate despite treatments, which likely explains the reduction and eventual loss of treatment efficacy after prolonged drug use. The loss of efficacy necessitates additional medications, surgical intervention, and even repeated surgical procedures. Without targeting these underlying pathological changes, any novel treatment methods, such as those being developed, i.e., Rho-associated coiled-coil protein kinase (ROCK) inhibitors, NO donors, and cytoskeleton modulators, probably will suffer from the same drawbacks and limitations, which likely lead to limited durations of efficacy after prolonged use.

Most importantly, glaucoma is diagnosed by the thinning of neural rim, and the deepening and the enlargement of the optic cup in the optic nerve head (ONH). In glaucomatous optic neuropathy, the thinning of neural tissue appears localized, expands to the neighbor rim area, and progresses to the disk margin. The reduction of nerve fiber layer thickness projects to the regional thinning of neural rim. This pattern is closely associated to the characteristic visual field loss in patients. The clinical and histological findings directly reflect the injury at the retinal ganglion cell (RGC) axons as these fibers exit the eye within the ONH and the topographical loss of RGC bodies in the retina [1, 2]. Although all current treatments are to lower IOP, glaucoma is widely accepted as a neurodegenerative disease that is related to many risk factors including IOP elevation as one of them.

To address these two unique and important developments of future therapies for glaucoma, this chapter will discuss disease modification treatment for trabecular abnormality and treatments aiming for neuroprotection and neuroregeneration. If proven successful, these approaches will provide fundamental breakthroughs for the management of this devastating disease.

7.2 Novel Therapeutic Targets for Trabecular Abnormality

7.2.1 Need for Disease Modification Treatment for Trabecular Abnormality

Based on the current understanding, abnormal reduction in aqueous outflow facility through the TM is the direct cause of IOP elevation, which is a major risk factor of POAG. Although complete networks of signaling pathways and the common initiating factor leading to the diminished TM outflow facility are yet to be fully elucidated, recent studies have produced several plausible, evidence-based mechanisms to explain the pathological changes observed in glaucoma patients. Treatment methods based on these observations and targeting the involved mechanisms should have a high likelihood of slowing down, halting, and/or even reversing the disease progression. In theory, such treatments that modify the disease progression may have two unique clinical features: (1) treatment efficacy will be maintained for a much longer duration since it is not undermined by the continuous worsening of the disease, which translates to minimizing or eliminating the need of prescribing additional drugs and eventually surgery to maintain the desired IOP and manage the disease; and (2) if the treatment can halt or reverse the disease progression, it is conceivable that the medication can be discontinued after a certain period of treatment, which will be a true case of "curing" the disease. Both of these unique features will be revolutionary in POAG therapy. Hence, disease modification treatment for TM abnormality is an important direction in new drug discovery and development for glaucoma.

7.2.2 Pathogenesis of Trabecular Abnormality

It is well established that IOP elevation in POAG patients is a direct result of a reduction in aqueous outflow through the TM, namely, a partial blockade of the trabecular outflow. The exact molecular and cellular mechanisms causing this change are not fully delineated. Morphological, histological, and biochemical studies in glaucoma patients show an excessive accumulation of extracellular matrix (ECM) in the juxtacanalicular region of the TM [3, 4], which can explain the blockade. The cytoskeleton of glaucomatous TM cells also appears to be organized differently from normal TM cells [5]. Since the TM cytoskeleton is closely linked to the ECM, these changes may synergize and alter cell rigidity and pliability [6], leading to changes of biomechanical properties of the outflow pathway and consequently outflow resistance [7, 8]. Some of the following potential therapeutic targets have been theorized to be an upstream cause of ECM accumulation, cytoskeleton reorganization, and/or cell rigidity. Other proposed targets likely affect additional pathogenesis pathways that await further clarification.

7.2.3 Therapeutic Targets

7.2.3.1 Myocilin

Myocilin and Glaucoma

Myocilin is the first confirmed gene in glaucoma, closely associated with juvenile glaucoma. Stone and colleagues reported that mutations of the myocilin gene occur in approximately 4% of glaucoma patients [9]. Subsequently, Alward et al. discovered the many different mutations related to glaucoma [10]. Various studies have corroborated that mutation of this gene is closely associated with glaucoma.

The myocilin gene (MYOC) is located in the GLC1A region of chromosome 1q. Its gene product is a glycoprotein. Dependent on the extent of glycosylation, myocilin can have two different molecular masses: 55 kDa and 57 kDa. This protein is expressed in most ocular tissues. In TM, myocilin is expressed at a high level, which is regulated by glucocorticoid, thus it is also named trabecular meshwork-inducible glucocorticoid response protein (TIGR). Despite it has been studied for many decades, its biological functions in normal TM are still unclear. Overexpression, gene knockout, or wild type myocilin does not affect IOP in the mouse [11, 12].

The exact biological function of myocilin in normal conditions is yet to be fully elucidated. However, based on studies using its mutants, we have learned how the protein may be involved in POAG. Jacobson et al. showed that disease-related mutations of myocilin prevent its secretion from cultured human TM cells [13]. Shepard et al. further reported that mutations induce conformational changes, leading to exposure of normally unexposed amino acids of the protein [14], which causes mutants to be mistakenly transported to and accumulated in peroxisomes. Accumulation of mutant myocilin activates endoplasmic reticulum stress response and interferes with TM functions. In the myocilin Y437H transgenic mouse, many POAG symptoms in human, such as ocular hypertension, optic neuropathy, RGC apoptosis, and abnormal pattern electroretinography (PERG), are observable. The TM tissues of these mice have increased the activity of endoplasmic reticulum associated protein degradation and unfolded protein response. These molecular mechanistic changes can affect the normal functions of TM. However, it is not clear if similar mechanistic changes also occur in POAG patients who do not have mutation in myocilin.

Therapeutic Strategies Targeting Myocilin Mutations

In addition to potential gene therapies that correct myocilin mutations, there is evidence that drug therapy is efficacious in correcting the pathological consequences of myocilin mutation. For example, Zode and coworkers reported the therapeutic effects of sodium 4-phenylbutyrate (4-PBA) in myocilin Y437H transgenic mice [15, 16]. 4-PBA is a commercially available, orally efficacious drug being used to treat urea metabolism disorder. In addition to this metabolic effect, it also functions as a molecular chaperone. Zode et al. found that oral or ocular topical administration of 4-PBA can significantly lower IOP, reduce optic nerve injury, and normalize PERG of the myocilin Y437H mouse. These findings indicate that molecular chaperone, by modifying protein secretion and by normalizing TM cell functions, may be a practical treatment method for glaucoma related to myocilin mutation. And not limited to only that, this mechanism of pharmacological action may even be generalizable to other types of glaucoma, regardless whether myocilin mutation is involved, since endoplasmic reticulum stress response has been shown in other TM abnormalities unrelated to myocilin.

7.2.3.2 Transforming Growth Factor (TGF)β2 and Related Factors

TGFβ2 and Glaucoma

TGFβ2 is one of the many growth factors and cytokines found in aqueous humor. Aqueous humor TGFβ2 levels are higher in POAG patients compared to non-glaucomatous individuals. Similarly, TM tissues derived from POAG patients have higher levels of TGFβ2 [17].

TGFβ2 has been hypothesized as a likely causative factor of glaucoma pathogenesis. In *ex vivo* human anterior segment perfusion organ culture, perfusion with TGFβ2 increases outflow resistance and IOP. Likewise, overexpression of biologically active TGFβ2 in the rat or mouse eye also increases outflow resistance and IOP [18, 19]. Binding of TGFβ2 to its receptor activates cytoplasmic Smad proteins, such as Smad2/3. The activated Smad proteins are translocated to the cell nucleus and induce or suppress expressions of a variety of genes. Changes in expressions of these genes translate to changes in cell functions, including cell survival, proliferation, migration, rearrangement of cytoskeleton, metabolism of ECM, and tissue fibrosis. These changes in the TM can directly or indirectly affect aqueous humor outflow and IOP.

TGFβ2-Related Proteins and Glaucoma

Other than TGFβ, the TGF protein superfamily also includes bone morphogenic protein (BMP). There are more than 20 BMP proteins found in mammals. Wordinger and colleagues discovered the presence of several BMPs and their receptors in human TM tissue and TM cells [20]. Binding of BMPs to their receptors also activates Smad proteins and consequently affects cell functions. BMP signaling pathways in the cells are very complex, influencing and being influenced by many other proteins, for example, secreted BMP antagonists, BMP and activin membrane-bound inhibitor (BAMBI), and cytoplasmic inhibitory proteins. Secreted BMP antagonists include chordin, gremlin, and follistatin. They bind to BMP receptors and prevent activation of the receptors. BAMBI is a trans-membrane glycoprotein lacking the intracellular kinase domain required for signal transduction. By binding BMP, it decreases the effective concentration of BMP available to activate the cognate BMP receptors. Hence, BAMBI is classified as a pseudo-receptor. Cytoplasmic inhibitory proteins consist of inhibitory Smad (I-Smad, e.g., Smad6 and Smad7). I-Smads interfere with the binding of R-Smad to BMP receptor and Co-Smad, preventing their entry into the cell nucleus, which in turn reduces the biological activity of TGFβ2. Consequently, overexpression of Smad7 decreases TM fibrosis induced by TGFβ2 [21].

Many of these proteins affect TM functions, aqueous humor outflow, and IOP. They are likely involved in glaucoma pathogenesis. For example, in glaucomatous TM tissue, expressions of gremlin and follistatin are significantly elevated [22, 23]. In *ex vivo* perfused human anterior segments, treatment with gremlin increases IOP [22]. BMP4, BMP7, and follistatin can reduce ECM accumulation induced by TGFβ2.

Therapeutic Strategies Targeting TGFβ2 and Related Proteins

Based on their mechanisms of actions, antiglaucoma therapeutic strategies targeting TGFβ2 and related proteins may focus on any of the TGFβ2 signaling steps. Some of the more theoretically feasible ones include: (a) downregulation of TGFβ2 expression using siRNA, shRNA, or CRSPR/cas9, (b) neutralizing TGFβ2 antibody, (c) inhibition of TGFβ2 receptor kinase, (d) overexpression of Smad7, (e) inhibitors of Smad2/3 functions, (f) overexpression of BMP4 or BMP7, and (g) reduction of BMP antagonists, such as gremlin and follistatin. A critical consideration of the development of these strategies is their selectivity on the TM. Because TGFβ2 is an important cytokine in regulating normal functions in many other ocular tissues, any therapeutic manipulation of these signaling pathways must be limited to and selective for the TM, lest they interfere with other ocular functions and produce short- or long-termed untoward pharmacological effects.

7.2.3.3 Secreted Frizzled-Related Protein-1 (sFRP-1)

sFRP-1 and Glaucoma

sFRP-1 is a component of the Wnt signaling pathways, which are present in many cells, including human TM cells [24, 25]. Under normal conditions, Wnt proteins bind to their receptors, Frizzled family receptors (Fz), and co-receptor lipoprotein receptor-related protein (LRP) 5/6. Upon activation of the receptor, the cytoplasmic phosphoprotein Dishevelled (Dsh) is activated. Activation of Dsh can further activate multiple possible pathways, of which the canonical pathway plays an important role in the regulation of outflow facility. The canonical pathway involves a destruction complex, including several proteins: Axin, adenomatosis polyposis coli (APC), protein phosphatase 2A (PP2A), glycogen synthase kinase 3β (GSK3β), and casein kinase 1α (CK1α). Prior to activation of Fz, the destruction complex targets β-catenin for ubiquitination and degrades it. Activation of Fz by Wnt disrupts this function of destruction complex by inhibiting the activity of GSK3β, which allows the accumulation of β-catenin and its subsequent translocation to the nucleus. In the nucleus, β-catenin serves as a transcriptional coactivator of transcription factors of the T-cell factor/lymphoid enhancing factor (TCF/LEF) family and induces cellular response via gene transduction.

In the TM tissue of POAG patients, sFRP-1 level is significantly higher than that of non-glaucoma donors [26]. sFRP-1 binds to Wnt, prevents the activation of Fz, and blocks the Wnt cellular signaling pathway [27]. Blockade of the signaling pathway allows the destruction complex to remain active and allows β-catenin to be degraded. Correspondingly, the β-catenin level in the TM of POAG patients is lower than normal. For the time being, the cause of sFRP-1 elevation has not been delineated. Nonetheless, sFRP-1 and other Wnt antagonists have been shown to cause stiffening of cultured human TM cells [28], which is expected to affect the compliance of the aqueous outflow pathway and may increase outflow resistance. In addition, it is interesting to note that in human TM cells, crosstalk exists between the Wnt and TGFβ2 signaling pathways [29].

In certain tumor cells, DNA methylation affects sFRP-1 expression. However, a study by Mao et al. showed that the sFRP-1 promotor is unmethylated in cultured TM cells derived from glaucoma and non-glaucoma human donors, even though the sFRP-1 level was higher in the glaucoma TM cells [30]. These results suggest that DNA methylation is unlikely a causative factor in sFRP-1 expression level in the TM cells.

In *ex vivo* perfused human anterior segments, sFRP-1 elevates IOP. Intravitreal injection of adenovirus encoding sFRP-1 (Ad5-sFRP-1) in the mouse increases sFRP-1 expression in the eye and increases IOP [25, 26]. Moreover, intravitreal injection of Ad5-Dkk1 also increases mouse IOP. Dkk1 is a selective inhibitory protein of the canonical Wnt signaling pathway, without affecting the non-canonical pathways. The exact molecular components and mechanisms involved in IOP regulation by sFRP-1 or Wnt are active foci of glaucoma research.

Therapeutic Strategies Targeting sFRP-1

Based on the observations that sFRP-1 is elevated and Wnt signaling activity is reduced in glaucoma TM, any means to normalize these changes can be useful in treating glaucoma. For example, small molecule inhibitors of GSK3β have been demonstrated to effectively ameliorate mouse ocular hypertensive induced by Ad5-sFRP-1 injection [26]. Therefore, inhibition of the many steps of the Wnt pathway can be, at least in theory, potential targets for modification of this disease. Nevertheless, Wnt signaling pathways play important roles in many biological functions of many cells. Minimizing untoward effects will be a critical concern for drug development targeting these pathways.

7.2.3.4 CD44

CD44 and Glaucoma

CD44 is a glycoprotein, present on the surface of a large number of mammalian cells, including TM cells. It interacts with hyaluronic acid, collagen, and matrix metalloproteinases (MMPs) and is involved in cell adhesion, cell–cell interaction, and migration. It affects tumor metastasis, lymphocyte activation, and homing.

CD44 can be hydrolyzed by a membrane-bound MMP, MT1-MMP, into a soluble 32 kDa sCD44. In the aqueous humor of POAG patients, Knepper et al. found that the sCD44 level was higher than non-glaucoma patients, and proposed that sCD44 may serve as a decoy receptor and reduce the biological functions of CD44 [31].

In the mouse, overexpression of either CD44 or sCD44 by viral vector transfection increases sCD44 level in aqueous humor and increases IOP for more than 50 days [32]. In the perfused porcine anterior segment, sCD44 significantly reduces aqueous outflow facility [32]. These findings indicate that sCD44 affects aqueous humor hydrodynamics and may contribute to the pathogenesis of glaucoma. However, the involved molecular mechanism and signaling pathway are still not clear, although sCD44 was shown to increase TM cell cross-linked actin network formation, which may lead to change in topography and pliability of the outflow pathway [32].

Therapeutic Strategy Targeting CD44

The intramembrane portion of CD44 is cleaved by γ-secretase. Knepper and coworkers found that a γ-secretase inhibitor could normalize aqueous outflow facility in the perfused porcine anterior segment. Topical ocular administration of the inhibitor reverses ocular hypertension induced by sCD44 overexpression in the mouse [32]. It is important to note that there are intensive research activities attempting to develop a clinically useful γ-secretase inhibitor to treat Alzheimer's disease. Some of these compounds may be useful in treating glaucoma in the future.

7.2.3.5 Serum Amyloid A (SAA)

SAA and Glaucoma

SAA is an inducible acute phase apolipoprotein. It is known for two major biological functions: regulation of cytokine expression and amyloid deposition. During inflammation and trauma, plasma concentration of SAA can rapidly increase to more than 1000-fold. By using microarray analysis comparing normal and glaucomatous TM tissues, Wang et al. identified that SAA expression was elevated in glaucoma patients. Subsequent qPCR and western blot studies validated these findings and further showed that the TM tissues and cells derived from glaucoma patients have higher levels of SAA.

SAA level in the TM tissue of POAG patients has been found to be higher than that of non-glaucoma donors: approximately fivefold higher in SAA mRNA levels, and threefold higher in SAA protein expression [33]. Similarly, SAA protein level in aqueous humor samples of POAG patients is approximately 12-fold higher than that in cataract patients [34]. It is interesting to note that the plasma SAA levels are not different between the two groups [33]. The source of elevated ocular SAA in POAG patients is not clear. However, it can be synthesized by TM cells. Cultured TM cells derived from POAG patients also have an elevated expression of SAA; its level can be as high as 25-fold of that of TM cells derived from non-glaucoma donors [33].

SAA levels in aqueous humor of POAG patients correlate with IOP elevation. In these samples, certain other cytokines, such as interleukin-8 (IL-8) and TGFβ, are also increased, suggesting that they may interact with each other, and perhaps many other yet-to-be-delineated factors, to effect pathological changes in the TM, leading to reduction in aqueous outflow facility and ocular hypertension [34–36]. Perfusion of human anterior segment with recombinant human SAA significantly increases IOP, and concomitantly IL-8 level [33]. These results collectively indicate that SAA likely plays an important role in the pathogenesis of glaucoma. Downregulation of SAA in the eye or inhibition of downstream signaling events of SAA may be meaningful targets for IOP therapy. At this time, no clear target has been identified yet. Future research in this area deserves attention.

7.2.3.6 Cochlin

Cochlin is a secreted, extracellular matrix-related protein. Little of its biological functions is understood. It is expressed in the inner ear, brain, kidney, lung, and eye. Bhattacharya and coworkers reported that its level in the TM of POAG patients is significantly higher than non-glaucomatous donors [37]. They also reported that in the DBA/2J mouse, concomitant with the onset of the spontaneous age-related elevation of IOP, cochlin protein level was increased in the TM tissue [37]. In *ex vivo* cultured monkey anterior segments, adenoviral vector mediated overexpression of cochlin led to a significant reduction in aqueous humor outflow facility [38]. The mechanism of cochlin's action on aqueous outflow is not yet fully elucidated at this time. However, in the TM, its expression can be induced by TGFβ2 [39]. Cochlin can further induce co-expression of TREK-1, a stretch-activated potassium channel leading to filopodia formation [40]. Interaction of cochlin and TREK-1 has been shown to induce TM cell architectural changes, which contributes to the regulation of aqueous humor outflow facility [41]. In addition, cochlin also stimulates the secretion of annexin A2, a protein involved in cytoskeletal remodeling [40]. These findings together suggest that cochlin may serve as a mechanosensor in the TM, play a role in regulating TM cell shape and motility, and affect aqueous outflow rate. Because many functions of this protein are still not fully understood, its related targets for medical intervention are yet to be identified. Nonetheless, it provides a novel and potential interesting direction for the future.

7.3 Novel Therapeutic Targets for Neuroprotection Treatment

7.3.1 Need for Neuroprotection and Neuroregeneration Treatment

As part of the central nervous system (CNS), RGC provides the final common pathway to transmit all visual information processed by the retina to the brain. Any damage or loss of RGCs would cause significant visual impact to glaucoma patients. In general, the visual damage is irreversible and advancing if conventional IOP-lowering treatment cannot achieve target pressure due to poor tolerance to medication or failed surgery. In some patients, visual deterioration cannot be stopped even when a low level of IOP is successfully maintained. A significant proportion of diagnosed patient will eventually become blind due to glaucoma progression [42, 43]. Clinical trials such as the Advanced Glaucoma Intervention Study [44], the Collaborative Normal Tension Glaucoma Study (CNTG) [45], the Collaborative Initial Glaucoma Treatment Study Trial (CIGT) [46], and the Early Manifest Glaucoma Trial (EMGT) [47] showed that lowering IOP reduces the risk of progressive RGC loss and visual function deficits in patients with newly diagnosed glaucoma, advanced glaucoma, normal-tension glaucoma, and ocular hypertension but no glaucoma. These clinical evidences clearly demonstrated that applying surgical/laser procedure, topical therapy, or both cannot completely prevent progression in all patients. Therefore, new therapy that targets neuroprotection or neuroregeneration is definitely needed. Neuroprotection aims to supplement the benefit provided by IOP-lowering treatment so that the rate of progression of RGC death can be slowed down, while neurorescue may reverse the visual dysfunction. Neuroregeneration is to restore the visual function by regrowing the body parts of the injured RGCs, replacing the lost RGCs by the new RGCs or reconnecting RGCs to target cells. The combined neuroprotection, neurorescue, and regeneration is also viewed as a potential approach to improve visual function for glaucoma in the future.

7.3.2 Mechanism of Pathogenesis of Glaucomatous Optic Neuropathy

Mechanisms involved in the initiation and progression of RGC degeneration in glaucoma are poorly understood because the available structural and functional testes are not sensitive enough to detect the onset of disease early or monitor the disease progression accurately. Limited supply of human specimens with clear medical history and multiple risk factors contributing to the development of glaucoma also make the investigation more challenging. There is a heterogeneous group of risk factors for glaucoma including elevated IOP and increased cup-to-disk ratio, older age, and thinner corneas [48]. The contribution of each risk factor to the rate of progression largely varies from individual to individual.

Increasing evidence supports the hypothesis that the process of glaucomatous RGC degeneration is compartmentalized at the subcellular level and various independent degenerative mechanisms are involved at different parts of a neuron such as the soma, axon, dendrite, and synapse [49, 50]. To completely preserve RGCs from degeneration, combinatory therapeutic approaches targeted at locations of degenerating

RGCs should be considered. Apoptosis has been found in human patients with glaucoma and in animal models of experimental glaucoma and is believed to be the final common cell death pathway [51, 52]. However, stimulation of apoptosis can be induced by a number of mechanisms which include excitotoxicity, free radical generation, ischemic injury, withdrawal of neurotrophins, mechanical stress, inflammation and immunoregulation, imbalance of ion transport, intracellular energy dysregulation, molecular apoptotic cascade, and protein misfolding, or combination of above [53, 54]. There is a need for understanding the pathophysiology of RGC degeneration under specified condition.

To highlight the potential of neuroprotective approaches for glaucoma, this chapter outlines the proposed mechanisms of RGC degeneration and briefly discusses the potential agents that have been explored in animal models of glaucoma. Previously published reviews are listed below for reference. In general, animals are believed to be more suitable for studying glaucomatous RGC degeneration because RGCs are immediately injured when the cells or retinal tissues are isolated. As a matter of fact, glaucoma describes a group of diseases, which can progress acutely or chronically and the disease mechanisms are complicated. It is widely accepted that there is no perfect model for glaucoma because the pathogenesis is largely unknown and combination of risk factors contributes to the rate of progression. For instance, once glaucomatous RGC degeneration is initiated, series of complicated events occur and individual RGCs are likely at different stage of injury processes at any given time. In addition, the interactions between neighboring cells and micro-environment play different roles in the pathogenesis. This chapter mainly describes the actions of neuroprotective targets that have been evaluated in animal models of glaucoma. The major reason is that these models are generally believed to be more relevant to human glaucoma. First, IOP elevation is known to be a major risk factor for glaucoma in humans and it is more logical to use animal models of glaucoma, which show moderately elevated IOP for a period of time. Second, animal models of glaucoma generate less acute and severe RGC loss than animal models of optic nerve axotomy/crush, retinal ischemia/reperfusion injury, and neurotoxicity, and the progressive RGC loss in animal model of glaucoma lasts for longer duration. Importantly, these models produce histological features that look similar to human glaucoma. These features include localized axonal damage at the ONH and sectorial loss of RGC bodies, which are the characteristics of glaucoma. The similarity of their histological features supports that the RGC degeneration in these animal models and humans may share similar cell death pathways, and the drug study data are expected to have greater potential for translation to the clinic setting. Although the findings obtained mainly from the animal models of glaucoma are focused in this chapter, the heterogeneity of the studies in terms of animal strains, sex and age, and different IOP induction methods are noted. These areas should be further addressed prior to the development of neuroprotection therapy [55, 56].

7.3.3 Therapeutic Targets

7.3.3.1 Excitotoxicity

Glutamate is a major neurotransmitter of fast excitation in the mammalian CNS. In the retina, glutamate-mediated neurotransmission is responsible to transmit visual signals from photoreceptors to intermediate retinal neurons, then to RGCs and onto brain targets. The receptors for glutamate are predominantly expressed in the outer plexiform layer and the inner plexiform layer which contains abundant glutamatergic synapses of different types of retinal neurons and also RGCs [57, 58].

The neurotoxic effect was noted as early as 1957 when Lucas and Newhouse reported that subcutaneous injection of glutamate caused severe damage to the inner retina in postnatal mice [59]. Excitotoxicity is a term used to describe the neuronal damage caused by excessive excitatory amino acids [60] and since then it has been linked to several neurodegenerative diseases such as amyotrophic lateral sclerosis, Huntington's disease, Alzheimer's disease, and glaucoma [61].

Excessive release of glutamate extracellularly and the imbalance of glutamate cycle may lead to neuronal death but under normal conditions, homeostatic mechanisms prevent overexpression of the glutamate receptors and the extracellular level of glutamate is tightly controlled by neighboring Muller cells. Accumulation of excessive glutamate results in overstimulation of ionotropic glutamate receptors such as *N*-methyl-D-aspartate (NMDA) receptor which triggers intracellular calcium influx leading to the activation of a complex cascade which destroys cell components and followed by programmed cell death. Whether the vitreal level of glutamate is increased in glaucoma is inconclusive. It is possible that glutamate is released in localized regions in retina or optic nerve during glaucomatous neurodegeneration and small fluctuation of extracellular glutamate level may contribute to the progressive RGC loss. In spite of that, the glutamate receptor antagonists have been most studied to show positive effects on preventing RGC loss.

The use of NMDA receptor antagonists for neuroprotection has been extensively investigated and has been reviewed elsewhere [62]. Memantine, a selective, non-competitive NMDA antagonist with moderate affinity, has been approved for treating Alzheimer's disease. Preclinical and experimental research with memantine appeared promising in protecting RGCs from glaucomatous damage. However, the phase III randomized, double masked, placebo-controlled clinical trial conducted to test the efficacy of memantine as a neuroprotective drug for glaucoma found no significant effect in preserving visual function. Whether it works in moderately high IOP or the beneficial effect could be observed in prolonged disease progression is yet to be studied. To further dissect the contributory role of glutamate to RGC death in glaucoma, in-depth examinations of non-NMDA glutamate receptors such as the AMPA-type channels and the uptake of excess glutamate via glutamate/aspartate transporters (GLAST or EAAT1) by Muller cells are also necessary [63].

Acetylcholine (ACh) and nicotine have been found to prevent glutamate-induced retinal toxicity. Pharmacological studies using pig- and rat-cultured RGCs have demonstrated that activation of α7 nicotinic acetylcholine receptors (α7 nAChRs) is associated with this neuroprotective effect. Although how activation of α7 nAChRs protects RGCs from glaucomatous loss is poorly known, the mediation of ACh receptors has been recently hypothesized as a potential neuroprotective pathway. Intravitreal injection of a specific α7 nAChR agonist, *N*-[(3*R*)-1-azabicyclo[2.2.2]oct-3-yl]-4-chlorobenzamide hydrochloride (PNU-282987) prevents RGC loss after episcleral injection of hypertonic saline [64]. Twice daily topical application of PNU-282987 was showed to provide neuroprotective effect against RGC loss in a dose-dependent fashion probably through the activation of α7 nAChRs since PNU-282987 was detected in the retina by mass spectrometry [65]. The protective effects of PNU-282987 in glaucoma models were demonstrated to be associated with the modulation of GABAergic synaptic transmission which causes de-excitation of ganglion cell circuits and suppresses excitotoxic processes and GABA receptor expression [66, 67]. Galantamine, a small molecule acetylcholinesterase inhibitor and allosteric ligand of nAChR, has been used to treat Alzheimer's disease. Galantamine was found to improve the cognitive deficits by its cholinergic boosting activity and its neuroprotective effects [68].

Calcium-channel blockers are believed to be a potential candidate for neuroprotection in glaucoma by preventing excessive calcium influx after overstimulation of NMDA receptor. Although improved visual functions such as sensitivity in the visual field test have been reported after administration of calcium-channel blockers, effects of calcium-channel blockers on blood flow and direct neuroprotection are hardly distinguished from each other.

7.3.3.2 Endothelins

Endothelin is a family of potent vasoactive peptides comprising endothelin (ET)-1, 2, and 3. These isoforms act through two classes of G-protein coupled receptors, namely, endothelin A (ETA) and endothelin B (ETB). Endothelin ligand binds to endothelin receptor and then activates different responses within tissues. The ETA receptor expresses in vasculature smooth-muscle cells and organs, whereas the ETB receptor is detected in brain and many epithelia. Both receptors are responsible for contraction in smooth-muscle cells. In addition to the endothelin receptors on the trabecular meshwork which links to IOP regulation, both receptors were found in the vascular smooth muscle of choroidal and retinal vessels [69]. ET-1 administration was demonstrated to cause a decrease in ocular blood flow in rabbits [70] and in healthy human subjects [71]. Upregulation of components of the endothelin system appears to be related to glaucoma in human and animal models. ET-1 may cause blood flow loss to the retina and optic nerve due to its potent vasoconstrictor effect. Whether the activation of ETB mediated by ET-1 causes neuronal damage is unclear [72]. Prior to significant axonal loss, ET-2 was to be upregulated early compared to non-glaucoma eyes.

Although both receptors are expressed in RGCs, ET-1 exerts a direct apoptotic effect on RGCs exclusively through the ETB receptor [73]. Ocular administration of ET-1 has been demonstrated to induce apoptosis of RGCs which was significantly diminished in ETB receptor-deficient rats.

Besides, there was a regulatory effect of ET-1 on anterograde axonal transport in the optic nerve through activation of the ETB receptor [74]. Intravitreal injection of ET-1 in rats led to biphasic change of anterograde transport with prolonged reduction and this dysregulation may directly contribute to subsequent loss of RGCs. The exposure to ET-1 caused astroglial proliferation in cultured human ONH astrocytes [75] but this effect could be blocked by a mixed ETA/B receptor antagonist suggesting that this treatment may be used to inhibit the adverse effects resulted from astroglial proliferation in glaucoma.

To elucidate the role of endothelin system during glaucoma, Howell et al. [76] recently demonstrated the expression of ET-2 in astrocytes and microglia/monocytes in the ONH in DBA/2J mice. Predominantly, the endothelin ETA receptor is expressed in vascular endothelial cells, while the ETB receptor is expressed in ONH astrocytes. The investigators found that oral administration of macitentan protects optic nerve axons from glaucomatous damage. Macitentan is a dual endothelin receptor antagonist that binds to both ETA and ETB receptors but has greater affinity, efficacy, and safety than previous antagonists such as bosentan. Howell and coworkers also showed that 80% of DBA/2J eyes treated with the combined targeting of the endothelin using bosentan and complement using C1qα mutation developed no detectable glaucoma, indicating that the combined inhibition of both systems protected RGCs better than any one of the mechanisms alone.

Specific and mixed antagonists have been developed for both receptors [77]. Peptide antagonists may have concerns on penetration across the blood–brain barrier and systemic bioavailability, while the non-peptide antagonist may have adverse effects such as major birth defects, liver toxicity, headache, nasopharyngitis, and peripheral oedema. Taken together, the effects of mixed ET receptor antagonists or specific ETB receptor antagonists used for neuroprotective therapy glaucoma have to be carefully evaluated.

7.3.3.3 Mitochondria

Mitochondria are cytoplasmic organelles which function as the main energy source in the form of ATP inside cells, regulate calcium homeostasis, and synthesize and metabolize key molecules such as fatty acid. It has been considered as the primary site of reactive oxygen species (ROS) production and detoxification, and therefore it becomes an important target for alleviating the oxidative stress. Mitochondria contain mitochondrial DNA and converts essential subunits of the respiratory chain leading to the flow of energy. Energy-dependent intracellular activities such as endocytosis, ion transport, and neurotransmitter biosynthesis help sustain mitochondria functions for metabolic and apoptotic signaling. Mitochondria dynamically change their shapes through fusion and fission and actively travel between soma, axon, and presynaptic vesicles. In humans and animals after IOP was elevated, large numbers of mitochondria were present in RGC unmyelinated axons but mitochondria were abnormally accumulated at the laminar region of ONH [78–80]. This finding strongly indicates the blockage of mitochondrial transport in the optic nerve axons and the site of injury at laminar cribrosa region. Other harmful conditions such as TNF-α, calcium influx, hypoxic, and oxidative stress may cause cell death cascades. These events trigger the release of apoptosis-inducing proteins such as cytochrome c and caspase 3 activators through opening the mitochondrial permeability transition pore and ultimately lead to apoptotic pathway of RGC death. Osborne et al. [81] hypothesized that initiation of glaucoma negatively affects RGC mitochondria resulting in oxidative stress, and the RGCs are gradually weakened and be more susceptible to damaging insults.

One of the potential neuroprotective strategies is to enhance the energy supply of neurons. Nicotinamide is a precursor of NADH, which is a substrate for the electron transport chain and a blocker of subsequent apoptotic response. Retinal level of nicotinamide adenine dinucleotide (NAD+), a key molecule in energy and redox metabolism, was decreased with age and the aging neurons became vulnerable to damages in DBA/2J mice [82]. This finding indicates that mitochondrial dysfunction occurs early during RGC degeneration and aging. The intake of vitamin B3 has shown to prevent RGC death, axonal loss, mitochondrial damage, and axonal transport deficient in DBA/2J mice with IOP elevation. AAV2-mediated overexpression of nicotinamide/nicotinic acid mononucleotide adenylyltransferase 1 (NMNAT1) has demonstrated RGC protection from glaucomatous damages in DBA/2J mice [82]. The protective effects of vitamin B3 intake and AAV-2-NMNAT1 were confirmed by RNA-Seq-detected gene expression supporting the essential role of vitamin B3. NMNAT1 is a key enzyme that converts B3 to NAD and this conversion plays a role in redox reactions. Williams et al. [82] hypothesized that the reduced level of NAD disrupts metabolism in the exposure to stress and, under IOP elevation, the mitochondrial function is negatively affected. The increased metabolism of fatty acids and production of free radicals subsequently leads to RGC loss. Whether glaucomatous neurodegeneration can be delayed by dietary supplementation with nicotinamide would require further study.

Compounds are used to enhance the available energy within the cell and prevent mitochondrial depolarization [81]. However, substances taken orally should reach mitochondria inside RGCs in sufficient quantities prior to exerting therapeutic effects. For instance, CoQ10, known as ubiquinone, carries electrons and facilitates ATP production. It shows protective effects in animal models of neurodegeneration such as Parkinson's disease and Huntington's disease. It also preserves RGCs by mediating electron transport, antioxidant properties, gene expression, and inhibition of the permeability transition pore. Of interest, the level of CoQ10 declines in the human retina by approximately 40% with age suggesting an association with age-related glaucomatous neurodegeneration [83].

Mitochondrial transcription factor A (Tfam) is a nucleus-encoded DNA-binding protein in mitochondria. It plays a role in mitochondrial gene expression and mtDNA maintenance. It is involved in oxidative phosphorylation (OXPHOS)-mediated ATP synthesis. Lee et al. [84] demonstrated that a diet supplemented with CoQ10 promoted RGC survival and preserved the axons in the ONH, as well as inhibited astroglial activation by preserving mtDNA content and Tfam/OXPHOS complex IV protein expression in the retina of glaucomatous DBA/2J mice.

To enhance the topical delivery and pharmacological effects of CoQ10, formulation of CoQ10 into micelles using the vitamin E derivative D-α-tocopherol polyethylene glycol 1000 succinate (TPGS) was administered to a rat model of hypertonic saline injection into episcleral vein [85]. The finding clearly demonstrated that CoQ10/TPGS provided a significant neuroprotective effect against RGC loss by preventing apoptosis as evaluated by *in vivo* imaging technique. Taken together, CoQ10 is a promising therapeutic strategy for ameliorating apoptosis, oxidative stress, and glutamate excitotoxicity in glaucomatous neurodegeneration by modulating mitochondrial function.

7.3.3.4 Antioxidants

Oxidative stress has long believed to play a key role in the pathogenesis of neurodegenerative diseases including glaucoma [86, 87]. ROS including superoxide anion, lipid radicals, hydroxyl radical, nitric oxide, and hydrogen peroxide significantly contribute to oxidative stress. ROS are primarily produced by the mitochondrial respiratory chain (oxidative phosphorylation). Excess ROS produces toxic by-product and results in oxidative stress. Oxidative stress causes cell death by damaging proteins, lipids, and nuclear/mitochondrial DNA [88, 89]. Normally several systems of superoxide dismutase, catalase, metallothioneins, glutathione transferase, as well as thioredoxin (Txn) reverse the adverse effects. Approaches that target at reducing accumulation of ROS, increasing antioxidants, enhancing cell defense systems, and neutralizing lipid peroxidation products may provide beneficial effects for neuroprotection in glaucoma.

Direct administration of antioxidants has been tested in animal models of glaucoma and human patients. The antioxidants that have been examined are resveratrol, flavonoids, vitamin E, vitamin C, glutathione, minocycline, CoQ10, lutein, Ginkgo biloba, Lycium barbarum, α-lipoic acid, and ghrelin. These antioxidants taken orally are aimed to achieve sufficient amount in mitochondria inside RGCs and reduce oxidative stress. They are expected to positively alter nutritional and physiological effects. It is important to note that they are non-toxic in general. Although recent studies of the patients with glaucoma [90] and Leber's hereditary optic neuropathy showed positive effect after the intake of antioxidants [91], there is still lacking evidence that oral antioxidants reduce mitochondria-related oxidative stress in disease status. For example, vitamins C and E have been taken as supplements in the treatment of glaucoma but the effects are unclear and the pharmacokinetics and metabolism of antioxidants remain unknown.

The use of the cell-permeable small-peptide based antioxidants SS02, SS-31, SS-19, and SS-20 or the triphenylphosphonium-based antioxidants such as MitoQs, MitoVitEs, and MitoPTNs, or the choline esters of glutathione and *N*-acetyl-cysteine [92, 93], is an option to supply antioxidants to RGC mitochondria for the treatment of glaucoma even though the delivery method of these substances may have concerns.

Several natural agents were reported to exert neuroprotective effects on RGCs in animal models of glaucoma by primarily acting as antioxidants. They are discussed below.

Wolfberry (fruit of *Lycium barbarum Linn*) is a red berry and tastes sweet. In Chinese medicine, it is used for improving vision and nourishing the kidney and liver functions. Active components in wolfberry mainly contain *Lycium barbarum polysaccharide* (LBP), zeaxanthine, betaine, and cerebroside. Those components have been shown to provide beneficial effects on photoreceptors against age-related macular degeneration [94, 95] and apoptosis oxidative stress [96, 97]. Chan et al. first reported that LBP protects RGCs in an experimental glaucoma [98]. The investigators from the same laboratory demonstrated that systemic administration of LBP decreases in the expression of ET-1 and ETA and increases the expression of ETB [99] and βB2-crystallin in inner retinal neurons [100], indicating that the underlying cellular mechanisms of LBP neuroprotection likely involves multiple pathways.

Ginkgo biloba, one of the commonly used traditional Chinese medicines, contains flavonoids. The extract of ginkgo biloba is used to reduce oxidative damage in glaucoma patients and animal models. Oral administration of EGb761 (a type of ginkgo extract) decreased RGC loss up to 5 months after exposed to IOP elevation in rats [101]. However, there is no consent on the beneficial effects of ginkgo extract on blood flow, visual field, and contrast sensitivity in normal-tension glaucoma patients.

Epigallocatechin-3-gallate (EGCG), the ester of catechin that belongs to the family of flavonoids and a type of polyphenol, is found in green tea. EGCG is a powerful antioxidant exhibiting multifunctional properties [102], including anti inflammatory and vasodilator effects, which all contribute to its neuroprotective action. In ocular tissue, intravitreal injection of EGCG inhibited lipid peroxidation in retinal degeneration. EGCG treatment downregulated the level of proapoptotic genes and proteins such as caspases 3 and 8 after retinal ischemia/reperfusion injury [103]. The activation of astrocytes and Muller cells in glaucoma was also reduced by administration of EGCG. Oral administration of EGCG promoted RGC survival in a mouse glaucoma model using microbead injection [104] supporting the idea that daily intake of EGCG may help reduce oxidative stress in individuals with retinal diseases.

Nitric oxide (NO), a free radical that is formed by NO synthase (NOS), is long believed to have a role in many neurodegenerative diseases including Alzheimer disease, multiple sclerosis, cerebral–cardiovascular diseases, and glaucoma. Three isoforms of NOS are classified as NOS-1 (neuronal), NOS-2 (an inducible enzyme), and NOS-3 (endothelial). It has been proposed that excessive NO production by reactive astrocytes and microglia damages RGC axons at the level of lamina cribrosa in the ONH. Excessive NOS-2 results in apoptosis and necrosis in RGCs. Increased levels of NO were noted in the rat retinas with glaucoma and particularly increased expression of NOS was shown in the ONH of glaucoma patients. Earlier studies reported conflicting data that oral administration of aminoguandine, a NOS-2 inhibitor, preserved RGCs from limbal veins cautery model [105] but did not protect RGC axons or induce NOS-2 expression in the retina or ONH of a rat model of episcleral vein injection with hypertonic saline and no significant increase in NOS-2 expression [106]. By contrast, Dai et al. [107] reported that aminoguandine treatment for 3 days immediately after IOP induction significantly protected RGCs and decreased NOS upregulation but not for the treatment lasted for entire period of IOP induction. Thus, the findings raised the possibility that a time-dependent design for aminoguanidine treatment may be implemented for neuroprotection in glaucoma.

In general, superoxide dismutase, glutathione, and thioredoxin (Txn) systems are responsible for protecting cells from damage caused by excessive ROS. The Txn system is a ubiquitous thiol-reducing system that includes Txn, Txnip, Txn reductase, and NADPH. The cycle of Txn reduction and oxidation in cytoplasm (Txn1) and mitochondria (Txn2) scavenges intracellular ROS resulted from oxidative stress. Txn reducing activity and its expression are negatively regulated by Txnip. Upregulation of Txnip reduces Txn interaction with apoptosis signal-regulating kinase 1 and increases toxicity to retinal neurons. In a rat glaucoma model, expression of Txn1 and Txn2 and Txnip was observed in nerve fiber layer, inner nuclear layer, and primarily in RGCs [108]. The use of electroporation to induce Txn1 and Txn2 expression in RGCs in vivo was demonstrated to enhance RGC survival in experimental glaucoma [109]. Collectively, *in vivo* transfection with Txn2 EGFP-Txn2 plasmid and electroporation protected RGCs against IOP elevation induced axonal degeneration by decreasing mitochondrial membrane potential and subsequent apoptosis-inducing factor translocation supporting that modulation of Txn system is a potential treatment strategy for neurodegenerative disease [108].

7.3.3.5 Chaperones

In human, protein misfolding and aggregation cause several neurodegenerative diseases including amyotrophic lateral sclerosis, prion diseases, Alzheimer's disease, Parkinson's disease, and Huntington's disease. The relationship between protein aggregation and glaucomatous RGC degeneration is yet to be investigated. However, stress proteins, and heat shock proteins (HSPs) in particular, are of interest in neuroprotection for glaucoma because they function as molecular chaperones. They enhance cell survival under stress, adverse environmental conditions, and disease insults [110]. These proteins are highly conserved and classified according to their molecular weight. There are six families including small HSP, HSP40, HSP60, HSP70, HSP90, and HSP110. They assist in folding, assembly and disassembly, repair, transport, subcellular localization, and organization of proteins. Under stressful conditions such as hyperthermia and ischemia, HSPs help refold the denatured proteins and facilitate the new protein synthesis. HSPs also inhibit apoptosis by suppressing signal transduction that leads to cell death. Stress-induced HSP expression requires that activation of heat shock factors (HSFs) is essential to the stress-induced HSP expression through binding to the heat shock promoter elements.

Geranylgeranylacetone (GGA) is an acylic polyisoprenoid and has been used for the treatment of gastric ulcers in Japan for years. Administration of GGA prevents oxidative stress in the liver, heart, brain, kidney, and retina in multiple animal models of ischemia and reperfusion. Induction of HSP70 and stimulation of the Txn system are the major contributors to the cytoprotective effect. Animals treated with daily intraperitoneal GGA increased HSP70 expression in RGCs almost immediately after drug administration and sustained to later days [111]. Five weeks after IOP elevation, the survival of RGCs was increased by almost 60% in the GGA-treated animals. Inhibition of HSP70 expression by co-administration of quercetin abolished the RGC protection offered by GGA. A neuroprotective effect of GGA was observed in a non-IOP elevation mouse model of RGC degeneration due to deficiency of a glutamate transporter GLAST [112]. These findings strongly suggest that the GGA administration induces HSP70 expression for RGC protection and this effect relates to the inhibition of neurotoxicity and oxidative stress.

17-AAG is a derivative of the antibiotic geldanamycin and known as a potent HSP90 inhibitor. It specifically binds to ATP-binding site of HSP90, executes the dissociation of HSF1, initiates heat shock response, and increases the production of HSPs. The HSP90 inhibitors-mediated heat shock response is associated with their cellular protection. A single intravitreal injection of 17-AAG promoted the survival of injured RGCs by approximately 50% with increased HSP70 expression [113]. An AAV2-HSP70 vector was used to induce HSP70 expression specifically in RGCs and the protein induction increased RGC survival by an average of 110% two weeks after optic nerve crush. These evidences support that HSP70-based gene therapy is useful to prevent axonal damage in RGCs.

The small HSP superfamily are the proteins with molecular mass between 12 and 43 kDa and characterized by a conserved sequence of 80–100 amino acids named as the "α-crystallin domain." They are known to function as chaperone and increase cell tolerance to apoptosis after exposed to stress insults. The small HSPs are ATP-independent chaperones and cooperate with ATP-dependent chaperones of the HSP70 family to prevent protein aggregation and reverse the misfolding of polypeptides [114].

Crystallins, particularly αA and αB, are generally upregulated in stressed or injured tissues and proposed to play an endogenous protective role in RGCs [115]. The observed downregulation of crystallin genes in retinas with chronic IOP elevation could weaken the survival ability of RGCs, and thus lead to cell death [116]. Overexpression of αA and αB crystallins by electroporation was found to significantly increase the number of survived RGCs 1 week and 2 weeks after optic nerve axotomy [117]. Beneficial effects of α crystallins on RGC survival against optic nerve crush and retinal ischemia/reperfusion injury may involve the inhibition of microglial activation, TNF-α or iNOS release, and caspase 3 expression. Of interest, members of the crystallin superfamily such as βB2 crystallin are implicated not only in enhancing the survival of RGCs against optic nerve injuries but also the regeneration of RGC axons [118].

Alzheimer's disease is characterized by the presence of amyloid-β (Aβ), a major constituent of senile plaques which is formed by abnormal processing of amyloid precursor protein. Recently, Aβ has been associated with the initiation of RGC apoptosis with evidence of increased Aβ expression in RGCs and abnormal amyloid precursor protein processing in experimental glaucoma [119]. Decreased vitreous Aβ levels were found to be consistent with retinal Aβ deposition in patients with glaucoma [120]. Previously, Guo et al. [121] showed the colocalization of Aβ with apoptotic RGCs in an established glaucoma model using hypertonic saline injection and a dose- and time-dependent effect of Aβ on RGC apoptosis as imaged by annexin-V technique. The investigators also evaluated three different approaches to targeting Aβ in experimental glaucoma and their combination effects. The treatments reduce Aβ formation by a β-secretase inhibitor, clear Aβ deposition by an anti-Aβ antibody, or inhibit Aβ aggregation and neurotoxic effects by Congo red. The findings demonstrated that combined therapy (three treatments) was the most effective approach. However, these compounds were not suitable for therapeutic use in patients. Later, a new Aβ aggregation modulator MRZ-99030 was discovered by Gazit [122] and this small molecule was shown to provide sufficient anti-Aβ effect and suitable toxicological and pharmacokinetic properties for human use. Salt et al. [123] observed a dose-dependent effect of MRZ-99030 against RGC apoptosis in rat glaucoma model, and a promising efficacy of the Aβ aggregation inhibitor MRZ-99030 after systemic administration as shown by pharmacokinetic experiments warranting further development of a topical neuroprotectant for glaucoma patients. The findings support the notion that Aβ is a promising target for neuroprotective intervention in glaucoma.

7.3.3.6 Inflammatory and Immune Response

In general, the immune response in the CNS is highly restricted, and the blood–brain barrier (BBB) limits the communication between the immune system and the CNS. However, accumulating evidences show that under diseases conditions, the immune and inflammatory reaction is regulated in response to a variety of insults and circulating peripheral immune cells can enter into the CNS. Neuroinflammation is found in both acute and chronic neurodegeneration involving the proliferation of microglia and astrocytes, and the release of inflammatory cytokines, neurotransmitters, chemokines, and ROS [124]. The final outcome depends on the severity and the duration of the neuro-inflammatory process and is related to various risk factors such as aging [125]. Similarly, the immune privilege of the retina and optic nerve in the eye is maintained by the presence of the blood–retina barrier [126]. When any early pathologic events take place at the ONH, many cell types and mechanism may respond to cellular stress and failures in regulation of immune system presumably cause the manifestation of glaucoma. However, the precise mechanisms underlying the complex interplay between immune privilege, protective immunity, and autoimmune in glaucomatous neurodegeneration remain largely unknown.

Increased titers of serum autoantibodies to retina and optic nerve proteins in glaucoma patients suggest that the immune system is involved in glaucoma [127–130]. Analysis of the blood samples showed increased serum cytokines and abnormal T-cell subsets and in turn the immune response with glial reaction may contribute to glaucomatous RGC damage. Additionally a topographical loss of RGCs resembling human glaucoma resulted from the immunization with HSPs in rats [131]. Besides, investigations demonstrated that the classical and lectin pathways of complement activation cascade are involved. Early elimination of dendritic synapses similar to glaucoma may require the complement components C1q or C3 [132]. Complement gene regulation was observed in the early stage of RGC degeneration in DBA/2J mice, and neuronal loss could be reduced by a mutation in complement component C1qa. Therapeutic approaches that targeted at immune and neuro-inflammatory responses and their signaling pathways for neuroprotection are discussed below.

Minocycline, a semi-synthetic tetracycline, demonstrates notable neuroprotection in inflammatory conditions because its lipophilic nature allows the molecules cross the BBB easily [133]. Consistently, minocycline treatment protects RGCs from degeneration following various injuries including ocular hypertension [134, 135] and in DBA/2J mice [136]. The findings support that minocycline prevents early microglial activation at retina and ONH, increases pro-survival genes expression, and decreases apoptotic genes regulation, thus shifting the balance toward the anti-apoptotic side in experimental glaucoma.

Cytokine TNF-α and its superfamily of receptors have been considered to contribute to glaucoma progression. TNF-α interacts with two receptors, TNF-R1 (p55) and TNF-R2 (p75), which are expressed by neurons, astrocytes, and microglia. TNF-R1 contains the death domain that is involved in cell apoptosis. Increased expression of TNF-R1A receptor was shown in a rat model of ocular hypertension induced by trabecular laser photocoagulation [137], and increased immunoreactivity for TNF-α and its receptor was noted in glaucomatous ocular tissues [138, 139]. Increased concentrations of TNF-α, subsequent microglial activation, and delayed loss of RGCs were found in the ocular hypertensive mouse retina. The deletion of genes coding for TNF-α or TNF-R2 receptor reduced RGC death under the condition of IOP elevation supporting that TNF-α also acts through the TNF-R2 receptor.

Etanercept is a fusion protein that consists of the ligand-binding domain of the TNF-R2. Etanercept competitively binds to the present TNF and acts as a TNF inhibitor. Hence, it minimizes the effect of TNF and has been used clinically for rheumatoid arthritis and other autoimmune diseases. The systemic use of etanercept did not affect IOP in episcleral vein cauterization model but significantly reduced microglial activation in ONH and TNF-α in retina, and prevented the loss of RGCs and axons, indicating the therapeutic potential of TNF-α inhibition for protecting RGCs in glaucoma [140].

Fas ligand (FasL) is a type II trans-membrane protein which belongs to the TNF family. While it has been identified to activate apoptosis in T-cell, increasing evidence shows that activation of the Fas receptor can also result in inflammation. Membrane-bound protein, membrane-bound Fas ligand (mFasL), is proapoptotic and proinflammatory, or it can be cleaved and released as a soluble isoform, soluble Fas ligand (sFasL). sFasL, the natural cleavage product, inhibits mFasL-mediated apoptosis and inflammation and, therefore, is considered as an mFasL antagonist. Recently, Krishnan et al. [141] showed that under homeostatic conditions, FasL in the eye is primarily cleaved to the soluble form and mFasL is definitely the pathogenic isoform. The investigators utilized genetic manipulation to stop FasL cleavage and observed accelerated and exacerbated destruction of retinal cells in both spontaneous and inducible models of glaucoma. Importantly, application of AAV2.sFasL was demonstrated to protect RGCs and axons in these models. These data point to a key role for mFasL in glaucoma pathogenesis and the protective role of sFasL in the development of glaucoma. Although it is not yet clear how sFasL attenuates mFasL activity, the therapeutic approach to modulate the balance between sFasL and mFasL under glaucomatous conditions has potential to treat glaucoma.

Activated T-lymphocytes that are primed to the constituents of the optic nerve would be attracted to the locations of injury and secret neuroprotective factors. Focal activation of the immune system in the optic nerve appears to be associated with the localized axonal damage in laser-induced ocular hypertension and vein cauterization models in rats [142–145]. Immune-mediated protection by glatiramer acetate (copolymer-1), a synthetic polypeptide, was observed and the potential for clinical use has to be further explored.

7.3.3.7 Neurotropic Factors

Neurotrophins are small secreted diffusible peptides. The binding of neurotrophic factors and their corresponding cell surface receptors activates signal transduction and enhances the survival effect on neurons in adult. They also induce proliferation, differentiation, axon elongation, as well as dendrite and synapse formation in the developing and mature neurons. Nerve growth factor (NGF), brain-derived neurotrophic factor (BDNF), neurotrophin-4/5, and neurotrophin-3 are the members of the classic neurotrophin family. The cell surface receptors include the tropomyosin-related kinases (Trk), TrkA and TrkB, and the p75 neurotrophin receptor (p75NTR). NGF and BDNF bind to TrkA and TrkB, respectively. p75NTR binds all neurotrophins with equal affinity and regulates apoptotic signaling cascades after injuries.

Deprivation of neurotrophic factors is one of the major hypotheses for the pathogenesis of glaucomatous optic neuropathy. Earlier studies demonstrated that both anterograde and retrograde transport were compromised in the ONH of humans and monkeys with high IOP elevation [78, 146, 147] and intra-axonal organelles were accumulated in the prelaminar and postlaminar regions of the ONH [148]. Similar disruption of axonal transport was reported in rodent models of experimental glaucoma and DBA/2J mice. The supply of neurotrophic factors from the brain to the RGC somas was proposed to be interrupted by this blockade. Accumulation of TrkB and altered transport of BDNF were reported in a rat model of experimental glaucoma [149, 150] and accumulation of dynein at the ONH indicated the blockage of dynein-mediated axonal transport in glaucoma [151]. Owing to the pro-survival effect of neurotrophins on RGCs, possible neuroprotective approaches involve supplying RGCs with exogenous neurotrophins, inducing endogenous expression of neurotrophins or modulating both Trk receptor and p75NTR systems.

The supply of sustained levels of neurotrophins by different viral vectors offers RGC protection [152]. Recently, the co-injection of an antagonist to leucine-rich repeat protein, LINGO-1, and BDNF was found to provide a greater neuroprotective effect on RGCs than with BDNF alone [153]. One laboratory evaluated the effect of NGF in eye drop in a rat model of glaucoma [154] and a few glaucoma patients [155] and confirmed the neuroprotective effect. Of interest, LINGO-1 is specific to the CNS and acts as a negative regulator of both survival of neuron and regeneration of axon [156, 157].

Several receptors of other trophic factors such as fibroblast growth factor receptor-1 (FGFR1), glial-cell-derived neurotrophic factor (GDNF) family receptor α 1 (Ret/GFRα1), hepatocyte growth factor receptor (HGFR), and granulocyte-macrophage colony-stimulating-factor receptor (GM-CSF-α-R) are found to be expressed in RGCs. Neurotrophins modulate many key processes during development and survival of RGCs, indicating the possible therapeutic potential for neuroprotection by direct application or activation of Trk signaling [158, 159]. Since Muller cells secret many neurotrophins including ciliary neurotrophic factor (CNTF) and become reactive during glaucomatous damage, further investigation identifying the beneficial effects of Muller cells to support RGC survival may help develop new therapeutic strategies. Human CNTF is a trophic factor showing neurotrophic effect on RGCs. A single intravitreal injection of CNTF protein protected RGCs from ocular hypertension [160]. Adenoviral vectors carrying CNTF gene preserved surviving RGCs from axotomy and reduced axonal loss by 15% from ocular hypertension in rats [161]. Other trophic factors or cytokines including artemin, basic fibroblast growth factor, interleukin-6, and erythropoietin also demonstrated neuroprotective effects. However, it is very challenging to maintain sustainable delivery, dosage, drug effectiveness, or life-long administration of neurotrophic factors in chronic condition.

7.3.3.8 Apoptotic Mediators

Apoptosis is a common form of programmed cell death. The cell commits suicide and undergoes the changes including in cell shrinkage, genomic fragmentation, nuclear pyknosis, and cell degradation. In contrast, necrosis causes cell membrane destruction and the spillage of cellular contents into the extracellular matrix leads to the damage and death of other cells. There are many initiating factors for apoptosis, classified as intrinsic and extrinsic pathways. The Bcl-2 family of mitochondrial membrane-bound proteins is considered as a principle class of intracellular apoptotic regulators. While some proteins in this family such as Bcl-2 and Bcl-XL inhibit apoptosis, other members such as Bax, Bad, and Bid promote the process. Evidences from knockout mice studies support the functional impact of Bcl-2 family proteins regulation on RGC soma susceptibility [49, 162]. Caspases are proteases that execute the dismantling and demolition of apoptotic cells. The initiator caspases such as caspases 8 and 9 activate other caspases, while the effector caspases such as caspases 3 and 7 cleave the substrates that are involved in cellular disassembly. In some experimental glaucoma models, inhibition of the effector caspases can be neuroprotective even though the initiator caspases are activated. Performing intravitreal injections of AAV vector carrying human baculoviral IAP repeat-containing protein-4 (BIRC4) has been shown to enhance RGC survival in experimental glaucoma [163]. Interestingly, emerging evidences show that inhibition or downregulation of other initiator caspases, caspase 3, or caspase 7 only provides partial protection against injury-induced RGC death, indicating the complexity of caspases regulation in RGC degeneration [164].

One approach for neuroprotection is to inhibit apoptosis by promoting survival pathways. For instance, brimonidine is administered to activate extracellular signal-regulated kinase (ERK) and Akt and leads to increased production of Bcl-2 and Bcl-XL. Another approach is to block the apoptotic cascades by administering caspase inhibitors. Although there are novel efficacies and improved pharmacokinetic properties of new peptidic and non-peptidic caspase inhibitors for the treatment of neurodegenerative and ocular diseases, no caspase inhibitory drugs are available for human mainly due to their toxicity, side effects, and poor pharmacokinetic properties. Recently, other cell death processes including autophagy and necrosis have been recently found to play a role in RGC death in experimental glaucoma [165]. Whether inhibition of apoptosis alone can completely prevent the progression of RGC death in glaucoma has to be clarified.

7.3.3.9 Scleral Remodeling

Peripapillary sclera (PPS) behavior has been shown to be a key factor in determining the effect of IOP on the ONH [166, 167]. Axial myopia and corneal thickness are known risk factors for glaucoma in human and these factors are associated with scleral physiology and anatomy. The sclera in rodent models of experimental glaucoma is significantly altered, while the sclera in glaucoma patients appears to be stiffer. In experimental glaucoma, the TGFβ pathways were regulated in ONH [168] and the expression of thrombospondins 1 and 4, which are activators of TGFβ, was increased more than twofold as demonstrated by proteomic analysis [169] suggesting a role of TGFβ in the remodeling of fibrous tissue. Quigley et al. [170] demonstrated that the administration of losartan, a selective angiotensin 1 receptor inhibitor, suppressed TGFβ signaling, decreased the blockage of axonal transport, and reduced axonal loss in a mouse glaucoma model. To consider whether alterations of the sclera as an approach to supplement IOP-lowering treatment in human, further investigations studying the drug effects on scleral structure and RGC survival in different types of mice after exposed to IOP elevation are required and the existing structural difference of sclera between rodents and humans will be the next challenge.

7.3.3.10 Transcription Factors

Many diseases are related to the dysregulation of transcription factors and the loss of function of transcription factors causes severe phenotypes of specific neurological disorders. The p38 MAPK signaling pathways lead to diverse cellular responses to external stimuli such as osmotic shock, pro-inflammatory cytokines, growth factors, and excitotoxic and oxidative injury. In neurodegenerative disorders, the p38 MAPK signaling affects activation of transcription factor 2 (ATF2), hyper-phosphorylation of tau neurofilaments, and upregulation of proapoptotic caspases [171, 172]. Increasing evidences support that p38 MAPK is a potential therapeutic target in glaucoma. For instance, topical administration of a selective inhibitor of the p38 MAPK (Ro3206145) promoted anterograde transport and prevented axonal degeneration of RGCs [173].

Other stress-activated cell signaling kinase pathways such as c-Jun N-terminal kinases (JNKs) and ERKs also play a key role in RGC degeneration. For example, NMDA-induced retinal excitotoxicity activates both JNK and p38 MAPK, and inhibitors for these signaling pathways protect RGCs in animal model [174, 175]. Similarly, SP600125, a broad-spectrum inhibitor for JNK phosphorylation, prevented RGC loss in IOP elevation models in dose-dependent manner [176, 177]. Syc-Mazurek et al. [178] observed that JUN, a target of pathological JNK signaling, was temporally and spatially expressed in RGCs of DBA/2J glaucoma mice. Genetic manipulation deleted the gene expression of JUN and in turn preserved RGC bodies from the injury related to IOP elevation but not RGC axons, indicating that a possible role of JNK–JUN signaling in somal degeneration.

Three members of Brn-3 family, namely, Brn3a, Brn3b, and Brn3c, share similar POU domain sequence and their transcription factors are expressed by restricted somatosensory neurons and RGCs. They play a major role in the development of CNS neurons. In the retina, both retinal ganglion precursor cells and mature RGCs express Brn3b [179]. The function of Brn3b is to regulate axon outgrowth, pathfinding, and proper polarization [180]. The expression of Brn-3b is critical to the survival of RGCs in mice during embryonic stage and birth, but not Brn3a or Brn3c [181] while the lack of Brn3b expression also caused the reduction of optic nerve fibers and thinning of the optic nerve. Stankowska et al. [182] demonstrated that intravitreal injection of AAV-2 coding for Brn3b promoted RGC protection, improved axonal integrity, and restored visual optomotor response in glaucoma model. The follow-up study elucidated that AAV-mediated Brn3b protein overexpression promoted neuroprotection of RGCs and their axons by modulating anti-apoptotic proteins such as p-AKT, Bcl-2, and Bcl-xL during ocular hypertension in rodents [183].

α-Adrenergic receptors are expressed in human retinas particularly in RGCs and the inner nuclear layer. Brimonidine, a selective α2-adrenergic receptor agonist, increases metabolism in retina and promoted growth in cultured retinal cells [184]. It has been shown to up-regulate endogenous level of BDNF in the RGCs after optic nerve crush [185] and reduce accumulation of extracellular glutamate and aspartate [186] and secondary degeneration [187]. In humans, brimonidine increases mean visual field sensitivity [188] and contrast sensitivity in POAG patients [189]. Patients with brimonidine treatment have superior preservation of RNFL than patients with timolol over a 12-month period [190]. However, a study in Singapore showed that there was no difference in the prevalence of visual field defects or rate of visual field progression between the angle closure glaucoma patients with brimonidine and timolol following initial laser peripheral iridotomy over 16 weeks [191]. Similarly, another study found no significant modification of the visual field indices by brimonidine treatment in primary open-angle glaucoma [192]. This discrepancy between clinical studies has to be addressed.

7.3.3.11 Stem Cell Transplant and Regenerative Signaling

Once injured, mature RGC axons are thought to be unable to regenerate through the optic nerve. Of importance, implantation of a peripheral nerve graft to the cut end of the optic nerve was found to promote the regeneration [193]. Subsequently, accumulating evidences show that experimental axonal regeneration requires reactivation of intrinsic growth capacity of mature RGCs and modification of extrinsic growth-inhibitory environment of the optic nerve.

During development, some suppressors of regeneration increase and associate with the decreased regenerative capacity in early postnatal period [194, 195]. Those suppressors include the transcription factor, Kruppel-like factor 4 (Klf-4) [196], phosphatase and tensin homologue (PTEN), a suppressor of cell signaling through the phosphoinositide-3-kinase (PI3 kinase)/activated protein kinase (Akt)/mammalian target of rapamycin (mTOR) pathway [197], and suppression of cytokine signaling 3 (SOCS3) [198]. Other Kruppel-like factor family transcription factors that promote regeneration decline during development [196]. Reactivation of growth capacity by suppressing a combination of these factors is shown to be more effective to regenerate RGC axons [199]. Axonal regeneration can be promoted by modifying the extrinsic growth-inhibitory environment of optic nerve by suppressing receptors to cell-extrinsic inhibitors such as neurite outgrowth inhibitor-A (Nogo-A), oligodendrocyte-myelin glycoprotein, and myelin-associated glycoprotein, inhibiting the Rho and ROCK pathway and mobile zinc in synaptic contacts between RGCs and amacrine cells after optic nerve injury. Apparently, there is no single target that is adequate to promote optic nerve regeneration. Manipulation of local glial, vascular, and inflammatory responses deserves additional attention and detailed evaluation on the quality of regenerative growth is definitely needed.

Although much advancement in axonal regeneration field has been made in the past 20 years, regenerative therapies still face many difficult problems in order to restore vision in glaucoma patients [200]. First, the regenerating axons have to pass optic nerve and reconnect to the right neurons at right targets in human brain. Simultaneously, RGCs have to make connections with various types of interneurons in the retina and restore specific retinal function. Second, the regenerating axons beyond the optic nerve head need remyelination through oligodendrocytes for conduction of electrical impulses. Considering glaucomatous RGC degeneration as compartmentalized [50], separate regenerative therapy targeting at different cellular compartments may be necessary.

Growth-associated protein-43 (GAP-43) is a protein kinase C substrate and is predominantly present in growing axons, synapses, and growth cones in association with actin cytoskeleton. After optic nerve injury, GAP-43 is highly expressed in regenerating RGCs and enhances axonal regeneration [201]. Importantly, intravitreal injection of BDNF has been reported to significantly increase GAP-43 regulation and induce neuronal survival. Recently, Huang et al. [202] examined whether AAV-mediated GAP-43 protected RGCs in laser-induced chronic IOP elevation injury. Surprisingly, AAV-GAP43 treatment led to more severe RGC death at 3 weeks after IOP elevation. Therefore, the use of regenerative agents should be cautious in disease conditions, and further clarification on mechanism and confirmation study is definitely needed.

Stem cells are thought to be able to replace degenerated RGC in glaucoma and recent evidences show the neuroprotective potential of stem cells. Since the nerve fiber of the olfactory system is the only part of the CNS that continues to grow and regenerate throughout adult life, olfactory ensheathing cells (OECs), a unique type of glial cells, were transplanted into the transected lesion site in the optic nerve of a cat model and the treatment induced regeneration of injured RGC axons dramatically. Dai et al. [203] found that the implantation of OECs into the region of the optic disk promoted RGC survival and the implanted OECs migrated into the dorsal area of the ONH where the optic nerve fibers with non-myelinated sheath.

Mesenchymal stromal cells (MSC) are multipotent self-replicating stromal cells. They secrete a wide array of neurotrophic factors and these factors may protect injured RGC and ultimately preserve vision. MSC can be isolated from a variety of adult tissues, such as adipose tissue (ADSC), bone marrow (BMSC), and MSC-like cells from the dental pulp (DPSC). DPSCs are multipotent cranial neural crest-derived stem cells that produce NGF, BDNF, and NT-3 than ADSC and BMSC. Mead et al. [204] compared the effects of transplanted BMSC, ADSC, and DPSC in the vitreous chamber of a rat model of TGF-β1-induced IOP elevation. Both BMSC and DPSC preserved RNFL thickness by retinal imaging using optical coherence tomography and enhanced RGC survival after exposed to IOP elevation for 35 days. The positive scotopic threshold response was measured by ERG to evaluate visual function in the rats. The visual function loss induced by IOP elevation was significantly reversed by DPSC treatment only but not BMSC and ADSC treatment.

Despite encouraging results, it should be noted that stem cells induce ocular complications such as neurotoxicity, reactive gliosis, and inflammation, and the implantation causes clumping of stem cells and thick epiretinal membrane. The adverse effects may be due in part to the inconsistency in the isolation and preparation of stem cells. Transplantation of stem cells is still considered as another promising strategy for protecting RGCs in glaucoma but clinical studies should be carefully regulated.

7.3.3.12 Multiple Mechanisms and Combinatory Therapy

Due to the multifactorial nature of the pathogenesis of glaucoma, enhancing the overall cell defense mechanisms, inhibiting multiple RGC degeneration mechanisms, or targeting at broad-spectrum neuroprotective effects rather than focusing on specific factors or single pathway is proposed as a viable strategy to promote RGC protection. Numerous agents that mediate diverse systemic effects have been tested for preserving RGC survival against glaucomatous damages. Some examples are shown below.

Erythropoietin (EPO) is a glycoprotein hormone secreted by kidney and liver and regulates erythropoiesis. The effects of EPO have been evaluated in animal models of neurodegenerative diseases and glaucoma. In systemic circulation, EPO binds and interacts with the EPO receptor to increase erythrocyte production by promoting cell survival through inhibiting apoptosis of erythroid progenitor cells. Nonhematopoietic tissue such as retina produces EPO and its receptor as well. Systemic administration of EPO is found to provide positive neuroprotective effect on cerebral neurons against stroke, mechanical trauma, excitotoxic injury, neuroinflammation, and 1,2,3,6-tetrahydropyridine (MPTP)-induced Parkinson syndrome in animal models. Treatment with EPO has also been demonstrated to prevent RGC damage from toxic insult with glutamate and nitric oxide or neurotrophic factor deprivation. Zhong et al. [205] showed that EPO injection to DBA/2J mice for 6 months starting from 5 months of age prevented the loss of RGCs but had no effect on IOP. A recent study indicated that systemic administration of rAAV2/8.mEpoR76E 1 month before and immediately after IOP elevation successfully rescued RGC axons and preserved axonal transport in both microbead occlusion model and DBA/2J mice [206]. In addition, rAAV2/8. mEpoR76E treatment was shown to preserve flash visual evoked potentials in DBA/2J mice. Subsequent study showed that rAAV2/8. mEpoR76E treatment preserved visual function in DBA/2J by multiple mechanisms: decreasing infiltration of peripheral immune cells, modulating microglial reactivity, and decreasing oxidative stress [207].

The renin–angiotensin system (RAS) plays a key role in the control of blood pressure and fluid balance. Renin, which is synthesized in the kidney, is secreted into blood. Angiotensinogen, which is released by the liver, is cleaved by plasma renin and results in angiotensin I. Subsequently, angiotensin I is converted to angiotensin II by the enzyme angiotensin-converting enzyme (ACE). The major functions of angiotensin II are mediated by the angiotensin II type 1 receptor (AT1-R) and its antagonists are widely used to treat hypertension and cardiovascular diseases. Interestingly, AT1-R antagonists are shown to attenuate inflammatory and oxidative stress in the retina [208, 209]. Daily oral administration of the AT1-R antagonist candesartan for 10 weeks increased RGC survival in experimental glaucoma in rats without affecting IOP or blood pressure [210]. The expression of AT1-R in the RGC layer cells was increased by candesartan treatment. Foureaux et al. [211] evaluated the effects of diminazene aceturate, an activator of endogenous ACE, in a glaucoma model and observed histological preservation of RGCs and axons, as well as reduced activation of caspase-3. However, both daily systemic or topical administration of the drug exerted IOP-lowering effects in the animal with experimental glaucoma. Since the long-term use of ACE inhibitors demonstrated beneficial effect on the visual fields in patients with normal-tension glaucoma [212], further investigations to understand the mechanism of actions in RGC survival may help develop new therapeutic target for neuroprotection.

The effects of opioids are mediated through activation of three opioid receptor subtypes: δ-opioid, κ-opioid, and μ-opioid receptors. These receptors are widely distributed in the CNS and their activations lead to modulation of many biological functions including pain perception, motivation, locomotion, hormone secretion, and reward. Husain et al. [213, 214] documented that morphine pretreatment significantly protects retinal neurons against acute ischemic injury and chronic glaucomatous damage. Systemic administration of a δ-opioid agonist SNC-121 protected against RGC loss due to IOP elevation, by suppressing TNF-α and p38 MAP activity in the retina [215]. A recent study suggests that SNC-121 treatment mediated its protective effect through the activation of PI3K/Akt pathway in ONH astrocytes and retina [216].

There are other neuroprotection agents that may involve multiple cellular or molecular mechanisms. For example, systemic administration of melatonin prevented visual dysfunction and RGC loss after chronic ocular hypertension, and this effect may be related to the inhibition of glutamate synaptic concentrations and NO levels, as well as increased retinal antioxidant defense system activity and GABA turnover rate and glutamic acid decarboxylase activity [217]. 17β-Estradiol and analogs were shown to protect RGC and optic nerve from various insults via a myriad of mechanisms and signaling cascades [218–224]. These interesting areas of development deserve careful investigation.

7.4 Concluding Remarks

Glaucoma therapy has existed for more than 100 years. From miotic agents to prostaglandin agonists and other novel drugs, achievements and improvements in IOP reduction efficacy with minimal adverse effects have been extraordinary. However, all of these current therapeutic approaches still cannot ameliorate, normalize, or reverse the underlying pathological mechanism(s). They also do not directly address the detrimental, degenerative effects of glaucoma on the retina and optic nerve. Under the current treatment methods, the disease continues to progress, and the RGC may continue to degenerate despite therapy. This chapter explores many novel concepts for the future treatment of glaucoma. These concepts are very different from the currently available symptomatic relief of ocular hypertension. They aim to modify the pathogenesis and pathophysiology at the TM, as well as protect, rescue, and regenerate the glaucomatous injuries at the retina and optic nerve.

In addition to treatment methods that only aim at one target, combined therapies or therapies that affect multiple targets may provide broad and superior beneficial effect. These types of approaches open exciting new avenues for glaucoma therapy.

These novel concepts are at various stages of drug development, some relatively early. The development process likely encounters many hurdles, including expected and unexpected difficulties. Their clinical usefulness requires much work for proof. However, continuous efforts will lead to continuous improvements. We anticipate excitement and revolution in the treatment of this devastating, blinding disease.

References

1. Quigley HA, Addicks EM. Regional differences in the structure of the lamina cribrosa and their relation to glaucomatous optic nerve damage. Arch Ophthalmol. 1981;99:137–43.
2. Quigley HA. Neuronal death in glaucoma. Prog Retin Eye Res. 1999;18:39–57.
3. Vranka JA, Kelley MJ, Acott TS, Keller KE. Extracellular matrix in the trabecular meshwork: intraocular pressure regulation and dysregulation in glaucoma. Exp Eye Res. 2015;133:112–25.
4. O'Callaghan J, Cassidy PS, Humphries P. Open-angle glaucoma: therapeutically targeting the extracellular matrix of the conventional outflow pathway. Expert Opin Ther Targets. 2017;21:1037–50.
5. Bermudez JY, Montecchi-Palmer M, Mao W, Clark AF. Cross-linked actin networks (CLANs) in glaucoma. Exp Eye Res. 2017;159:16–22.
6. Wang K, Read AT, Sulchek T, Ethier CR. Trabecular meshwork stiffness in glaucoma. Exp Eye Res. 2017;158:3–12.
7. Tamm ER, Braunger BM, Fuchshofer R. Intraocular pressure and the mechanisms involved in resistance of the aqueous humor flow in the trabecular meshwork outflow pathways. Prog Mol Biol Transl Sci. 2015;134:301–14.
8. Braunger BM, Fuchshofer R, Tamm ER. The aqueous humor outflow pathways in glaucoma: a unifying concept of disease mechanisms and causative treatment. Eur J Pharm Biopharm. 2015;95:173–81.
9. Stone EM, Fingert JH, Alward WL, et al. Identification of a gene that causes primary open angle glaucoma. Science. 1997;275:668–70.
10. Alward WL, Fingert JH, Coote MA, et al. Clinical features associated with mutations in the chromosome 1 open-angle glaucoma gene (GLC1A). N Engl J Med. 1998;338:1022–7.
11. Gould DB, Miceli-Libby L, Savinova OV, et al. Genetically increasing Myoc expression supports a necessary pathologic role of abnormal proteins in glaucoma. Mol Cell Biol. 2004;24:9019–25.
12. Kim BS, Savinova OV, Reedy MV, et al. Targeted disruption of the myocilin gene (Myoc) suggests that human glaucoma-causing mutations are gain of function. Mol Cell Biol. 2001;21:7707–13.
13. Jacobson N, Andrews M, Shepard AR, et al. Non-secretion of mutant proteins of the glaucoma gene myocilin in cultured trabecular meshwork cells and in aqueous humor. Hum Mol Genet. 2001;10:117–25.
14. Shepard AR, Jacobson N, Millar JC, et al. Glaucoma-causing myocilin mutants require the Peroxisomal targeting signal-1 receptor (PTS1R) to elevate intraocular pressure. Hum Mol Genet. 2007;16:609–17.
15. Zode GS, Bugge KE, Mohan K, et al. Topical ocular sodium 4-phenylbutyrate rescues glaucoma in a myocilin mouse model of primary open-angle glaucoma. Invest Ophthalmol Vis Sci. 2012;53:1557–65.

16. Zode GS, Kuehn MH, Nishimura DY, et al. Reduction of ER stress via a chemical chaperone prevents disease phenotypes in a mouse model of primary open angle glaucoma. J Clin Invest. 2011;121:3542–53.
17. Ozcan AA, Ozdemir N, Canataroglu A. The aqueous levels of TGF-beta2 in patients with glaucoma. Int Ophthalmol. 2004;25:19–22.
18. Shepard AR, Millar JC, Pang IH, Jacobson N, Wang WH, Clark AF. Adenoviral gene transfer of active human transforming growth factor-{beta}2 elevates intraocular pressure and reduces outflow facility in rodent eyes. Invest Ophthalmol Vis Sci. 2010;51:2067–76.
19. Gottanka J, Chan D, Eichhorn M, Lutjen-Drecoll E, Ethier CR. Effects of TGF-beta2 in perfused human eyes. Invest Ophthalmol Vis Sci. 2004;45:153–8.
20. Wordinger RJ, Clark AF. Bone morphogenetic proteins and their receptors in the eye. Exp Biol Med (Maywood). 2007;232:979–92.
21. Fuchshofer R, Stephan DA, Russell P, Tamm ER. Gene expression profiling of TGFbeta2- and/or BMP7-treated trabecular meshwork cells: identification of Smad7 as a critical inhibitor of TGF-beta2 signaling. Exp Eye Res. 2009;88:1020–32.
22. Wordinger RJ, Fleenor DL, Hellberg PE, et al. Effects of TGF-beta2, BMP-4, and gremlin in the trabecular meshwork: implications for glaucoma. Invest Ophthalmol Vis Sci. 2007;48:1191–200.
23. Fitzgerald AM, Benz C, Clark AF, Wordinger RJ. The effects of transforming growth factor-beta2 on the expression of follistatin and activin A in normal and glaucomatous human trabecular meshwork cells and tissues. Invest Ophthalmol Vis Sci. 2012;53:7358–69.
24. Logan CY, Nusse R. The Wnt signaling pathway in development and disease. Annu Rev Cell Dev Biol. 2004;20:781–810.
25. Mao W, Millar JC, Wang WH, et al. Existence of the canonical Wnt signaling pathway in the human trabecular meshwork. Invest Ophthalmol Vis Sci. 2012;53:7043–51.
26. Wang WH, McNatt LG, Pang IH, et al. Increased expression of the WNT antagonist sFRP-1 in glaucoma elevates intraocular pressure. J Clin Invest. 2008;118:1056–64.
27. Finch PW, He X, Kelley MJ, et al. Purification and molecular cloning of a secreted, Frizzled-related antagonist of Wnt action. Proc Natl Acad Sci U S A. 1997;94:6770–5.
28. Morgan JT, Raghunathan VK, Chang YR, Murphy CJ, Russell P. Wnt inhibition induces persistent increases in intrinsic stiffness of human trabecular meshwork cells. Exp Eye Res. 2015;132:174–8.
29. Webber HC, Bermudez JY, Sethi A, Clark AF, Mao W. Crosstalk between TGFbeta and Wnt signaling pathways in the human trabecular meshwork. Exp Eye Res. 2016;148:97–102.
30. Mao W, Rubin JS, Anoruo N, Wordinger RJ, Clark AF. SFRP1 promoter methylation and expression in human trabecular meshwork cells. Exp Eye Res. 2012;97:130–6.
31. Knepper PA, Goossens W, Mayanil CS. CD44H localization in primary open-angle glaucoma. Invest Ophthalmol Vis Sci. 1998;39:673–80.
32. Giovingo M, Nolan M, McCarty R, et al. sCD44 overexpression increases intraocular pressure and aqueous outflow resistance. Mol Vis. 2013;19:2151–64.
33. Wang WH, McNatt LG, Pang IH, et al. Increased expression of serum amyloid A in glaucoma and its effect on intraocular pressure. Invest Ophthalmol Vis Sci. 2008;49:1916–23.
34. Takai Y, Tanito M, Ohira A. Multiplex cytokine analysis of aqueous humor in eyes with primary open-angle glaucoma, exfoliation glaucoma, and cataract. Invest Ophthalmol Vis Sci. 2012;53:241–7.
35. Furlaneto CJ, Campa A. A novel function of serum amyloid A: a potent stimulus for the release of tumor necrosis factor-alpha, interleukin-1beta, and interleukin-8 by human blood neutrophil. Biochem Biophys Res Commun. 2000;268:405–8.
36. Ribeiro FP, Furlaneto CJ, Hatanaka E, et al. mRNA expression and release of interleukin-8 induced by serum amyloid A in neutrophils and monocytes. Mediators Inflamm. 2003;12:173–8.
37. Bhattacharya SK, Rockwood EJ, Smith SD, et al. Proteomics reveal Cochlin deposits associated with glaucomatous trabecular meshwork. J Biol Chem. 2005;280:6080–4.
38. Lee ES, Gabelt BT, Faralli JA, et al. COCH transgene expression in cultured human trabecular meshwork cells and its effect on outflow facility in monkey organ cultured anterior segments. Invest Ophthalmol Vis Sci. 2010;51:2060–6.
39. Bhattacharya SK, Gabelt BT, Ruiz J, Picciani R, Kaufman PL. Cochlin expression in anterior segment organ culture models after TGFbeta2 treatment. Invest Ophthalmol Vis Sci. 2009;50:551–9.
40. Goel M, Sienkiewicz AE, Picciani R, Lee RK, Bhattacharya SK. Cochlin induced TREK-1 co-expression and annexin A2 secretion: role in trabecular meshwork cell elongation and motility. PLoS One. 2011;6:e23070.
41. Carreon TA, Castellanos A, Gasull X, Bhattacharya SK. Erratum: interaction of cochlin and mechanosensitive channel TREK-1 in trabecular meshwork cells influences the regulation of intraocular pressure. Sci Rep. 2017;7:6430.
42. Peters D, Bengtsson B, Heijl A. Factors associated with lifetime risk of open-angle glaucoma blindness. Acta Ophthalmol. 2014;92:421–5.
43. Malihi M, Moura Filho ER, Hodge DO, Sit AJ. Long-term trends in glaucoma-related blindness in Olmsted County, Minnesota. Ophthalmology. 2014;121:134–41.
44. AGIS. The Advanced Glaucoma Intervention Study (AGIS): 7. The relationship between control of intraocular pressure and visual field deterioration. The AGIS Investigators. Am J Ophthalmol. 2000;130:429–40.
45. CNTG. Comparison of glaucomatous progression between untreated patients with normal-tension

glaucoma and patients with therapeutically reduced intraocular pressures. Collaborative Normal-Tension Glaucoma Study Group. Am J Ophthalmol. 1998;126:487–97.
46. Lichter PR, Musch DC, Gillespie BW, et al. Interim clinical outcomes in the Collaborative Initial Glaucoma Treatment Study comparing initial treatment randomized to medications or surgery. Ophthalmology. 2001;108:1943–53.
47. Heijl A, Leske MC, Bengtsson B, Hyman L, Bengtsson B, Hussein M. Reduction of intraocular pressure and glaucoma progression: results from the Early Manifest Glaucoma Trial. Arch Ophthalmol. 2002;120:1268–79.
48. Friedman DS, Wilson MR, Liebmann JM, Fechtner RD, Weinreb RN. An evidence-based assessment of risk factors for the progression of ocular hypertension and glaucoma. Am J Ophthalmol. 2004;138:S19–31.
49. Nickells RW. The cell and molecular biology of glaucoma: mechanisms of retinal ganglion cell death. Invest Ophthalmol Vis Sci. 2012;53:2476–81.
50. Whitmore AV, Libby RT, John SW. Glaucoma: thinking in new ways-a role for autonomous axonal self-destruction and other compartmentalised processes? Prog Retin Eye Res. 2005;24:639–62.
51. Garcia-Valenzuela E, Shareef S, Walsh J, Sharma SC. Programmed cell death of retinal ganglion cells during experimental glaucoma. Exp Eye Res. 1995;61:33–44.
52. Kerrigan LA, Zack DJ, Quigley HA, Smith SD, Pease ME. TUNEL-positive ganglion cells in human primary open-angle glaucoma. Arch Ophthalmol. 1997;115:1031–5.
53. Almasieh M, Wilson AM, Morquette B, et al. The molecular basis of retinal ganglion cell death in glaucoma. Prog Retin Eye Res. 2012;31:152–81.
54. Baltmr A, Duggan J, Nizari S, Salt TE, Cordeiro MF. Neuroprotection in glaucoma - is there a future role? Exp Eye Res. 2010;91:554–66.
55. Quigley HA. Clinical trials for glaucoma neuroprotection are not impossible. Curr Opin Ophthalmol. 2012;23:144–54.
56. Liu Y, Pang IH. Challenges in the development of glaucoma neuroprotection therapy. Cell Tissue Res. 2013;353:253–60.
57. Lukasiewicz PD. Synaptic mechanisms that shape visual signaling at the inner retina. Prog Brain Res. 2005;147:205–18.
58. Peng YW, Blackstone CD, Huganir RL, Yau KW. Distribution of glutamate receptor subtypes in the vertebrate retina. Neuroscience. 1995;66:483–97.
59. Lucas DR, Newhouse JP. The toxic effect of sodium L-glutamate on the inner layers of the retina. AMA Arch Ophthalmol. 1957;58:193–201.
60. Olney JW. Brain lesions, obesity, and other disturbances in mice treated with monosodium glutamate. Science. 1969;164:719–21.
61. Meldrum B, Garthwaite J. Excitatory amino acid neurotoxicity and neurodegenerative disease. Trends Pharmacol Sci. 1990;11:379–87.
62. Lipton SA. Paradigm shift in neuroprotection by NMDA receptor blockade: memantine and beyond. Nat Rev Drug Discov. 2006;5:160–70.
63. Derouiche A, Rauen T. Coincidence of L-glutamate/L-aspartate transporter (GLAST) and glutamine synthetase (GS) immunoreactions in retinal glia: evidence for coupling of GLAST and GS in transmitter clearance. J Neurosci Res. 1995;42:131–43.
64. Iwamoto K, Birkholz P, Schipper A, Mata D, Linn DM, Linn CL. A nicotinic acetylcholine receptor agonist prevents loss of retinal ganglion cells in a glaucoma model. Invest Ophthalmol Vis Sci. 2014;55:1078–87.
65. Mata D, Linn DM, Linn CL. Retinal ganglion cell neuroprotection induced by activation of alpha7 nicotinic acetylcholine receptors. Neuropharmacology. 2015;99:337–46.
66. Zhou X, Cheng Y, Zhang R, et al. Alpha7 nicotinic acetylcholine receptor agonist promotes retinal ganglion cell function via modulating GABAergic presynaptic activity in a chronic glaucomatous model. Sci Rep. 2017;7:1734.
67. Zhou X, Zong Y, Zhang R, et al. Differential modulation of GABAA and NMDA receptors by an alpha7-nicotinic acetylcholine receptor agonist in chronic glaucoma. Front Mol Neurosci. 2017;10:422.
68. Almasieh M, Zhou Y, Kelly ME, Casanova C, Di Polo A. Structural and functional neuroprotection in glaucoma: role of galantamine-mediated activation of muscarinic acetylcholine receptors. Cell Death Dis. 2010;1:e27.
69. Stitt AW, Chakravarthy U, Gardiner TA, Archer DB. Endothelin-like immunoreactivity and receptor binding in the choroid and retina. Curr Eye Res. 1996;15:111–7.
70. Sugiyama T, Moriya S, Oku H, Azuma I. Association of endothelin-1 with normal tension glaucoma: clinical and fundamental studies. Surv Ophthalmol. 1995;39(Suppl 1):S49–56.
71. Polak K, Petternel V, Luksch A, et al. Effect of endothelin and BQ123 on ocular blood flow parameters in healthy subjects. Invest Ophthalmol Vis Sci. 2001;42:2949–56.
72. Cioffi GA, Wang L, Fortune B, et al. Chronic ischemia induces regional axonal damage in experimental primate optic neuropathy. Arch Ophthalmol. 2004;122:1517–25.
73. MacCumber MW, D'Anna SA. Endothelin receptor-binding subtypes in the human retina and choroid. Arch Ophthalmol. 1994;112:1231–5.
74. Stokely ME, Brady ST, Yorio T. Effects of endothelin-1 on components of anterograde axonal transport in optic nerve. Invest Ophthalmol Vis Sci. 2002;43:3223–30.
75. Prasanna G, Krishnamoorthy R, Clark AF, Wordinger RJ, Yorio T. Human optic nerve head astrocytes as a target for endothelin-1. Invest Ophthalmol Vis Sci. 2002;43:2704–13.
76. Howell GR, MacNicoll KH, Braine CE, et al. Combinatorial targeting of early pathways profoundly

inhibits neurodegeneration in a mouse model of glaucoma. Neurobiol Dis. 2014;71:44–52.
77. Rosenthal R, Fromm M. Endothelin antagonism as an active principle for glaucoma therapy. Br J Pharmacol. 2011;162:806–16.
78. Anderson DR, Hendrickson A. Effect of intraocular pressure on rapid axoplasmic transport in monkey optic nerve. Invest Ophthalmol. 1974;13:771–83.
79. Quigley HA, Guy J, Anderson DR. Blockade of rapid axonal transport. Effect of intraocular pressure elevation in primate optic nerve. Arch Ophthalmol. 1979;97:525–31.
80. Quigley HA, Addicks EM, Green WR, Maumenee AE. Optic nerve damage in human glaucoma. II. The site of injury and susceptibility to damage. Arch Ophthalmol. 1981;99:635–49.
81. Osborne NN, Nunez-Alvarez C, Joglar B, Del Olmo-Aguado S. Glaucoma: focus on mitochondria in relation to pathogenesis and neuroprotection. Eur J Pharmacol. 2016;787:127–33.
82. Williams PA, Harder JM, Foxworth NE, et al. Vitamin B3 modulates mitochondrial vulnerability and prevents glaucoma in aged mice. Science. 2017;355:756–60.
83. Qu J, Kaufman Y, Washington I. Coenzyme Q10 in the human retina. Invest Ophthalmol Vis Sci. 2009;50:1814–8.
84. Lee D, Shim MS, Kim KY, et al. Coenzyme Q10 inhibits glutamate excitotoxicity and oxidative stress-mediated mitochondrial alteration in a mouse model of glaucoma. Invest Ophthalmol Vis Sci. 2014;55:993–1005.
85. Davis BM, Tian K, Pahlitzsch M, et al. Topical Coenzyme Q10 demonstrates mitochondrial-mediated neuroprotection in a rodent model of ocular hypertension. Mitochondrion. 2017;36:114–23.
86. Tezel G. Oxidative stress in glaucomatous neurodegeneration: mechanisms and consequences. Prog Retin Eye Res. 2006;25:490–513.
87. Osborne NN, del Olmo-Aguado S. Maintenance of retinal ganglion cell mitochondrial functions as a neuroprotective strategy in glaucoma. Curr Opin Pharmacol. 2013;13:16–22.
88. Osborne NN, Chidlow G, Layton CJ, Wood JP, Casson RJ, Melena J. Optic nerve and neuroprotection strategies. Eye (Lond). 2004;18:1075–84.
89. Lascaratos G, Garway-Heath DF, Willoughby CE, Chau KY, Schapira AH. Mitochondrial dysfunction in glaucoma: understanding genetic influences. Mitochondrion. 2012;12:202–12.
90. Ramdas WD, Wolfs RC, Kiefte-de Jong JC, et al. Nutrient intake and risk of open-angle glaucoma: the Rotterdam Study. Eur J Epidemiol. 2012;27:385–93.
91. Carelli V, La Morgia C, Valentino ML, et al. Idebenone treatment in Leber's hereditary optic neuropathy. Brain. 2011;134:e188.
92. Murphy MP, Smith RA. Targeting antioxidants to mitochondria by conjugation to lipophilic cations. Annu Rev Pharmacol Toxicol. 2007;47:629–56.
93. Reddy PH. Mitochondrial medicine for aging and neurodegenerative diseases. Neuromolecular Med. 2008;10:291–315.
94. Moeller SM, Jacques PF, Blumberg JB. The potential role of dietary xanthophylls in cataract and age-related macular degeneration. J Am Coll Nutr. 2000;19:522S–7S.
95. Gale CR, Hall NF, Phillips DI, Martyn CN. Lutein and zeaxanthin status and risk of age-related macular degeneration. Invest Ophthalmol Vis Sci. 2003;44:2461–5.
96. Thomson LR, Toyoda Y, Langner A, et al. Elevated retinal zeaxanthin and prevention of light-induced photoreceptor cell death in quail. Invest Ophthalmol Vis Sci. 2002;43:3538–49.
97. Chucair AJ, Rotstein NP, Sangiovanni JP, During A, Chew EY, Politi LE. Lutein and zeaxanthin protect photoreceptors from apoptosis induced by oxidative stress: relation with docosahexaenoic acid. Invest Ophthalmol Vis Sci. 2007;48:5168–77.
98. Chan HC, Chang RC, Koon-Ching Ip A, et al. Neuroprotective effects of Lycium barbarum Lynn on protecting retinal ganglion cells in an ocular hypertension model of glaucoma. Exp Neurol. 2007;203:269–73.
99. Mi XS, Chiu K, Van G, et al. Effect of Lycium barbarum polysaccharides on the expression of endothelin-1 and its receptors in an ocular hypertension model of rat glaucoma. Neural Regen Res. 2012;7:645–51.
100. Chiu K, Zhou Y, Yeung SC, et al. Up-regulation of crystallins is involved in the neuroprotective effect of wolfberry on survival of retinal ganglion cells in rat ocular hypertension model. J Cell Biochem. 2010;110:311–20.
101. Hirooka K, Tokuda M, Miyamoto O, Itano T, Baba T, Shiraga F. The Ginkgo biloba extract (EGb 761) provides a neuroprotective effect on retinal ganglion cells in a rat model of chronic glaucoma. Curr Eye Res. 2004;28:153–7.
102. Zhang B, Osborne NN. Oxidative-induced retinal degeneration is attenuated by epigallocatechin gallate. Brain Res. 2006;1124:176–87.
103. Zhang B, Rusciano D, Osborne NN. Orally administered epigallocatechin gallate attenuates retinal neuronal death in vivo and light-induced apoptosis in vitro. Brain Res. 2008;1198:141–52.
104. Shen C, Chen L, Jiang L, Lai TY. Neuroprotective effect of epigallocatechin-3-gallate in a mouse model of chronic glaucoma. Neurosci Lett. 2015;600:132–6.
105. Neufeld AH, Sawada A, Becker B. Inhibition of nitric-oxide synthase 2 by aminoguanidine provides neuroprotection of retinal ganglion cells in a rat model of chronic glaucoma. Proc Natl Acad Sci U S A. 1999;96:9944–8.
106. Pang IH, Johnson EC, Jia L, et al. Evaluation of inducible nitric oxide synthase in glaucomatous optic neuropathy and pressure-induced optic nerve damage. Invest Ophthalmol Vis Sci. 2005;46:1313–21.

107. Dai Y, Weinreb RN, Kim KY, et al. Inducible nitric oxide synthase-mediated alteration of mitochondrial OPA1 expression in ocular hypertensive rats. Invest Ophthalmol Vis Sci. 2011;52:2468–76.
108. Munemasa Y, Kwong JM, Kim SH, Ahn JH, Caprioli J, Piri N. Thioredoxins 1 and 2 protect retinal ganglion cells from pharmacologically induced oxidative stress, optic nerve transection and ocular hypertension. Adv Exp Med Biol. 2010;664: 355–63.
109. Munemasa Y, Ahn JH, Kwong JM, Caprioli J, Piri N. Redox proteins thioredoxin 1 and thioredoxin 2 support retinal ganglion cell survival in experimental glaucoma. Gene Ther. 2009;16:17–25.
110. Piri N, Kwong JM, Gu L, Caprioli J. Heat shock proteins in the retina: focus on HSP70 and alpha crystallins in ganglion cell survival. Prog Retin Eye Res. 2016;52:22–46.
111. Ishii Y, Kwong JM, Caprioli J. Retinal ganglion cell protection with geranylgeranylacetone, a heat shock protein inducer, in a rat glaucoma model. Invest Ophthalmol Vis Sci. 2003;44:1982–92.
112. Dong Z, Shinmei Y, Dong Y, et al. Effect of geranylgeranylacetone on the protection of retinal ganglion cells in a mouse model of normal tension glaucoma. Heliyon. 2016;2:e00191.
113. Kwong JM, Gu L, Nassiri N, et al. AAV-mediated and pharmacological induction of Hsp70 expression stimulates survival of retinal ganglion cells following axonal injury. Gene Ther. 2015;22:138–45.
114. Horwitz J. Alpha-crystallin can function as a molecular chaperone. Proc Natl Acad Sci U S A. 1992;89:10449–53.
115. Piri N, Kwong JM, Caprioli J. Crystallins in retinal ganglion cell survival and regeneration. Mol Neurobiol. 2013;48:819–28.
116. Piri N, Song M, Kwong JM, Caprioli J. Modulation of alpha and beta crystallin expression in rat retinas with ocular hypertension-induced ganglion cell degeneration. Brain Res. 2007;1141:1–9.
117. Munemasa Y, Kwong JM, Caprioli J, Piri N. The role of alphaA- and alphaB-crystallins in the survival of retinal ganglion cells after optic nerve axotomy. Invest Ophthalmol Vis Sci. 2009;50:3869–75.
118. Thanos S, Bohm MR, Schallenberg M, Oellers P. Traumatology of the optic nerve and contribution of crystallins to axonal regeneration. Cell Tissue Res. 2012;349:49–69.
119. McKinnon SJ. Glaucoma: ocular Alzheimer's disease? Front Biosci. 2003;8:s1140–56.
120. Yoneda S, Hara H, Hirata A, Fukushima M, Inomata Y, Tanihara H. Vitreous fluid levels of beta-amyloid((1-42)) and tau in patients with retinal diseases. Jpn J Ophthalmol. 2005;49:106–8.
121. Guo L, Salt TE, Luong V, et al. Targeting amyloid-beta in glaucoma treatment. Proc Natl Acad Sci U S A. 2007;104:13444–9.
122. Gazit E. Mechanisms of amyloid fibril self-assembly and inhibition. Model short peptides as a key research tool. FEBS J. 2005;272:5971–8.
123. Salt TE, Nizari S, Cordeiro MF, Russ H, Danysz W. Effect of the Abeta aggregation modulator MRZ-99030 on retinal damage in an animal model of glaucoma. Neurotox Res. 2014;26:440–6.
124. Amor S, Peferoen LA, Vogel DY, et al. Inflammation in neurodegenerative diseases--an update. Immunology. 2014;142:151–66.
125. Vivekanantham S, Shah S, Dewji R, Dewji A, Khatri C, Ologunde R. Neuroinflammation in Parkinson's disease: role in neurodegeneration and tissue repair. Int J Neurosci. 2015;125:717–25.
126. Benhar I, London A, Schwartz M. The privileged immunity of immune privileged organs: the case of the eye. Front Immunol. 2012;3:296.
127. Wax MB, Barrett DA, Pestronk A. Increased incidence of paraproteinemia and autoantibodies in patients with normal-pressure glaucoma. Am J Ophthalmol. 1994;117:561–8.
128. Tezel G, Seigel GM, Wax MB. Autoantibodies to small heat shock proteins in glaucoma. Invest Ophthalmol Vis Sci. 1998;39:2277–87.
129. Yang J, Tezel G, Patil RV, Romano C, Wax MB. Serum autoantibody against glutathione S-transferase in patients with glaucoma. Invest Ophthalmol Vis Sci. 2001;42:1273–6.
130. Wax MB, Yang J, Tezel G. Serum autoantibodies in patients with glaucoma. J Glaucoma. 2001;10:S22–4.
131. Wax MB, Tezel G, Yang J, et al. Induced autoimmunity to heat shock proteins elicits glaucomatous loss of retinal ganglion cell neurons via activated T-cell-derived fas-ligand. J Neurosci. 2008;28:12085–96.
132. Howell GR, Macalinao DG, Sousa GL, et al. Molecular clustering identifies complement and endothelin induction as early events in a mouse model of glaucoma. J Clin Invest. 2011;121:1429–44.
133. Kim HS, Suh YH. Minocycline and neurodegenerative diseases. Behav Brain Res. 2009;196:168–79.
134. Levkovitch-Verbin H, Waserzoog Y, Vander S, Makarovsky D, Piven I. Minocycline upregulates pro-survival genes and downregulates pro-apoptotic genes in experimental glaucoma. Graefes Arch Clin Exp Ophthalmol. 2014;252:761–72.
135. Bordone MP, Gonzalez Fleitas MF, Pasquini LA, et al. Involvement of microglia in early axoglial alterations of the optic nerve induced by experimental glaucoma. J Neurochem. 2017;142:323–37.
136. Bosco A, Inman DM, Steele MR, et al. Reduced retina microglial activation and improved optic nerve integrity with minocycline treatment in the DBA/2J mouse model of glaucoma. Invest Ophthalmol Vis Sci. 2008;49:1437–46.
137. Yang Z, Quigley HA, Pease ME, et al. Changes in gene expression in experimental glaucoma and optic nerve transection: the equilibrium between protective and detrimental mechanisms. Invest Ophthalmol Vis Sci. 2007;48:5539–48.
138. Yuan L, Neufeld AH. Tumor necrosis factor-alpha: a potentially neurodestructive cytokine produced by glia in the human glaucomatous optic nerve head. Glia. 2000;32:42–50.

139. Yang X, Luo C, Cai J, et al. Neurodegenerative and inflammatory pathway components linked to TNF-alpha/TNFR1 signaling in the glaucomatous human retina. Invest Ophthalmol Vis Sci. 2011;52: 8442–54.
140. Roh M, Zhang Y, Murakami Y, et al. Etanercept, a widely used inhibitor of tumor necrosis factor-alpha (TNF-alpha), prevents retinal ganglion cell loss in a rat model of glaucoma. PLoS One. 2012;7:e40065.
141. Krishnan A, Fei F, Jones A, et al. Overexpression of soluble Fas ligand following adeno-associated virus gene therapy prevents retinal ganglion cell death in chronic and acute murine models of glaucoma. J Immunol. 2016;197:4626–38.
142. Bakalash S, Kessler A, Mizrahi T, Nussenblatt R, Schwartz M. Antigenic specificity of immunoprotective therapeutic vaccination for glaucoma. Invest Ophthalmol Vis Sci. 2003;44:3374–81.
143. Bakalash S, Ben-Shlomo G, Aloni E, et al. T-cell-based vaccination for morphological and functional neuroprotection in a rat model of chronically elevated intraocular pressure. J Mol Med (Berl). 2005;83:904–16.
144. Bakalash S, Pham M, Koronyo Y, et al. Egr1 expression is induced following glatiramer acetate immunotherapy in rodent models of glaucoma and Alzheimer's disease. Invest Ophthalmol Vis Sci. 2011;52:9033–46.
145. Schori H, Kipnis J, Yoles E, et al. Vaccination for protection of retinal ganglion cells against death from glutamate cytotoxicity and ocular hypertension: implications for glaucoma. Proc Natl Acad Sci U S A. 2001;98:3398–403.
146. Radius RL, Anderson DR. Rapid axonal transport in primate optic nerve. Distribution of pressure-induced interruption. Arch Ophthalmol. 1981;99:650–4.
147. Dandona L, Hendrickson A, Quigley HA. Selective effects of experimental glaucoma on axonal transport by retinal ganglion cells to the dorsal lateral geniculate nucleus. Invest Ophthalmol Vis Sci. 1991;32:1593–9.
148. Gaasterland D, Tanishima T, Kuwabara T. Axoplasmic flow during chronic experimental glaucoma. 1. Light and electron microscopic studies of the monkey optic nervehead during development of glaucomatous cupping. Invest Ophthalmol Vis Sci. 1978;17:838–46.
149. Pease ME, McKinnon SJ, Quigley HA, Kerrigan-Baumrind LA, Zack DJ. Obstructed axonal transport of BDNF and its receptor TrkB in experimental glaucoma. Invest Ophthalmol Vis Sci. 2000;41:764–74.
150. Quigley HA, McKinnon SJ, Zack DJ, et al. Retrograde axonal transport of BDNF in retinal ganglion cells is blocked by acute IOP elevation in rats. Invest Ophthalmol Vis Sci. 2000;41:3460–6.
151. Martin KR, Quigley HA, Valenta D, Kielczewski J, Pease ME. Optic nerve dynein motor protein distribution changes with intraocular pressure elevation in a rat model of glaucoma. Exp Eye Res. 2006;83:255–62.
152. Martin KR, Quigley HA, Zack DJ, et al. Gene therapy with brain-derived neurotrophic factor as a protection: retinal ganglion cells in a rat glaucoma model. Invest Ophthalmol Vis Sci. 2003;44:4357–65.
153. Fu QL, Li X, Yip HK, et al. Combined effect of brain-derived neurotrophic factor and LINGO-1 fusion protein on long-term survival of retinal ganglion cells in chronic glaucoma. Neuroscience. 2009;162:375–82.
154. Colafrancesco V, Parisi V, Sposato V, et al. Ocular application of nerve growth factor protects degenerating retinal ganglion cells in a rat model of glaucoma. J Glaucoma. 2011;20:100–8.
155. Lambiase A, Aloe L, Centofanti M, et al. Experimental and clinical evidence of neuroprotection by nerve growth factor eye drops: implications for glaucoma. Proc Natl Acad Sci U S A. 2009;106:13469–74.
156. Mi S, Lee X, Shao Z, et al. LINGO-1 is a component of the Nogo-66 receptor/p75 signaling complex. Nat Neurosci. 2004;7:221–8.
157. Shao Z, Browning JL, Lee X, et al. TAJ/TROY, an orphan TNF receptor family member, binds Nogo-66 receptor 1 and regulates axonal regeneration. Neuron. 2005;45:353–9.
158. Johnson TV, Bull ND, Martin KR. Neurotrophic factor delivery as a protective treatment for glaucoma. Exp Eye Res. 2011;93:196–203.
159. Kimura A, Namekata K, Guo X, Harada C, Harada T. Neuroprotection, growth factors and BDNF-TrkB signalling in retinal degeneration. Int J Mol Sci. 2016;17:1584.
160. Ji JZ, Elyaman W, Yip HK, et al. CNTF promotes survival of retinal ganglion cells after induction of ocular hypertension in rats: the possible involvement of STAT3 pathway. Eur J Neurosci. 2004;19:265–72.
161. Pease ME, Zack DJ, Berlinicke C, et al. Effect of CNTF on retinal ganglion cell survival in experimental glaucoma. Invest Ophthalmol Vis Sci. 2009;50:2194–200.
162. Maes ME, Schlamp CL, Nickells RW. BAX to basics: how the BCL2 gene family controls the death of retinal ganglion cells. Prog Retin Eye Res. 2017;57:1–25.
163. McKinnon SJ, Lehman DM, Tahzib NG, et al. Baculoviral IAP repeat-containing-4 protects optic nerve axons in a rat glaucoma model. Mol Ther. 2002;5:780–7.
164. Choudhury S, Liu Y, Clark AF, Pang IH. Caspase-7: a critical mediator of optic nerve injury-induced retinal ganglion cell death. Mol Neurodegener. 2015;10:40.
165. Kitaoka Y, Munemasa Y, Kojima K, Hirano A, Ueno S, Takagi H. Axonal protection by Nmnat3 overexpression with involvement of autophagy in optic nerve degeneration. Cell Death Dis. 2013;4:e860.
166. Stowell C, Burgoyne CF, Tamm ER, Ethier CR. Biomechanical aspects of axonal damage in glaucoma: a brief review. Exp Eye Res. 2017;157:13–9.

167. Yang H, Reynaud J, Lockwood H, et al. The connective tissue phenotype of glaucomatous cupping in the monkey eye - clinical and research implications. Prog Retin Eye Res. 2017;59:1–52.
168. Johnson EC, Jia L, Cepurna WO, Doser TA, Morrison JC. Global changes in optic nerve head gene expression after exposure to elevated intraocular pressure in a rat glaucoma model. Invest Ophthalmol Vis Sci. 2007;48:3161–77.
169. Oglesby EN, Tezel G, Cone-Kimball E, et al. Scleral fibroblast response to experimental glaucoma in mice. Mol Vis. 2016;22:82–99.
170. Quigley HA, Pitha IF, Welsbie DS, et al. Losartan treatment protects retinal ganglion cells and alters scleral remodeling in experimental glaucoma. PLoS One. 2015;10:e0141137.
171. Ackerley S, Grierson AJ, Banner S, et al. p38alpha stress-activated protein kinase phosphorylates neurofilaments and is associated with neurofilament pathology in amyotrophic lateral sclerosis. Mol Cell Neurosci. 2004;26:354–64.
172. Munoz L, Ammit AJ. Targeting p38 MAPK pathway for the treatment of Alzheimer's disease. Neuropharmacology. 2010;58:561–8.
173. Dapper JD, Crish SD, Pang IH, Calkins DJ. Proximal inhibition of p38 MAPK stress signaling prevents distal axonopathy. Neurobiol Dis. 2013;59:26–37.
174. Munemasa Y, Ohtani-Kaneko R, Kitaoka Y, et al. Contribution of mitogen-activated protein kinases to NMDA-induced neurotoxicity in the rat retina. Brain Res. 2005;1044:227–40.
175. Munemasa Y, Ohtani-Kaneko R, Kitaoka Y, et al. Pro-apoptotic role of c-Jun in NMDA-induced neurotoxicity in the rat retina. J Neurosci Res. 2006;83:907–18.
176. Sun H, Wang Y, Pang IH, et al. Protective effect of a JNK inhibitor against retinal ganglion cell loss induced by acute moderate ocular hypertension. Mol Vis. 2011;17:864–75.
177. Kim BJ, Silverman SM, Liu Y, Wordinger RJ, Pang IH, Clark AF. In vitro and in vivo neuroprotective effects of cJun N-terminal kinase inhibitors on retinal ganglion cells. Mol Neurodegener. 2016;11:30.
178. Syc-Mazurek SB, Fernandes KA, Libby RT. JUN is important for ocular hypertension-induced retinal ganglion cell degeneration. Cell Death Dis. 2017;8:e2945.
179. Xiang M, Zhou L, Macke JP, et al. The Brn-3 family of POU-domain factors: primary structure, binding specificity, and expression in subsets of retinal ganglion cells and somatosensory neurons. J Neurosci. 1995;15:4762–85.
180. Wang SW, Gan L, Martin SE, Klein WH. Abnormal polarization and axon outgrowth in retinal ganglion cells lacking the POU-domain transcription factor Brn-3b. Mol Cell Neurosci. 2000;16:141–56.
181. Gan L, Xiang M, Zhou L, Wagner DS, Klein WH, Nathans J. POU domain factor Brn-3b is required for the development of a large set of retinal ganglion cells. Proc Natl Acad Sci U S A. 1996;93:3920–5.
182. Stankowska DL, Minton AZ, Rutledge MA, et al. Neuroprotective effects of transcription factor Brn3b in an ocular hypertension rat model of glaucoma. Invest Ophthalmol Vis Sci. 2015;56:893–907.
183. Phatak NR, Stankowska DL, Krishnamoorthy RR. Bcl-2, Bcl-xL, and p-AKT are involved in neuroprotective effects of transcription factor Brn3b in an ocular hypertension rat model of glaucoma. Mol Vis. 2016;22:1048–61.
184. Prokosch V, Panagis L, Volk GF, Dermon C, Thanos S. Alpha2-adrenergic receptors and their core involvement in the process of axonal growth in retinal explants. Invest Ophthalmol Vis Sci. 2010;51:6688–99.
185. Gao H, Qiao X, Cantor LB, WuDunn D. Up-regulation of brain-derived neurotrophic factor expression by brimonidine in rat retinal ganglion cells. Arch Ophthalmol. 2002;120:797–803.
186. Donello JE, Padillo EU, Webster ML, Wheeler LA, Gil DW. alpha(2)-Adrenoceptor agonists inhibit vitreal glutamate and aspartate accumulation and preserve retinal function after transient ischemia. J Pharmacol Exp Ther. 2001;296:216–23.
187. Yoles E, Wheeler LA, Schwartz M. Alpha2-adrenoreceptor agonists are neuroprotective in a rat model of optic nerve degeneration. Invest Ophthalmol Vis Sci. 1999;40:65–73.
188. Ruiz Lapuente C, Ruiz Lapuente A, Link B. Influence of topical brimonidine on visual field in glaucoma. Eur J Ophthalmol. 2001;11(Suppl 2):S67–71.
189. Evans DW, Hosking SL, Gherghel D, Bartlett JD. Contrast sensitivity improves after brimonidine therapy in primary open angle glaucoma: a case for neuroprotection. Br J Ophthalmol. 2003;87:1463–5.
190. Tsai JC, Chang HW. Comparison of the effects of brimonidine 0.2% and timolol 0.5% on retinal nerve fiber layer thickness in ocular hypertensive patients: a prospective, unmasked study. J Ocul Pharmacol Ther. 2005;21:475–82.
191. Aung T, Oen FT, Wong HT, et al. Randomised controlled trial comparing the effect of brimonidine and timolol on visual field loss after acute primary angle closure. Br J Ophthalmol. 2004;88:88–94.
192. Sebastiani A, Parmeggiani F, Costagliola C, Ciancaglini M, D'Oronzo E, Mastropasqua L. Effects of acute topical administration of clonidine 0.125%, apraclonidine 1.0% and brimonidine 0.2% on visual field parameters and ocular perfusion pressure in patients with primary open-angle glaucoma. Acta Ophthalmol Scand Suppl. 2002;236:29–30.
193. So KF, Aguayo AJ. Lengthy regrowth of cut axons from ganglion cells after peripheral nerve transplantation into the retina of adult rats. Brain Res. 1985;328:349–54.
194. Wang JT, Kunzevitzky NJ, Dugas JC, Cameron M, Barres BA, Goldberg JL. Disease gene candidates revealed by expression profiling of retinal ganglion cell development. J Neurosci. 2007;27:8593–603.
195. Park KK, Hu Y, Muhling J, et al. Cytokine-induced SOCS expression is inhibited by cAMP analogue:

impact on regeneration in injured retina. Mol Cell Neurosci. 2009;41:313–24.
196. Moore DL, Blackmore MG, Hu Y, et al. KLF family members regulate intrinsic axon regeneration ability. Science. 2009;326:298–301.
197. Park KK, Liu K, Hu Y, et al. Promoting axon regeneration in the adult CNS by modulation of the PTEN/mTOR pathway. Science. 2008;322:963–6.
198. Smith PD, Sun F, Park KK, et al. SOCS3 deletion promotes optic nerve regeneration in vivo. Neuron. 2009;64:617–23.
199. Fischer D, Leibinger M. Promoting optic nerve regeneration. Prog Retin Eye Res. 2012;31:688–701.
200. Calkins DJ, Pekny M, Cooper ML, Benowitz L. The challenge of regenerative therapies for the optic nerve in glaucoma. Exp Eye Res. 2017;157:28–33.
201. Doster SK, Lozano AM, Aguayo AJ, Willard MB. Expression of the growth-associated protein GAP-43 in adult rat retinal ganglion cells following axon injury. Neuron. 1991;6:635–47.
202. Huang C, Cen LP, Liu L, et al. Adeno-associated virus-mediated expression of growth-associated protein-43 aggravates retinal ganglion cell death in experimental chronic glaucomatous injury. Mol Vis. 2013;19:1422–32.
203. Dai C, Khaw PT, Yin ZQ, Li D, Raisman G, Li Y. Olfactory ensheathing cells rescue optic nerve fibers in a rat glaucoma model. Transl Vis Sci Technol. 2012;1:3.
204. Mead B, Hill LJ, Blanch RJ, et al. Mesenchymal stromal cell-mediated neuroprotection and functional preservation of retinal ganglion cells in a rodent model of glaucoma. Cytotherapy. 2016;18:487–96.
205. Zhong L, Bradley J, Schubert W, et al. Erythropoietin promotes survival of retinal ganglion cells in DBA/2J glaucoma mice. Invest Ophthalmol Vis Sci. 2007;48:1212–8.
206. Bond WS, Hines-Beard J, GoldenMerry YL, et al. Virus-mediated EpoR76E therapy slows optic nerve axonopathy in experimental glaucoma. Mol Ther. 2016;24:230–9.
207. Hines-Beard J, Bond WS, Backstrom JR, Rex TS. Virus-mediated EpoR76E gene therapy preserves vision in a glaucoma model by modulating neuroinflammation and decreasing oxidative stress. J Neuroinflammation. 2016;13:39.
208. Nagai N, Noda K, Urano T, et al. Selective suppression of pathologic, but not physiologic, retinal neovascularization by blocking the angiotensin II type 1 receptor. Invest Ophthalmol Vis Sci. 2005;46:1078–84.
209. Downie LE, Pianta MJ, Vingrys AJ, Wilkinson-Berka JL, Fletcher EL. AT1 receptor inhibition prevents astrocyte degeneration and restores vascular growth in oxygen-induced retinopathy. Glia. 2008;56:1076–90.
210. Yang H, Hirooka K, Fukuda K, Shiraga F. Neuroprotective effects of angiotensin II type 1 receptor blocker in a rat model of chronic glaucoma. Invest Ophthalmol Vis Sci. 2009;50:5800–4.
211. Foureaux G, Nogueira JC, Nogueira BS, et al. Antiglaucomatous effects of the activation of intrinsic Angiotensin-converting enzyme 2. Invest Ophthalmol Vis Sci. 2013;54:4296–306.
212. Hirooka K, Baba T, Fujimura T, Shiraga F. Prevention of visual field defect progression with angiotensin-converting enzyme inhibitor in eyes with normal-tension glaucoma. Am J Ophthalmol. 2006;142:523–5.
213. Husain S, Potter DE, Crosson CE. Opioid receptor-activation: retina protected from ischemic injury. Invest Ophthalmol Vis Sci. 2009;50:3853–9.
214. Husain S, Abdul Y, Crosson CE. Preservation of retina ganglion cell function by morphine in a chronic ocular-hypertensive rat model. Invest Ophthalmol Vis Sci. 2012;53:4289–98.
215. Abdul Y, Akhter N, Husain S. Delta-opioid agonist SNC-121 protects retinal ganglion cell function in a chronic ocular hypertensive rat model. Invest Ophthalmol Vis Sci. 2013;54:1816–28.
216. Husain S, Ahmad A, Singh S, Peterseim C, Abdul Y, Nutaitis MJ. PI3K/Akt pathway: a role in delta-opioid receptor-mediated RGC neuroprotection. Invest Ophthalmol Vis Sci. 2017;58:6489–99.
217. Belforte NA, Moreno MC, de Zavalia N, et al. Melatonin: a novel neuroprotectant for the treatment of glaucoma. J Pineal Res. 2010;48:353–64.
218. Kumar DM, Perez E, Cai ZY, et al. Role of nonfeminizing estrogen analogues in neuroprotection of rat retinal ganglion cells against glutamate-induced cytotoxicity. Free Radic Biol Med. 2005;38:1152–63.
219. Nakazawa T, Takahashi H, Shimura M. Estrogen has a neuroprotective effect on axotomized RGCs through ERK signal transduction pathway. Brain Res. 2006;1093:141–9.
220. Zhou X, Li F, Ge J, et al. Retinal ganglion cell protection by 17-beta-estradiol in a mouse model of inherited glaucoma. Dev Neurobiol. 2007;67:603–16.
221. Russo R, Cavaliere F, Watanabe C, et al. 17Beta-estradiol prevents retinal ganglion cell loss induced by acute rise of intraocular pressure in rat. Prog Brain Res. 2008;173:583–90.
222. Yamashita H, Yamada-Nakayama C, Sugihara K, et al. Functional and morphological effects of beta-estradiol in eyes with N-methyl-D-Aspartate-induced retinal neurotoxicity in rats. Exp Eye Res. 2011;93:75–81.
223. Li H, Wang B, Zhu C, et al. 17beta-estradiol impedes Bax-involved mitochondrial apoptosis of retinal nerve cells induced by oxidative damage via the phosphatidylinositol 3-kinase/Akt signal pathway. J Mol Neurosci. 2013;50:482–93.
224. Prokai-Tatrai K, Xin H, Nguyen V, et al. 17beta-estradiol eye drops protect the retinal ganglion cell layer and preserve visual function in an in vivo model of glaucoma. Mol Pharm. 2013;10:3253–61.

8 Clinical Practice Considerations

Xueli Chen and Yi Dai

Abstract

Glaucoma is a group of eye conditions which result in characteristic damage to the optic nerve. The pathogenesis and management of primary angle closure glaucoma are different from that of primary open-angle glaucoma. The main types of secondary glaucoma and their underlying causes, treatment principles, and medication options are discussed in this chapter. Treatment of secondary glaucoma should be directed at blocking the underlying disease process and lowering the IOP. Glaucoma therapy related ocular surface disease and drug tolerance are important issues that need more attention. Medical management of the children or pregnant with glaucoma is challenging with respect to balancing disease progression while minimizing systemic risks. Both ophthalmologists and health care providers should be aware of the necessity of careful monitoring and avoiding the potentially dangerous side effects of anti-glaucoma medications.

X. Chen · Y. Dai (✉)
Department of Ophthalmology and Visual Science, Eye and ENT Hospital, Shanghai Medical College, Fudan University, Shanghai, China

NHC Key Laboratory of Myopia (Fudan University), Key Laboratory of Myopia, Chinese Academy of Medical Sciences, Shanghai, China

Shanghai Key Laboratory of Visual Impairment and Restoration (Fudan University), Shanghai, China
e-mail: ydai@fudan.edu.cn

Keywords

Primary angle closure glaucoma · Secondary glaucoma · Drug tolerance · Ocular surface disease · Pregnancy · Breast-feeding

8.1 Primary Angle Closure Glaucoma

Primary angle closure glaucoma (PACG) is a common cause of blindness. The estimated rate of bilateral blindness in PACG will remain high in 2020 (about 22.6% in 23.36 million patients). The fundamental pathologic change is angle closure in PACG. Therapeutic strategies aiming to open the angle are proving their effectiveness. Compared with primary open-angle glaucoma (POAG), PACG is a more intraocular pressure (IOP)-dependent disease. While growing body of evidence is available on how to set target IOPs when treating POAG, no consensus is available on what IOP levels are required to prevent progression of glaucomatous optic neuropathy in PACG [1].

Pilocarpine is one of the cholinergic agents widely used in Asian countries for patients with PACG, as it is effective and inexpensive. Pilocarpine is a direct muscarinic agonist. It contracts the pupillary sphincter, pulling the peripheral iris away from the trabecular meshwork and therefore reopening the drainage angle.

X. Sun, Y. Dai (eds.), *Medical Treatment of Glaucoma*,
https://doi.org/10.1007/978-981-13-2733-9_8

However, frequently used pilocarpine may cause ocular adverse effects, such as synechial miosis, ciliary muscle spasm to induce malignant glaucoma, and tearing the peripheral retina in some cases. Partly due to these side effects, the commonly used concentrations of pilocarpine are 0.5% and 1%, while the concentrations of 4% are rarely used. In addition, pilocarpine has not been shown to lower IOP in these eyes which had whole angle closed because of permanent synechial formation [2, 3].

Medications used in POAG to reduce IOP are also used in cases of PACG. The mechanism of beta-blockers, alpha-agonists, and carbonic anhydrase inhibitors for IOP reduction is decreasing the secretion of aqueous humor. They can be utilized in all types of glaucoma, irrespective of the state of the anterior chamber angle. On the other hand, the main mechanism of prostaglandin analogs (PGAs) for IOP reduction is increasing uveoscleral outflow. They have no effects on the aqueous humor production. Studies have suggested that PGAs provide a significant IOP-lowering efficacy in eyes with chronic angle closure glaucoma and are as effective as timolol [4]. However, the mechanism of action of PGAs in eyes with angle closure remains elusive. Further studies are needed to elucidate the effect of PGAs in PACG.

PACG can be divided into acute PACG or chronic PACG according to the timing or suddenness of onset. The developmental course of acute PACG can be further divided into preclinical, attack (including acute and mild attacks), intermittent, chronic, and absolute stages. The mild attacks are present with small IOP spikes due to partial angle closure. It usually can be relieved after topical pilocarpine administration or good rest such as sleep during which physiological miosis is achieved by parasympathetic nerve excitation. However, acute angle closure attack is an ophthalmic emergency. A sudden IOP elevation higher than 60–70 mmHg may occur due to complete angle closure. Treatments to lower the IOP should be initiated as soon as possible. Systemically administered hyperosmotic agents, such as intravenous mannitol, along with oral carbonic anhydrase inhibitor and topical aqueous suppressants, can be used in combination if necessary. Frequent pilocarpine dosing may be more effective after IOP has been lowered to below 50 mmHg, in which the iris ischemia were reduced and pupillary sphincter may respond to the miotics. Topical steroid application is also important to control the inflammation of anterior segment, restrain the formation of peripheral anterior synechiae, and protect the microstructure and outflow function of angle drainage [1].

8.2 Secondary Glaucoma

Secondary glaucoma refers to certain form of glaucoma with an identifiable ocular or systemic cause of IOP elevation, resulting in optic nerve damage. Treatment of secondary glaucoma should be directed at blocking the underlying disease process and lowering the IOP.

8.2.1 Steroid-Induced Glaucoma

Glucocorticoid therapy, whether given by the topical, periocular, or systemic route, can cause IOP elevation and glaucomatous optic neuropathy in a subset of patients. There is highly individualized response to glucocorticoid application, including adverse ocular effects in susceptible patients. Individuals with POAG or a family history of the disease are more likely to be high steroid responders. High myopes, diabetics, and patients with connective tissue diseases (especially rheumatoid arthritis) have a similar predisposition. The pathogenesis of steroid-induced glaucoma is not well understood, but reduction in trabecular meshwork outflow is regarded as the main reason of IOP elevation [5].

Pharmacogenomics is the study of the role of genome on a person's response to drugs, which may identify genetic variants affecting glucocorticoid sensitivity. The trabecular meshwork-inducible glucocorticoid response (TIGR) gene product was the first gene reported to be associated with POAG. The gene is now called MYOC (myocilin). The function of MYOC protein in normal biology was not known when its causative role in POAG was discovered, and its normal function in cells remains elusive so far. MYOC is reported to be linked to activation of signaling pathways altered in both POAG and steroid-induced glaucoma. With the rapid development of epigenetics, effective approaches based on precision medicine may be developed to monitor the judicious use of glucocorticoids [6].

As for the management, discontinuation of the glucocorticoids is the first choice. The IOP usually returns to normal within a few weeks, although a few patients may have a sustained elevation of IOP. Several studies have showed that the incidence of steroid-induced glaucoma and the reversibility of the IOP elevation depend upon the glucocorticoid potency, formulation (which influences ocular penetration), dosing frequency, and duration of exposure. All available IOP-lowering medications can be used in these patients, beginning with aqueous humor suppressants. These include beta-blockers, followed by either alpha2-agonists or topical carbonic anhydrase inhibitors. Monotherapy with PGA is mostly safe and effective in patients with steroid-induced glaucoma [7]. However, in patients who have developed IOP elevation after using glucocorticoids to control uveitis, PGAs are relatively contraindicated.

8.2.2 Uveitic Glaucoma

Uveitic glaucoma is a common complication of uveitis affecting up to 20% of patients. Intraocular inflammation, secondary corticosteroid response, and varying types and degrees of angle closure contribute to its pathogenesis. The form of uveitis that most frequently produces IOP elevation is anterior uveitis and chronic forms of uveitis [8].

Treatment is targeted at reducing the inflammation and lowering the IOP. Control of the ocular inflammation alone frequently leads to normalization of the IOP. Topical administration is preferred for anterior segment disease and commonly used corticosteroids include 1.0% prednisolone and 0.1% dexamethasone. It may also be treated with medications that modulate the immune system. As for management of IOP elevation, aqueous humor suppressants including beta-blockers, alpha2-agonists, or topical carbonic anhydrase are the first-line hypotensive agents in the treatment of uveitic glaucoma. PGAs and miotics are generally contraindicated in the inflamed eyes.

Posner–Schlossman syndrome (also known as glaucomatocyclitic crisis) and Fuchs heterochromic iridocyclitis are uveitic glaucoma that were previously believed to be idiopathic. Recent studies have highlighted the role of viruses, such as cytomegalovirus, herpes simplex virus, and rubella virus in the pathogenesis of these diseases [9]. Antiviral therapy including systemic administration and intravitreal injection may be beneficial in eyes with detectable viral DNA. Su et al. reported that topical 2% ganciclovir treatment was effective for clearing the aqueous viral load and assisting the IOP control of CMV-positive anterior uveitis patients [10].

8.2.3 Traumatic Glaucoma

Blunt or penetrating ocular trauma is a common cause of ocular morbidity and occurs most often in young adults and children. Causes of IOP elevation after trauma include a variety of clinical presentations. Hyphema is the most common sign in the anterior segment after blunt trauma. As the blood gradually clears in the anterior segment, the IOP may remain elevated most commonly due to angle recession and trabecular meshwork damage. Other mechanisms of elevated IOP after blunt trauma include traumatic iritis, angle closure due to dislocation of the lens and injury to the zonular fibers, vitreous filling in the anterior chamber, vitreous hemorrhage, Schwartz–Matsuo syndrome, etc. Elevated IOP resulted from blunt ocular injury may occur in hours to years, so it is important to follow these patients indefinitely [11–14].

Traumatic glaucoma was usually defined as long-term glaucoma medication use (at least 3 months) or need for glaucoma surgery. Medications that reduced aqueous production are the first-line choices in the treatment of traumatic glaucoma. Corticosteroids may be helpful if an ocular inflammatory component is present. Chronic IOP elevation due to trabecular damage and angle recession does not respond well to miotic therapy, while PGAs have a theoretical benefit in these cases [15].

8.2.4 Neovascular Glaucoma

Neovascular glaucoma (NVG) is a severe form of secondary glaucoma characterized by rubeosis iridis and proliferation of fibrovascular tissue in the anterior chamber angle. Retinal ischemic diseases including diabetic retinopathy and occlusion of central retinal vessels account for nearly two-thirds of all cases of NVG. Other ocular and extraocular vascular disorders, such as choroidal melanoma, uveitis, and carotid artery obstructive disease, have also been recognized to induce rubeosis iridis and NVG [16].

The management of NVG involves both reducing elevated IOP and treating the underlying disease. Panretinal photocoagulation is the standard treatment for ablation of the ischemic retina. With the advent of the anti-VEGF agents, the success in controlling active neovascularization has been greatly enhanced. NVG can be divided into preglaucoma stage (rubeosis iridis), open-angle stage, and angle-closure stage. When the anti-VEGF treatment was applied before the angle-closure stage, the neovascular located at the anterior chamber angle and iris may fade rapidly and IOP elevation can be reversed. Following panretinal photocoagulation, stimulus for neovascularization of the anterior segment can be mostly reduced. Once the angle is synechial closed exceeding about 270°, IOP elevation cannot be reduced even with the regression of neovascularization. But the anti-VEGF therapy may facilitate the initial surgical management of NVG [17–20].

Aqueous suppressants including beta-blockers, alpha-agonists, and carbonic anhydrase inhibitors are usually the main choices of IOP-lowering medications. PGAs may be effective in open-angle stage but may also exacerbate ocular inflammation. Osmotic agents may provide acute but transient lowering of IOP to clear the cornea for treatment or diagnosis. Topical corticosteroids can be used to control ocular inflammation, and cycloplegic agents can be used to alleviate pains. Miotics should be avoided since they can increase inflammation and discomfort. Most cases of NVG in angle-closure stage are refractory to pharmacological treatment and require surgical intervention. Further studies are needed to demonstrate whether combined anti-VEGF therapy can improve the long-term outcome of NVG.

8.2.5 Pigmentary Glaucoma

Pigmentary glaucoma is a specific form of open-angle glaucoma that occurs in eyes with pigment dispersion syndrome. Its prevalence is predominantly high in Caucasians, particularly men. The pathogenesis of pigment dispersion syndrome and pigmentary glaucoma is not totally understood. The classic diagnostic triad in pigment dispersion syndrome consists of (1) a Krukenberg spindle (pigmented iris cells deposited on the posterior surface of the cornea); (2) slit-like, radial, mid-peripheral iris transillumination defects; and (3) dense pigmentation on the trabecular meshwork. The deposited iris pigment (melanin granules) released largely due to iridozonular friction contributes to damage to the trabecular meshwork over time and impede the conventional outflow of aqueous humor [21, 22].

Treatment may be targeted at relieving reverse pupillary block and lowering the IOP. Laser peripheral iridotomy can be considered as a prophylactic and effective treatment, which has been shown to reverse the posteriorly bowed iris configuration, and prevent further pigment liberation. Miotics such as pilocarpine could stretch the iris, relieve iridozonular contact, and diminish pigment dispersion, while at the same time lowering IOP by the direct effect on aqueous outflow. However, pilocarpine is often not tolerated by young patients because of the accommodative spasm and further induced myopia. It has been recommended to take pilocarpine only once daily at bedtime. Long-term pilocarpine use may also increase the risk of retinal detachment in the young myopic population and induce the formation of posterior synechiae. PGAs and aqueous suppressants (beta-blockers, alpha-agonists, and carbonic anhydrase inhibitors) can effectively reduce IOP in patients with pigmentary glaucoma. Prostaglandin analogs may be preferred over aqueous suppressants as treatment with aqueous suppressants slows down the clearance of pigment from the trabecular meshwork. However, it also has been proposed that the long-term use of PGAs may exacerbate this condition by increasing iridal pigmentation [23, 24].

8.2.6 Pseudoexfoliation Glaucoma

Pseudoexfoliation syndrome (XFS) is a systemic disorder with ocular manifestations, including open- and closed-angle glaucoma and cataract with zonular weakness. The pseudoexfoliative material may be seen as white flecks on the anterior lens capsule, pupillary margin of the iris, ciliary process, zonule, and the trabecular meshwork. The prevalence of XFS increases considerably with age and varies significantly across geographic regions and ethnic groups. Population-based studies have identified mutations on the lysyl-oxidase-like 1 (LOXL1) gene as a risk factor for XFS. Environmental factors, such as latitude of residence and caffeine consumption, have been reported to be associated with XFS in genetically predisposed individuals. It is suggested that mutations in LOXL1 gene may cause accumulation of pseudoexfoliative material in the trabecular meshwork, leading to IOP elevation. LOXL1 deficiency may also affect the biomechanical properties of optic nerve head, particularly lamina cribrosa, making it more vulnerable to IOP elevation. It is estimated that about 30% XFS eyes develop pseudoexfoliation glaucoma (XFG) within their lifetime [25–27].

XFG has been reported to be responsible for about 20–25% of cases of open-angle glaucoma worldwide. When XFG is unilateral, it is recommended that careful follow-up of the fellow eye is necessary since there is a high probability of XFG development over time. Treatment for XFG is similar to the treatment of POAG. However, compared with POAG patients, XFG patients often present with higher baseline IOP and poor response to medical treatment. A combination of topical IOP-lowering medications is often required to achieve the target IOP in XFG patients. PGAs are usually the first-line choice for initial medical treatment, which has been proven to be more effective than aqueous suppressants in IOP-lowering and diurnal IOP control. Aqueous suppressants, including beta-blockers, alpha-agonists, and carbonic anhydrase inhibitors, can be prescribed as adjunctive medications. Fixed combination PGA/timolol eye drops have shown better diurnal IOP control than PGA monotherapy in XFG. Miotics such as pilocarpine may also be useful to XFG patients. Miotics could inhibit pupillary movement, relieve iridozonular contact, and diminish pigment and exfoliation material liberation, while lowering IOP by enhancing aqueous outflow in trabecular meshwork. But in practice, pilocarpine is used infrequently, largely due to its ocular side effects, such as dim vision and posterior synechiae. It is also possible that pilocarpine may induce pupillary block and angle closure in XFG patients due to zonular weakness, increased lens thickness, and anterior movement of the lens–iris diaphragm [28, 29].

8.2.7 Malignant Glaucoma

Malignant glaucoma is a rare but serious form of glaucoma that typically encountered after glaucoma surgery in eyes with chronic angle closure glaucoma, although it has been reported to occur spontaneously, under miotic therapy, or after any ophthalmic procedure. The concept of malignant glaucoma includes various clinical conditions, which have these common features: shallowing or flattening of the central and peripheral anterior chambers, elevation of the intraocular pressure (IOP), and unresponsiveness to or aggravation by use of miotics but frequent relief with cycloplegic–mydriatic treatment. The classic cause of malignant glaucoma is believed to be aqueous humor misdirection due to ciliary block. But the exact etiology of this group of conditions is not fully understood [30].

Pharmacological management is usually tried for several days before surgical intervention is attempted. First-line agents include mydriatic–cycloplegic agents and aqueous suppressants. Cycloplegics can tighten the lens zonules by relaxing the ciliary muscle, pulling the anteriorly displaced lens backwards, and alleviating the ciliary block. The aqueous suppressants can decrease the posterior pooling of the aqueous humor by reducing its production. Osmotic agents are used to dehydrate the vitreous and reduce vitreous volume, allowing posterior movement of the lens–iris diaphragm with expansion of anterior chamber space. Topical corticosteroids can also be used to alleviate ocular inflammation. Medical therapy is reported to be effective in about 50% patients within a 5-day period. When the anterior chamber deepens and the IOP normalizes, medical treatment can be slowly withdrawn in most cases. However, indefinite cycloplegia with topical atropine may still be required to prevent recurrence of malignant glaucoma in some cases [31, 32].

8.3 Long-Term Usage

Glaucoma is a chronic disease that requires long-term and even lifetime treatment. Several important issues have received specific attentions during the long-term usage of IOP-lowering medications.

8.3.1 Drug Tolerance

Drug tolerance is a patient's diminished response to a drug following its repeated use. The process of tolerance development is sometimes reversible (e.g., through a drug holiday) and can involve both physiological and psychological factors.

The topic use of timolol, a beta-blocker, has been the first-line therapy in the treatment of glaucoma during the 1980s and early 1990s. Several studies have reported the diminishing IOP reduction during treatment with timolol. Boger reviewed the subject and introduced the term "long-term drift" and "short-term escape" which describe the reduction of timolol's efficacy over a few days and over months and years, respectively [33]. The incidence of loss of efficacy has been reported as 10% of patients for each year of non-selective beta-blocker treatment in several long-term clinical trials. This means that only 50% patients will show a clinically relevant response after 5 year treatment of timolol. In about 10% cases, the efficacy of beta-blockers in IOP reduction may decrease over time. It has been reported that in the "timolol holiday" lasting 30–60 days, using dipivefrin 0.1% twice daily can better help restore the sensitivity to timolol [34].

Prostaglandin analogs (PGAs) have become the most frequently prescribed initial eye drops for lowering IOP in POAG patients during the last decade. Many studies have focused on comparisons between prostaglandin analogs and timolol. The results suggested that prostaglandin analogs have better IOP-lowering effects than timolol. PGAs also showed progressive IOP reduction and absence of long-term drift up to 5 years. In glaucoma patients whose IOP is not adequately controlled with timolol, a good effect on IOP reduction was achieved by switching from timolol to PGAs [35]. In practice, patients who showed the diminishing efficacy of IOP reduction to PGA monotherapy during long time follow-up are not rare. The mechanism underlying these phenomena remains largely unknown. One should also consider that worsening of disease severity per se could lead to loss of effect in PGAs. Quite a few studies suggested that glaucoma patients on one PGA who experienced IOP elevation during the course of therapy may benefit from switching to other kind of PGAs [36].

8.3.2 Ocular Surface Disease

Patients with glaucoma who were taking one or more ocular IOP-lowering medications have been shown to suffer from a higher prevalence of ocular surface disease (OSD) than age related controls. Recent studies suggest that OSD demonstrates an overall prevalence in 42% (range 20–59%) of glaucoma patients and is severe in 36% (range 14–66%). Glaucoma therapy related

OSD can be defined as an imbalance of the ocular surface homeostasis caused by the toxic effect of chronic topical medication, which leads to tear film instability, epithelial damage, and inflammation [37–39].

The cause of OSD in glaucoma patients is thought to be multifactorial: both conditions are common in the elderly patients; the presence of additional anterior segment ocular disorders (e.g., blepharitis, allergy, dry eye, or eyelid anatomical abnormalities) may further contribute to the onset of OSD. More importantly, topical IOP-lowering eye drops can trigger or exacerbate OSD if they contain preservatives, particularly benzalkonium chloride (BAK). Human corneal and conjunctival cell cultures exhibited a dose-dependent decrease in cell survival when treated with solutions containing increasing BAK concentrations. Adverse effects induced by BAK, including conjunctival inflammation and fibrosis, tear film instability, corneal cytotoxicity, anterior chamber inflammation, trabecular meshwork cell apoptosis, cataract development, macular edema, and even systemic effects, have been documented. Aside from the BAK as the main cause, the active hypotensive agents in IOP-lowering eye drops may also play a role in glaucoma therapy related OSD [40–42].

To reduce the occurrence rate and severity of OSD, the use of preservative-free or non-BAK-preserved IOP-lowering agents is a good option. A preservative-free formulation of timolol and PGAs, as well as fixed combinations, such dorzolamide/timolol and prostaglandin/timolol, has become commercially available in some countries or regions. The efficacy and safety of these medications have been proved, while the higher cost of current preservative-free therapies needs to be reduced. Alternative ophthalmic preservatives have also been developed (e.g., Purite®, [Allergan, Irvine, CA] and Polyquad® preservative [Alcon, Fort Worth, TX]) to reformulate the BAK-preserved IOP-lowering medications. This advancement can offer glaucoma patients alternate therapies that can reduce their exposure to BAK. It is especially critical to help preserve the ocular surface homeostasis of patients where preservative-free anti-glaucoma agents are currently unavailable.

In addition, medical therapy to manage the OSD in glaucoma patients is important. Artificial tears (preservative free or BAK free) are often prescribed to alleviate the symptoms and signs of glaucoma therapy related OSD. A study reported that strategies to control the OSD in patients with glaucoma, including twice-daily lid hygiene measures, a 3-month course of 50 mg daily oral doxycycline, topical carmellose sodium (celluvisc) 0.5% 4–6 times daily, and preservative-free equivalents of topical anti-glaucoma medications as deemed appropriate, may improve the IOP control and the management of glaucoma [43].

8.3.3 Effect on Cornea

The relationship between IOP measurements and central corneal thickness (CCT) has long been recognized. Recent study suggested that long-term PGAs monotherapy has the influence on the cornea of POAG patients. Topical PGAs may change the biomechanical properties of cornea, further influence IOP measurements and patient follow-up. The outcomes include reduction in corneal hysteresis, corneal resistance factor, and CCT in patients with POAG. These changes may contribute to underestimation of the IOP measured by Goldmann applanation tonometry and warrant caution when assessing response to PGA treatment. The effects are reversible. Once cessation of the PGAs, the corneal parameters may reverse to the baseline [44, 45].

8.4 Special Patients

8.4.1 For Children and Teenagers

During the medical treatment of infants and young children with glaucoma, one should bear in mind that children are not small adults. Systemic adverse reactions rarely seen in adults can occur in young children. Topical carbonic anhydrase inhibitors are generally safe and effective for infants and children [46]. It was reported that oral carbonic anhydrase inhibitor administration may cause growth retardation and metabolic acidosis [47]. Topical beta-blockers should be avoided in premature infants or neonates [48]. When timolol is used in younger children, treatment should be better to begin with 0.25% concentrations, excluding those with a history of asthma or bradycardia. Selective beta-blocker, betaxolol, is safer than timolol. PGAs are less effective in children than in adults, and are more likely to be effective in older children and those with juvenile-onset open-angle glaucoma. Systemic and ocular side effects in children on latanoprost are infrequent and mild [49]. Brimonidine is absolutely contraindicated in neonates and infants (under the age of 2 year). Because of risks of pronounced central nervous system depression, such as apnea, brimonidine should be used with great caution in children younger than 8 years [50].

Surgery intervention is the primary treatment strategy for primary congenital glaucoma. Medical therapies are the options only when surgery has to be delayed or surgical procedures can't adequately control the IOP. Open-angle juvenile glaucoma patients often have better response to hypotensive treatment than primary congenital glaucoma, possibly due to the former has a relatively developed anterior chamber angle approximating that in the adult, while the latter often exhibited a developmental abnormality of the anterior chamber angle leading to obstruction of aqueous outflow.

Topical beta-blockers and carbonic anhydrase inhibitors are the first-line hypotensive agents in the treatment of congenital glaucoma, and then the PGAs. Miotics have limited value in treating children with glaucoma, except for its routine use after trabeculotomy or goniotomy to pull the peripheral iris away from the trabecular meshwork for congenital glaucoma. For juvenile-onset open-angle glaucoma, PGAs would be the first choice. Beta-blockers would be the second choice, followed by carbonic hydrase inhibitors in fixed combination with beta-blockers. Adrenergic agonists would be the last choice.

8.4.2 For Pregnant and Breast-Feeding Women

Medical management of the pregnant or nursing patients is challenging with respect to balancing disease progression in the mother while minimizing risks to the fetus or infants. Data are limited on this topic due to ethical and legal constraints in this patient population. The FDA has established drug pregnancy categories of A, B, C, D, and X based on human or animal studies. Pregnancy Category A (controlled studies show no risk) is the safest one. Brimonidine has a Pregnancy Category B rating (presumed safety based on animal studies). All other ocular hypotensive agents have a Pregnancy Category C rating (uncertain safety; no human or animal studies).

Brimonidine is generally the preferred first-line drug in the first, second, and early third trimester. Late in the third trimester, brimonidine should be discontinued because it can induce central nervous system depression in newborns wherein topical carbonic anhydrase inhibitors may be the optimal choice. The beta-blockers tend to be used during pregnancy because there is long-term experience with this drug class. But it also has the potential to reduce fetal respiration in late pregnancy. Very few data exist on the risk of taking prostaglandin analogs in pregnancy, although some small case series of subjects who took it while pregnant revealed no adverse effects on pregnancy and no birth defects. Some ophthalmologists choose avoiding the prostaglandins during the third trimester because of the theoretical risk of premature labor. Argon laser trabeculoplasty or selective laser trabeculoplasty is an alternative treatment that can be performed in all trimesters.

Special attention should also be paid during breast-feeding. Carbonic anhydrase inhibitors are suggested to use in nursing mother by American Academy of Pediatrics. PGAs may also be considered to use during breast-feeding. The data are controversial as to whether timolol poses a threat to the breast-feeding infant. EGS Guideline [53] suggests that beta-blockers could be used in nursing mother, while the Preferred Practice Pattern

[54] from American Academy of Ophthalmology suggests not. Since timolol and carbonic anhydrase inhibitors have been detected in breast milk, low doses of these medications should be considered and the infant should be carefully monitored when ocular hypotensive agents are used in the breast-feeding period [51–54].

8.4.3 Depression and Cognitive Impairment

Brimonidine should be used with caution in patients with depression as illustrated by the prescribing information for ALPHAGAN P. Tricyclic antidepressants can affect the metabolism and uptake of circulating amine. Though data on brimonidine is rare, tricyclic antidepressants have been reported to blunt the hypotensive effect of systemic clonidine, which is an alpha-adrenergic agonist. Brimonidine can pass through the blood–brain barrier and potentially cause central nervous system depression; however, published reports on the occurrence of psychological depression after brimonidine administration are rare.

Depressive symptoms were reported in 17/165 patients after taking timolol eye drops about 40 years ago. Later on, several reports further suggest the linking between timolol to depression. Cases were also reported about the occurrence of clinical depression following topical betaxolol administration. However, these cases are uncommon and doubts remains. A study suggested that ongoing beta-blockers use was not causally related to markers of depression [55–57].

On the other hand, some antidepressants and antianxiety agents can precipitate angle closure glaucoma in susceptible eyes, mainly by pupillary effect of mydriasis [58, 59]. Preventive laser peripheral iridotomy is effective in eliminating pupillary block and preventing acute attacks.

Cognitive impairment may also become common in elderly patients with glaucoma. This has important implications for adherence to treatment, as difficulties in understanding and remembering information may largely increase the nonadherence to treatments prescribed by physicians. It is crucial that physicians and caregivers are aware of the prevalence of such conditions, as they are among the first to interact with such patients [60].

Given the relatively high prevalence of depression and anxiety disorders, as well as cognitive impairment, both ophthalmologists and psychiatrists should be aware of the necessity of careful monitoring and avoiding the potentially dangerous drug interactions.

References

1. Sun X, Dai Y, Chen Y, et al. Primary angle closure glaucoma: what we know and what we don't know. Prog Retin Eye Res. 2017;57:26–45.
2. Pape LG, Forbes M. Retinal detachment and miotic therapy. Am J Ophthalmol. 1978;85:558e566.
3. Stocker FW. Experimental studies on the blood-aqueous barrier; electrophotometric measurements of fluorescein content of aqueous after intravenous injection of fluorescein, the eye being under the influence of physostigmine, pilocarpine, neostigmine or atropine. Arch Ophthalmol. 1947;37:583e5.
4. Aung T, Wong HT, Yip CC, Leong JY, Chan YH, Chew PT. Comparison of the intraocular pressure-lowering effect of Latanoprost and timolol in patients with chronic angle closure glaucoma: a preliminary study. Ophthalmology. 2000;107:1178–83.
5. Razeghinejad R, Katz L. Steroid-induced iatrogenic glaucoma. Ophthalmic Res. 2012;47:66–80.
6. Fini ME, Schwartz SG, Gao X, et al. Steroid-induced ocular hypertension/glaucoma: focus on pharmacogenomics and implications for precision medicine. Prog Retin Eye Res. 2017;56:58–83.
7. Scherer WJ, Hauber FA. Effect of latanoprost on intraocular pressure in steroid-induced glaucoma. J Glaucoma. 2000;9(2):179–82.
8. Sng CC, Ang M, Barton K. Uveitis and glaucoma: new insights in the pathogenesis and treatment. Prog Brain Res. 2015;221:243–69.
9. Van Gelder RN. Idiopathic no more: clues to the pathogenesis of Fuchs heterochromic iridocyclitis and glaucomatocyclitic crisis. Am J Ophthalmol. 2008;145(5):769–71.
10. Su C, Hu F, Wang T, et al. Clinical outcomes in cytomegalovirus-positive Posner-Schlossman syndrome patients treated with topical ganciclovir therapy. Am J Ophthalmol. 2014;158:1024–31.
11. Bojikian KD, Stein AL, Slabaugh MA, et al. Incidence and risk factors for traumatic intraocular pressure elevation and traumatic glaucoma after open-globe injury. Eye. 2015;29:1579–84.

12. Ng DS, Ching RH, Chan CW. Angle-recession glaucoma: long-term clinical outcomes over a 10-year period in traumatic microhyphema. Int Ophthalmol. 2015;35:107–13.
13. Sihota R, Kumar S, Gupta V, et al. Early predictors of traumatic glaucoma after closed globe injury: trabecular pigmentation, widened angle recess, and higher baseline intraocular pressure. Arch Ophthalmol. 2008;126:921–6.
14. Turalba AV, Shah AS, Andreoli MT, et al. Predictors and outcomes of ocular hypertension after open-globe injury. J Glaucoma. 2014;23:5–10.
15. Bleiman BS, Schwartz A. Paradoxical intraocular pressure response to pilocarpine: a proposed mechanism and treatment. Arch Ophthalmol. 1979;97:1305.
16. Brown GC, Magargal LE, Schachat A, et al. Neovascular glaucoma: etiologic considerations. Ophthalmology. 1984;91:315.
17. Ehlers JP, Spirn MJ, Lam A, et al. Combination intravitreal bevacizumab/panretinal photocoagulation versus panretinal photocoagulation alone in the treatment of neovascular glaucoma. Retina. 2008;28:696–702.
18. Yazdani S, Hendi K, Pakravan M, et al. Intravitreal bevacizumab for neovascular glaucoma: a randomized controlled trial. J Glaucoma. 2009;18:632–7.
19. Wolf A, von Jagow B, Ulbig M, Haritoglou C. Intracameral injection of bevacizumab for the treatment of neovascular glaucoma. Ophthalmologica. 2011;226:51–6.
20. Ha JY, Lee TH, Sung MS, Park SW. Efficacy and safety of intracameral bevacizumab for treatment of neovascular glaucoma. Korean J Ophthalmol. 2017;31(6):538–47.
21. Allingham R, et al. Pigmentary glaucomas and other glaucomas associated with disorders of the iris and ciliary body. In: Shield's textbook of glaucoma. 5th ed. Philadelphia: Lippincott Williams & Wilkins; 2005. p. 303–17.
22. Michelessi M, Lindsley K. Peripheral iridotomy for pigmentary glaucoma. Cochrane Database Syst Rev. 2016;2:CD005655.
23. Anderson MG, Smith RS, Hawes NL, et al. Mutations in genes encoding melanosomal proteins cause pigmentary glaucoma in DBA/2J mice. Nat Genet. 2002;30:81–5.
24. Haynes WL, Johnson AT, Alward WL. Inhibition of exercise-induced pigment dispersion in a patient with the pigmentary dispersion syndrome. Am J Ophthalmol. 1990;109(5):601–2.
25. Tarkkanen A. Exfoliation syndrome: a historical perspective. J Glaucoma. 2018;27:S1–3.
26. Miglior S, Bertuzzi F. Exfoliative glaucoma: new evidence in the pathogenesis and treatment. Prog Brain Res. 2015;221:233–41.
27. Schlötzer-Schrehardt U, Hammer CM, Krysta AW, et al. LOXL1 deficiency in the lamina cribrosa as candidate susceptibility factor for a pseudoexfoliation-specific risk of glaucoma. Ophthalmology. 2012;119(9):1832–43.
28. Schlötzer-Schrehardt U, Naumann GO. Ocular and systemic pseudoexfoliation syndrome. Am J Ophthalmol. 2006;141:921–37.
29. Michalik A, Kaufman P. Medical management of glaucoma in exfoliation syndrome. J Glaucoma. 2018;27:S87–90.
30. Foreman-Larkin J, Netland PA, Salim S. Clinical management of malignant glaucoma. J Ophthalmol. 2015;2015:283707.
31. Simmons J. Malignant glaucoma. Br J Ophthalmol. 1972;56:263–72.
32. Ruben S, Tsai J, Hitchings R. Malignant glaucoma and its management. Br J Ophthalmol. 1997;81:163–7.
33. Boger WP. Short-term "escape" and long-term "drift". The dissipation effects of the beta adrenergic blocking agents. Surv Ophthalmol. 1983;28(Suppl):235–42.
34. Gandolfi SA. Restoring sensitivity to timolol after long-term drift in primary open-angle glaucoma. Invest Ophthalmol Vis Sci. 1990;31:354–8.
35. Bron AM, Denis P, Nordmann JP, et al. Additive IOP-reducing effect of latanoprost in patients insufficiently controlled on timolol. Acta Ophthalmol Scand. 2001;79(3):289–93.
36. Germano RA, Susanna R, De Moraes CG, et al. Effect of switching from latanoprost to bimatoprost in primary open-angle glaucoma patients who experienced intraocular pressure elevation during treatment. J Glaucoma. 2016;25(4):e359–66.
37. Leung EW, Medeiros FA, Weinreb RN. Prevalence of ocular surface disease in glaucoma patients. J Glaucoma. 2008;17(5):350–5.
38. Stewart WC, Stewart JA, Nelson LA. Ocular surface disease in patients with ocular hypertension and glaucoma. Curr Eye Res. 2011;36(5):391–8.
39. Holló G, Katsanos A, Boboridis KG, Irkec M, Konstas AGP. Preservative-free prostaglandin analogs and prostaglandin/timolol fixed combinations in the treatment of glaucoma: efficacy, safety and potential advantages. Drugs. 2017;78(1):39–64. https://doi.org/10.1007/s40265-017-0843-9.
40. Ammar DA, Noecker RJ, Kahook MY. Effects of benzalkonium chloride-preserved, polyquad-preserved, and sofZia-preserved topical glaucoma medications on human ocular epithelial cells. Adv Ther. 2010;27:837–45.
41. Rouland J-F, Traverso CE, Stalmans I, Fekih LE, Delval L, Renault D, et al. Efficacy and safety of preservative-free latanoprost eyed drops, compared with BAK-preserved latanoprost in patients with ocular hypertension or glaucoma. Br J Ophthalmol. 2013;97:196–200.
42. Shedden A, Adamsons IA, Getson AJ, Laurence JK, Lines CR, Hewitt DJ, Ho TW. Comparison of the efficacy and tolerability of preservative-free and preservative-containing formulations of the dorzolamide/timolol fixed combination (COSOPTTM) in patients with elevated intraocular pressure in a randomized clinical trial. Graefes Arch Clin Exp Ophthalmol. 2010;248:1757–64.

43. Batra R, Tailor R, Mohamed S. Ocular surface disease exacerbated glaucoma: optimizing the ocular surface improves intraocular pressure control. J Glaucoma. 2014;23(1):56–60.
44. Meda R, Wang Q, Paoloni D, et al. The impact of chronic use of prostaglandin analogues on the biomechanical properties of the cornea in patients with primary open-angle glaucoma. Br J Ophthalmol. 2017;101:120–5.
45. Wu N, Chen Y, Yu X, Li M, Wen W, Sun X. Changes in corneal biomechanical properties after long-term topical prostaglandin therapy. PLoS One. 2016;11:e0155527.
46. Whitson JT, Roarty JD, Vijayal L, et al. Efficacy of brinzolamide and levobetaxolol in pediatric glaucomas: a randomized clinical trial. J AAPOS. 2008;12:239–46 e3.
47. Futagi Y, Otani K, Abe J. Growth suppression in children receiving acetazolamide with antiepileptic drugs. Pediatr Neurol. 1996;15:323–6.
48. Passo MS, Palmer EA, Van Buskirk EM. Plasma timolol in glaucoma patients. Ophthalmology. 1984;91:1361–3.
49. Enyedi LB, Freedman SF. Latanoprost for the treatment of pediatric glaucoma. Surv Ophthalmol. 2002;47(Suppl1):S129–32.
50. Enyedi L, Freedman S. Safety and efficacy of brimonidine in children with glaucoma. J AAPOS. 2001;5:281.
51. Salim S. Glaucoma in pregnancy. Curr Opin Ophthalmol. 2014;25:93–7.
52. Razeghinejad MR, Tania Tai TY, Fudemberg SJ, Katz LJ. Pregnancy and glaucoma. Surv Ophthalmol. 2011;56:324–35.
53. European Glaucoma Society. Terminology and guidelines for glaucoma. 4th ed. Mainz: European Glaucoma Society; 2014.
54. American Academy of Ophthalmology. Preferred practice pattern. 3rd ed. San Francisco: American Academy of Ophthalmology; 2015.
55. McMahon CD, Shaffer RN, Hoskins HD, Hetherington J. Adverse effects experienced by patients taking timolol. Am J Ophthalmol. 1979;88:736–8.
56. Schweitzer I, Maguire K, Tuckwell V. Antiglaucoma medication and clinical depression. Aust N Z J Psychiatry. 2001;35:569–71.
57. Bright R, Everitt D. Beta-blockers and depression. Evidence against an association. JAMA. 1992;267(13):1783–7.
58. Lachkar Y, Bouassida W. Drug-induced acute angle closure glaucoma. Curr Opin Ophthalmol. 2007;18:129–33.
59. Kadoi C, Hayasaka S, Tsukamoto E, et al. Bilateral angle closure glaucoma and visual loss precipitated by antidepressant and antianxiety agents in a patient with depression. Ophthalmologica. 2000;214(5):360–1.
60. Yochim BP, Mueller AE, Kane KD, et al. Prevalence of cognitive impairment, depression, and anxiety symptoms among older adults with glaucoma. J Glaucoma. 2012;21:250–4.

Patient Management

9

Enping Chen, Behrad Samadi,
and Laurence Quérat

Abstract

Glaucoma care is a great challenge. Our aim as caregivers is, often with limited resources, to provide lifelong care to an ever-increasing number of patients suffering from a vision-threatening disease. To achieve this, we not only need to mobilize the available resources in the healthcare system but also must cooperate with our patients. Furthermore, we should discuss the importance of glaucoma care with policy makers and healthcare payers so that adequate resources are allocated to glaucoma care. Patient-centered cost-effective glaucoma management should be carried out at both the individual level and at group levels, covering those patients yet to be diagnosed. At present, elevated intraocular pressure (IOP) is the only factor we can modify in our daily clinical practice. However, our care should not be limited to this. We should bear in mind throughout the care process that our goal is to ensure a good quality of life for glaucoma patients at a sustainable cost. This chapter discusses the glaucoma care process at different stages of the disease, from early detection to low-vision rehabilitation. We feel that it is essential to establish a good cooperation with the patient, and ensure that the patient understands the importance of glaucoma treatment and adheres to the treatment regimen. This chapter ends with a brief discussion on "big data" analysis. Big data analysis with standardized criteria for diagnosing different types of glaucoma, well-defined patient-related outcome measures, and relevant hypotheses may provide us with insight into key areas of interest, such as vision-related quality of life, care quality, and effectiveness of treatment regimens.

Keywords

Vision-related quality of life · Quality of care Cooperation with patients · Patient information · Compliance · Sustainable glaucoma care

9.1 Patient Management

Bian Que was a well-known physician who lived over 2500 years ago during the Spring and Autumn period in China [1]. Legend says that one day King Wen of Kingdom Wei asked Bian Que: "I have heard that you and your brothers are all physicians, and I want to know who the best is?" Bian Que answered: "My oldest brother is the best, and my second oldest brother is better than me." The King Wen was surprised: "But everyone talks only about you, not your brothers!" Bian Que answered: "My oldest brother can prevent diseases and treat them before the

E. Chen (✉) · B. Samadi · L. Quérat
Glaucoma Service, St. Erik Eye Hospital, Karolinska Institutet, Stockholm, Sweden
e-mail: enping.chen@sll.se

X. Sun, Y. Dai (eds.), *Medical Treatment of Glaucoma*, https://doi.org/10.1007/978-981-13-2733-9_9

patients have any symptoms and his patients are not aware how much he has done for them, so only my family understands his skills. My second oldest brother can detect early signs of diseases and treat the patients when they have minor symptoms. People believe he can only treat minor diseases and he is known in my village. I diagnose diseases when the patients are very ill and treat them with strong medicine. Sometimes I succeed in saving a patient, and people believe that I can make miracles, so I am well known."

9.1.1 Pre-glaucoma

9.1.1.1 Screening

The goal of glaucoma care is to maintain the patient's visual function and related quality of life at a sustainable cost (EGS guidelines, 3rd edition, 2008). As glaucoma is a progressive and potentially blinding disease [2, 3], we should try to prevent its progress so that glaucoma patients can have a good vision-related quality of life throughout their lifetimes.

Several studies have shown that general screening is not cost-effective for society [4–6, 7, 8], as only approximately 2–4% of the population above 40 years of age suffers from glaucoma [9] and there is no single effective method with good enough sensitivity and specificity for screening [10]. Screening based solely on intraocular pressure (IOP) measurement is not accurate [11] and risks missing approximately 50% of cases, as several studies have found that approximately 50% of glaucoma patients do not have high IOP [12–14]. Visual field screening using frequency doubling technology (FDT) can sometimes miss advanced glaucoma damage [15]. Optical coherence tomography (OCT) has good sensitivity and specificity only at a late stage of the disease [15]. A recent meta-analysis showed that imaging methods were significantly influenced by the degree of glaucoma damage. These methods had poorer results in early stages of glaucoma and the risk of bias due to patient selection was high; in other words, the diagnostic accuracy of population screening could be lower than that shown by studies including pre-diagnosed subjects [16]. It is important to realize the limitation of these instruments to avoid over- and underdiagnosis. We sometimes encounter patients whose healthy eyes are wrongly classified as glaucomatous based on imaging results mistakenly indicating a defect in the retinal nerve fiber layer; these results are often attributable to artifacts or to limitations of the imaging device. As the thinning of the retinal nerve fiber layer is shown in red, this false diagnosis is called the "red disease" [17]. Moreover, these misdiagnosed patients often receive IOP-lowering medication. Combining several examination methods with an expert system may increase the accuracy of the diagnosis [18], but this approach is time consuming. A recent study reported that a single wide-field OCT with a hybrid deep learning method protocol had better accuracy than the 24-2 or 10-2 visual field tests or standard OCT in differentiating glaucomatous eyes from healthy eyes and could probably be used for screening [19]. However, this method is still under development and needs to be verified. As previously mentioned, because glaucoma damage is currently irreversible with today's treatment and there is a high risk of blindness among glaucoma patients [2, 3], we should try to reduce the risk of visual handicap by detecting glaucoma at an early stage. In addition, early detection of the disease would reduce the cost of treatment, as treating advanced glaucoma is reportedly more expensive than treating early stage disease [20–22].

As most types of glaucoma are symptomless at an early stage, many patients wish to have screening for their biological relatives. Yet publicly financed screening for open-angle glaucoma is currently not cost-effective and is therefore not recommended [23]. A feasible alternative is to recommend that high-risk individuals seek care [23–26] for the detection of the disease. For example, the Swedish Glaucoma Society has recommended that glaucoma patients encourage their biological children and siblings to have regular examinations for glaucoma after the age of 50 years. In addition, the Swedish Guidelines recommend that an optic disc examination should be included in ophthalmic examinations, for example, before cataract operations, for patients above

60 years of age, given the risk of glaucoma [23]. Examinations to detect glaucoma should include visual field examination, examination of the optic disc and retinal fiber layer, and tonometry [23]. If the result is normal, a follow-up visit is recommended every 5 years. This interval is adjusted according to the number of family members suffering from glaucoma and the ages at which they were diagnosed [23]. In areas with high prevalence of angle-closure glaucoma, gonioscopy should be an integral part of the examination to identify eyes at risk of angle closure and angle-closure glaucoma.

Many studies have demonstrated that approximately 50% of glaucoma patients go undiagnosed, a figure that could be even higher in developing countries [27–29] due to unawareness of glaucoma or the unavailability of eye care [29, 30]. Poor awareness and lack of knowledge of glaucoma [31], including by those suffering from this disease, is common in some developing countries [9, 28, 32–34]. However, even in developed countries there is a lack of awareness of glaucoma [35]. To test public knowledge of glaucoma in Stockholm, Sweden, *Ögontrycket*, the official magazine of Svenska Glaukomförbundet, the Swedish glaucoma patients' association, held interviews with one hundred pedestrians in three communes of Stockholm County. Most of the interviewees were approximately 65 years old or older. They were asked a short question, "What is glaucoma?," while looking at a card with the word "Glaucoma" written on it in bold letters. If the interviewee did not know the word "glaucoma," they could guess what it was. The survey results were disappointing, as only 20% of the interviewees had any knowledge of glaucoma. For the participants who did not know what glaucoma was, their guesses ranged from something related to "glad," as glaucoma began with "gla," to a new technical gadget or an exotic dish [36]. People also very commonly confuse cataracts with glaucoma [23]. Public education about glaucoma could promote general awareness of this disease and its detrimental consequences, hopefully encouraging high-risk people to seek glaucoma care [37, 38]. Such education would also be an important channel for informing policy makers of the severe consequences of glaucoma damage, not only to patients but also to society, to remind them to allocate adequate resources for glaucoma care. Great efforts have been made in recent years to spread information about glaucoma, initiated by the World Glaucoma Association and local glaucoma societies. An important event for this purpose is the annual World Glaucoma Week in March, which involves public lectures, media coverage, IOP measurement, and screening, attracting many members of the public ranging from glaucoma patients and their relatives to policy makers.

9.1.1.2 Ocular Hypertension

Ocular hypertension is defined as an eye with an IOP exceeding the upper limit of the statistically normal range [39], without necessarily being accompanied by any functional or structural defects. Studies of ocular hypertension have revealed that the risk factors for conversion to glaucoma in this group are high IOP and thin corneas [40, 41]. There are many local variations in the treatment of ocular hypertension, and the glaucoma guidelines of the Swedish Ophthalmological Society recommend that patients with an IOP exceeding 25 mmHg measured on several occasions should be followed up annually or biannually. Pressure-lowering treatment is recommended if the IOP exceeds 28–30 mmHg or if exfoliation exists [23]. The decision to treat should be discussed with the patient and weighed individually with regard to benefits and risks, taking account of the patient's age, health status, risk of side effects, quality of life, and eventually the cost of treatment. Unnecessary treatment should be avoided, as eyes with high IOP only have a potential risk of glaucoma and are otherwise healthy.

9.1.1.3 Suspected or Confirmed Angle Closure

The risk factors for angle closure are Asian descent, female, hyperopia, increasing age, positive family history, short axial length, the size, shape, or position of the crystalline lens [42], and the other eye having angle closure/angle-closure glaucoma. Patients with these risk factors should be informed of the risk and symptoms of acute attack and be encouraged to seek an ophthalmic examination. Suspected or confirmed angle closure is potentially curable if we can maintain an open chamber angle and if the trabecular meshwork is not damaged.

9.1.2 Glaucoma

9.1.2.1 Glaucoma Diagnosis and Patient Evaluation

Glaucoma diagnosis is based on damage to the optic disc and the retinal nerve fiber layer and on corresponding glaucomatous visual field defects. In difficult cases, the two-out-of-three rule is recommended by the Finnish evidence-based guidelines for open-angle glaucoma [43]. It is important to avoid both over- and underdiagnosis and related mistreatment. It is also advisable to avoid giving a diagnosis before all related examinations are completed, as it is known that receiving a glaucoma diagnosis has a negative influence on quality of life [44]. Providing sufficient information about glaucoma and glaucoma treatment is therefore essential to reducing the patient's worries while giving a glaucoma diagnosis to the patient.

Glaucoma can be classified as open-angle or angle-closure glaucoma according to gonioscopy findings. Examination of cornea, lens, chamber angle, iris, signs of inflammation, and retinal circulation may help us identify the subtype of the disease.

When diagnosing glaucoma, it is important to document baseline information such as race, family history, previous maximum IOP, concomitant diseases (including other eye diseases), and concomitant medication.

Staging

There are several methods for staging glaucoma damage based on visual field examination. The most commonly used method is classification according to the mean deviation (MD) score.

Humphrey Perimetry

In Humphrey perimetry, Stage 0 is ocular hypertension or earliest glaucoma with an MD score of >0.00 dB, Stage 1 is early glaucoma with an MD score of –0.01 to –5.00 dB, Stage 2 is moderate glaucoma with an MD score of –5.01 to –12.00 dB, Stage 3 is advanced glaucoma with an MD score of –12.01 to –20.00 dB, and Stage 4 is severe glaucoma with an MD score of –20.01 dB or worse. Stage 5 is end-stage glaucoma, in which visual field examination by Humphrey perimetry is impossible due to visual acuity of 0.1 or worse caused by glaucoma [45].

To stage the vision-related quality of life, a threshold is estimated, i.e., a visual field index (VFI) of 50%, corresponding to an MD score of approximately –18 dB in the best eye. A VFI value of less than 50% or an MD score of lower than –18 dB in the best eye indicates visual handicap with severely reduced vision-related quality of life [46]. The advantage of staging using VFI is that it takes the location of the scotoma into account.

Octopus Perimetry

In octopus perimetry, Stage 0 is ocular hypertension or earliest glaucoma with an MD score of ≤–0.8 dB, Stage 1 is early glaucoma with an MD score of –0.7 to 4.4 dB, Stage 2 is moderate glaucoma with an MD score of 4.5 to 9.5 dB, Stage 3 is advanced glaucoma with an MD score of 9.5 to 15.3 dB, Stage 4 is severe glaucoma with an MD score of 15.4 to 23.1 dB, and Stage 5 is end-stage glaucoma with an MD score of ≥23.2 dB [45].

Risk Factors for Blindness

The World Health Organization (WHO) program Vision 2020: The Right to Sight estimated that 80 million patients will suffer from glaucoma in 2020, 11 million of whom will be blind due to glaucoma [31]. Peters et al. [3] found the risk of blindness in treated glaucoma patients 15 years after glaucoma diagnosis to be approximately 50% in one eye and 20% in both eyes. Similar results were obtained by a Finnish group [2]. It is therefore crucial to, at glaucoma diagnosis, identify those patients at risk of blindness.

High IOP, late stage of glaucoma damage at diagnosis, and old age are identified as risk factors of glaucoma-related blindness [47]; moreover, patients of African origin have a high risk of blindness [48].

Discussion and Consideration of Treatment Options

After giving the patient initial information at diagnosis, we should then discuss various treatment alternatives and evaluate the need for rehabilitation. It is important to discuss the possible outcomes of the treatment regimens with the patient, to listen actively to the patient's opinions and preferences, and, together with the patient, to plan future care considering the patient's quality of life as well as the efficacy, safety, and cost-effectiveness of the treatment. When pressure-lowering treatment is needed, the benefits and risks of each treatment alternative should be weighed and discussed with the patient. A treatment decision should be reached based on medical judgment, respect for patient autonomy, ethical considerations, and the available resources.

Patient Behavior in Interaction with Care Providers

A report of the Swedish Association of Local Authorities and Regions classified patients into four groups according to their behavior in interaction with care providers: "independent and engaged," "worried and engaged," "traditional and indifferent," and "vulnerable and worried" [49]. Identification of patient behavior may help us adapt the information, treatment, and low-vision care to the patient.

9.1.2.2 Treatment

The goal of treatment, according to European Glaucoma Society Guidelines, is to maintain the patient's visual function and related quality of life at a sustainable cost [50]. Because medical and surgical treatments have been identified as factors significantly predictive of indirect disability [51, 52], it is essential to keep in mind that the treatment should "do no harm" and to balance the benefits and risks of treatment against the quality of life of each individual patient.

Information as Part of the Treatment

Receiving a glaucoma diagnosis has a negative influence on the patient's quality of life [44]. Patients usually become anxious about their vision after the diagnosis, so information about glaucoma presented in a way understandable to the patient [53], together with written material on glaucoma, may ease their anxiety. The patients should not only be well informed about and motivated to adhere to treatment but also take part in deciding on the treatment regimen. Moreover, we should also adapt the method of information provision and quantity of information according to the type of patient behavior. For the traditional and indifferent and the vulnerable and worried patients [49], we might need to repeat small amounts of information on several occasions. The discussion should balance sympathy for the patient against the medical facts; we should also bear in mind that glaucoma patients and healthcare providers might have different views on the purpose of treatment. It is not unusual for clinicians to be satisfied with successfully lowering the IOP, while patients are less enthusiastic, wondering why their vision has not improved at all. Informing the patients and discussing the possible effects of treatment may narrow the gap between different viewpoints.

Target IOP

Studies have shown that the rate of disease progression is slower at a lower IOP level [54–56]. The target IOP is an estimate of the IOP at which glaucoma progression may be prevented and its clinical effectiveness confirmed retrospectively. The concept of target pressure is useful for understanding the principle of glaucoma treatment: In eyes with more glaucoma damage, a high rate of progression, and more risk factors, a relatively lower IOP should be targeted. However, how to apply target IOPs clinically is still controversial [57]. In clinical practice, the target IOP is often calculated from a single IOP measurement. However, IOP can fluctuate considerably over the course of a day and patterns of IOP variation can even differ between days [58, 59]. Therefore, a target IOP based on a single IOP value would be misleading. Furthermore, even if several IOP values are obtained during a given period, it is not clear whether the target pressure should be estimated according to the highest IOP or to the mean or median of these values. In addition, there are several formulas and recommendations for target IOP calculation [43, 60, 61] and so far there is no clinical evidence of the validity of these formulas. Consequently, it is common for different target IOPs to be estimated by different care providers for the same eye. The uncertainty of the target IOP should be explained to the care personnel and the patient to prevent misunderstanding and misinterpretation. The target IOP should be adjusted continuously according to the rate of progression during the care process. Striving to achieve a certain target IOP at all costs is sometimes inadvisable, as the target IOP is an approximation and the final goal of glaucoma care is the patient's well-being.

Avoidance of Overtreatment

We should avoid treating patients with an uncertain glaucoma diagnosis, such as an unconfirmed high IOP, a first-time visual field defect not corresponding to optic disc alteration, or a deviation in nerve fiber thickness caused by artifacts ("red disease"). Sometimes we may just monitor patients without starting treatment. For example, we can follow up a low-risk angle-closure suspect if the patient is not motivated to commence preventive treatment, especially if the patient is living in an area where medical care is easily accessible. Another example would be a patient with short life expectancy or a weak, multiple-diseased patient with minor glaucoma damage, especially if the other eye is healthy.

The guidelines of the European Glaucoma Society recommend starting with monotherapy and then waiting and evaluating the treatment effect [50]. Beginning with multiple topical treatments is related to a risk of overtreatment, increased risk of side effects, reduced adherence, and increased cost. Preservative-free topical treatment is recommended in eyes with ocular surface disease or sensitivity to preservatives [62].

To ensure sustainable glaucoma care, European Glaucoma Society guidelines also recommend taking account of economic factors [50]. The frequency of follow-up visits should be scheduled according to the severity of damage, rate of progression, general eye status, general health status, and available resources. If the patient has several risk factors, then more frequent follow-up visits are indicated. Standardization of care for low-risk patients [63] could reduce frequent unjustified follow-up visits. Moreover, frequent visits may be a factor that negatively affects patient quality of life [64], implying that more care is not always better care [65].

There are different administrative systems for managing follow-up appointments. In the system in which the patients themselves keep the schedule and make the appointments at the right time, it was found that reduced clinic waiting times, simplified appointment scheduling, appropriate education, and counseling could improve patient adherence to the recommended follow-up schedule [66].

It is generally recommended that functionally stable patients be followed up in private clinics and unstable patients in public hospitals [63]. Which patients should be followed up, and how this should be done, varies among clinics depending on the available resources, tradition, and culture of the local healthcare system. Frequent follow-up visits are not always related to greater patient satisfaction. A survey organized by Glaukomförbundet, the Swedish glaucoma patients' association, found that glaucoma patients in Sweden visited eye clinics on average three times per year, with great regional variation. For example, patients in Region G made five visits annually while in neighboring Region U patients visited the clinic only once a year [67]. The patients were more satisfied with the glaucoma care in Region U, even though they made less frequent follow-up visits to the eye clinic in this region, supporting the theory that more care is not always better [65].

Avoidance of Undertreatment

Undertreatment is also common in glaucoma care, because at least 50% of glaucoma patients are undiscovered [4, 13, 14, 27, 68–71] and approximately 25–50% of patients do not take their eye drops [72–74]. It is important to inform and motivate our glaucoma patients to improve their adherence to the glaucoma treatment. Ways to improve adherence include identification of risk factors [75, 76], reduction of side effects, and a trusting patient–physician relationship [77–79].

Information can be provided to patients through various channels and should be conveyed in a way understandable to them [53]. Public education, patient magazines, and information brochures are just a few examples of possible means of information dissemination. Newly diagnosed glaucoma patients may appreciate a "Glaucoma School," i.e., a discussion meeting involving a small group of patients, their relatives, and healthcare professionals, which would be an excellent forum for further education and idea exchange. The annual World Glaucoma Week is an example of an occasion when the public is informed about glaucoma and its consequences.

It is also very important to spread information about glaucoma and its treatment to various medical specialties and medical professional groups in the healthcare system, as glaucoma medications tend to be ignored and not administered during hospitalization by other specialties [80]. Of course, spreading such information in the healthcare system is also important in view of systemic side effects. Even in developed countries, personnel sometimes do not realize the importance of glaucoma medication and may not know how to administer the eye drops (personal communication with glaucoma patients).

Compliance, Adherence, Persistence, and Patient Education

By now, we know that the risk of developing glaucoma and the progression of the disease are reduced by lowering IOP through using medication in the form of eye drops [41, 55, 81].

However, for the medical treatment of glaucoma to be successful, compliance, otherwise known as adherence, is of the essence. *Compliance* can generally be described as taking a medication or following treatment as prescribed by the doctor, while *adherence* is a more active and dedicated form of compliance. Measures of compliance are not standardized and, clinically, compliance is often vaguely described as being good or poor, or in binary terms such as patients being compliant or non-compliant.

In research, various methods have been used to measure compliance, such as interviews, patient self-reports, medication possession ratio, and electronic monitoring. Electronic monitoring started in the late 1970s following previous compliance studies carried out through interviews and self-reports. In an article from 1980, Norell and Granström described their method of connecting a micro-switch to the cap of the eye drop bottle, thereby recording the date and hour each time the bottle was opened and used [82]. They also studied the patient's instillation technique by measuring the amount of residual fluorescein in the fornix after the patients themselves had topically administered the drops. They concluded that 41% of patients missed six or more doses over a 20-day period and that 43% exceeded an 8-h dose interval at least 20% of the time [82].

Irrespective of the method of measuring compliance, studies have repeatedly shown that patients often fail to adhere to the treatment prescribed by their ophthalmologist [83–85]. One review article reported noncompliance rates ranging from 5% to 80%, and another publications found noncompliance rates of at least 25% [74, 86, 87].

Numerous studies have also examined medication persistence, defined as the total time on therapy [85, 88]. Like compliance, the measurement methods for persistence are not standardized, though they all indicate the degree of non-persistence, for example, a patient who takes eye drops every other day is fully persistent with the treatment but only 50% compliant [74]. Doubtless, non-adherent/non-compliant and/or non-persistent patients, irrespective of the measurement methods or exact definitions, will fail to achieve the intended or full treatment effects, having a negative effect on the patient's glaucoma progression, quality of life, and cost of healthcare. Lacks of adherence and persistence have been shown to be common among glaucoma patients in various countries [72, 73, 89–91] and might be related to unnecessary increases in the cost of care [74]. Because glaucoma often requires lifelong treatment, the matter of long-term compliance is particularly challenging for both patients and ophthalmologists.

Identifying Non-Compliance

Compliance can be defined as how well a patient's dosing history corresponds to the prescribed regimen. However, identifying poor compliance is difficult, because glaucoma patients tend to overestimate their adherence and ophthalmologists often have difficulties detecting and predicting non-adherence in their clinical practice [84, 92]. What makes it even more difficult is that some patients employ "white coat compliance," meaning that they adhere to treatment when consultation is approaching and then scale down afterward. This all indicates that patients generally want to be thought of as good patients by their doctors and therefore might conceal their non-adherence.

There is no easy way of identifying non-adherent patients, though a proper adherence assessment interview by the physician might be helpful. First, starting with an open-ended question about taking their medications will reveal the patient's understanding of their medications. For example one might simply ask "How is it going with your eye drop/drops?" The answer would then hopefully provide us with information on the patients perception of which eye drops they are using, the dosage, adverse effects, compliance and so forth. However the answers are not always given so easily and therefore the patient needs to understand that the success of their medical regimen is dependent on their physician's accurate knowledge of how they use their eye drops. If the patient falsely claims to be compliant despite a high IOP, the doctor might mistakenly intensify the treatment. At the same time, it is very important to acknowledge the difficulties of taking medication and that patients sometimes miss or forget to take it. By this time, the patient should feel comfortable enough to acknowledge whether they are having adherence problems, and as a final step, the doctor should directly ask about compliance [93].

Risk Factors

Multiple risk factors for poor adherence with glaucoma therapy have been described. These risk factors can be grouped into four major categories: medication-related factors, patient factors, provider factors, and environmental factors [94].

Medication Regimen

Complicated treatment regimens, especially a dose frequency of more than twice daily, may adversely affect adherence [87]. Likewise, cost of medicine and side effects, such as redness, burning, and itching, may have similar impacts [95–97].

Patient Factors

When it comes to self-administering drops, common obstacles to adherence are forgetfulness and physical barriers, such as difficulties reading prescription labels and manipulating bottles [98]. Comorbidity may exacerbate these factors. These characteristics are more common in older patients, who as a group may display less compliance. However, at the same time, low disease severity with lack of symptoms is associated with less adherence, which has been described in younger patients [85, 99]. Although results regarding gender differences in glaucoma adherence are inconsistent, some studies have shown that men are more likely to be non-adherent than women [87]. Patients with lower education and lower socioeconomic status are less likely to adhere to treatment [87]. These factors may be linked to the amount of knowledge of glaucoma, because it has been shown that a lack of knowledge of the disease and poor understanding of treatment benefits are also associated with lower adherence [95, 100].

Provider Factors

Self-reported compliance studies have shown that a poor patient–doctor relationship negatively affects adherence and that issues of trust and communication are crucial in this [96, 100]. Failing to convey the risk of vision loss has been shown to be a critical element of such communication problems.

Environmental Factors

The nature of these factors is specific to individuals, implying that situations making it difficult for patients to adhere to the treatment regime, such as a major event in the patient's life, frequent traveling, or just a change in routine [75, 100], may come into play.

Improving Adherence

There are several different approaches to improving patient adherence [93]. As in any functional relationship, proper patient–doctor communication is key. Patients need to understand their illness, their medication, and how adherence relates to disease control. This comprehensive information, which will motivate the patient to cooperate, needs to be regularly reinforced at follow-up visits. Also, doctors should ensure that the information is conveyed to a partner, relative, or a friend who might accompany the patient, assuming there is patient consent. Skillful communication with patients [101] and an individualized approach are essential to achieving good adherence.

The Glaucoma Service of St. Erik Eye Hospital, Stockholm, Sweden, provides glaucoma patients with both verbal information and a brochure that briefly explains the disease (Figs. 9.1 and 9.2). The brochure, also available on the Internet, contains information about symptoms (including pictures illustrating visual field loss), how the diagnosis is established, various available treatments, and how the disease progresses. The importance of lowering IOP and attending follow-up visits is emphasized throughout the text. In addition, all newly diagnosed patients are invited to attend a much-appreciated "Glaucoma School," at which a lecture on the subject is given by a glaucoma specialist, followed by a discussion session.

To further increase awareness of glaucoma in Sweden, Glaukomförbundet, the Swedish glaucoma patients' association, has an excellent website with information about the disease. In addition, anyone may post questions concerning glaucoma on the website, which will then be answered by a glaucoma specialist. The association also produces the popular scientific magazine *Ögontrycket* four times a year, presenting relevant information about glaucoma and recent treatment advances.

Next, the treatment regimen needs to be optimized and fit the patient's lifestyle. This means simplifying the therapy by reducing dosing frequency and using combination eye drops when possible and indicated, thereby reducing polypharmacy [101].

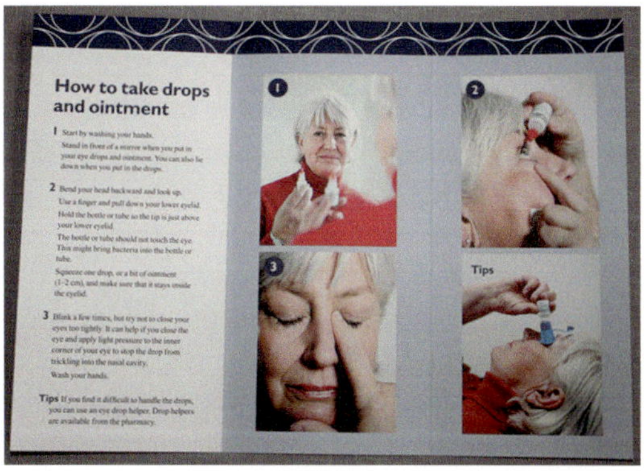

Fig. 9.1 Patient information brochure from St. Erik Eye Hospital (Reproduced with permission)

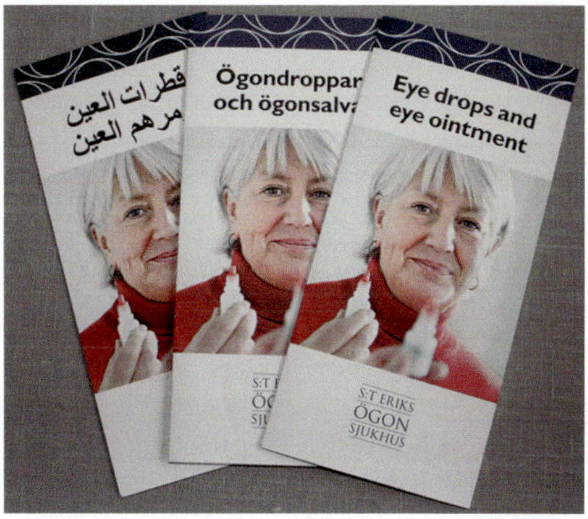

Fig. 9.2 Patient information brochures in different languages from St. Erik Eye Hospital (Reproduced with permission)

Furthermore, adherence will be improved by using well-tolerated drugs with side effects kept as low as possible. If the cost of medications is an issue that cannot be resolved by choosing different medications, which are lower in cost or covered by the patient's medical insurance, one might consider changing the treatment.

It is important to keep in mind that despite good compliance, patients may still not receive the correct dose of glaucoma medication due to problems with the technique of instilling the eye drops [102], which the patients themselves might be unaware of. Studies have shown that approximately 40–50% of patients have difficulties instilling eye drops [102, 103]. Some examples of poor technique are completely missing the eye, delivering a higher dose than necessary, and ocular trauma or bottle contamination due to contact between the bottle tip and the eye globe or lid. Unfortunately, poor technique is commonly associated with old age and poor vision, both of which are strongly associated with glaucoma [104, 105]. We must always ensure that the patient correctly instills the eye drops, and instructions on the matter should be given whenever needed, especially when starting on drops for the first time (Fig. 9.1). Different patients have different needs, so the individual capabilities of the glaucoma patient must be taken into account. With age, muscle strength weakens and difficulties aiming the bottle correctly might become an issue [106], so care must be taken to choose an ergonomically appropriate bottle or eye drop aid. Eye drop aids are commonly available free from pharmaceutical companies and should be available at the clinic and provided to glaucoma patients when necessary. Another option might be to arrange for someone else to help with instillation. If the possibility of an eye drop scheme is limited, then one might consider switching from medication to laser or surgery.

If forgetfulness is an issue, it might help the patient to have printed treatment plans, reminder aids, or even to relate the dosing to another activity, for example, taking eye drops after toothbrushing or taking another medication. Also, advise patients who frequently travel or work to have an extra bottle with them or at their worksite.

Conclusion

Adherence to medical treatment is a significant problem in the care of glaucoma patients and one of the greater challenges in preventing vision loss from glaucoma. Risk factors for non-adherence are based on various patient-specific factors such as cost, instillation difficulties, denial, lack of information/education, forgetfulness, complicated treatment regimens, schedule, tolerability, and side effects. By improving patient adherence to glaucoma medication regimens, we may significantly delay disease progression and subsequent vision loss, thereby increasing quality of life. The most important approach to reinforcing adherence is to improve the patient's knowledge of the disease and of his or her medications.

9.1.2.3 Following Up Open-Angle Glaucoma and Angle-Closure Glaucoma

Glaucoma care is resource intensive. A survey revealed that one quarter of visits to eye clinics in Sweden are glaucoma related [107]. Due to the vast number of patients and limited available resources, glaucoma care should be effective, sustainable, and affordable to society, and it is important to ensure that the "right patient gets the right service at the right time and right place from the right caregivers" [63].

Glaucoma care should entail more than simply checking visual fields, monitoring optic nerves, writing prescriptions, and performing laser or surgical procedures. It is important that we maintain good communication and meaningful cooperation with our patients [108, 109]. Follow-up visits are the most essential part of glaucoma care. During these visits, we should monitor: (1) the vision-related quality of life of the patient (patient-evaluated effect of treatment), (2) the effects of treatment on the optic nerve, visual field, and IOP (care-provider-evaluated effects of treatment), and (3) side effects of treatment (evaluation by both care providers and patients).

It is important to emphasize to the patients that we cannot cure glaucoma and that they must live with the disease and receive lifelong IOP-lowering treatment. What we can do is to try to slow the reduction of their visual field with medication, laser treatment, or pressure-lowering surgery. The purpose of all these treatment alternatives is the same, that is, to lower the IOP, which is currently the only valid way of slowing progression of glaucoma. To achieve this, we need good cooperation between the healthcare receiver and provider. This information should be discussed with patients at diagnosis and should be repeated during follow-up visits.

During this process, we should also recheck the diagnosis to avoid over- and underdiagnosis and adjust the treatment to avoid under- and over-treatment, in order to provide care that is suitable for patients and affordable to society. During follow-ups, we should estimate the therapeutic effect and balance the benefits and side effects of the treatment regimen. Most importantly, we must evaluate the vision-related quality of life over the course of glaucoma progression, and make efforts to compensate for the visual disabilities caused by glaucoma by providing aids of various kinds. Suitable vision aids should be considered throughout the care process, not only at the end stage of the disease.

Follow-up visits should include checking the general health status to find out whether there is any worsening of the patient's general condition caused by the glaucoma or its treatment, or whether the patient is taking new medications that may interfere with the glaucoma treatment. Any new symptoms possibly related to the side effects of glaucoma medication should be noted.

Risk Factors for Glaucoma Progression

Many risk factors may be related to the reduction of the visual field. High IOP is a major risk factor and maintaining a lower IOP may prevent visual field deterioration [110, 111]. Many studies have shown that each additional mmHg of elevated IOP is related to at least a 10% risk of glaucoma progression [40, 110, 112–116]. With this knowledge in mind, we can estimate the target pressure and reduce the IOP to a level that might reduce the rate of disease progression and maintain lifelong useful vision for the patient [114, 117, 118]. A lower target IOP should be set in eyes with exfoliation, as this is known to relate to a higher rate of progression [110, 111, 119–122]. It is also reported that disc hemorrhage, worse baseline visual field, thinner cornea, older age, African origin, and family history are related to rapid progression [110, 111, 122–125]. Many studies have suggested that low diastolic perfusion is a risk factor for glaucoma progression [126–132], though the clinical ability to adjust this factor is limited [23]. If it is needed, we may consult patient's family physician for a 24-hour blood pressure measurement and to optimize blood pressure medication.

Several other possible risk factors are still controversial, for example, fluctuation in IOP [121, 133–140] and the influence of cardiovascular diseases [112, 115, 122, 141–144]. At the moment, there is no conclusive evidence that diabetes or high blood pressure are related to the progression of glaucoma [23].

Follow-Up Visits and Detection of Rapid Progression

As glaucoma reduces the size of the visual field, monitoring this parameter is the most relevant action in following the visual quality of life of the patient, so the visual field examination should be the basis of all follow-ups. With visual field examinations, we can estimate whether the disease is functionally stable or worsening and, if so, calculate the rate of worsening. The European Glaucoma Guidelines and Swedish Glaucoma Guidelines recommend that patients on average receive six visual field examinations in the first 2 years after diagnosis to detect a worsening of 4 dB (mean deviation) depending on the variability of visual field examinations [112]. The intervals may be adjusted according to the level of worsening we wish to detect and to the available resources. The United Kingdom Glaucoma Treatment Study showed that reliable baseline visual fields and frequent examinations might increase the possibility of early detection of disease progression [113].

Reduction of the visual field can be captured using both event analysis and trend analysis, with the latter showing rate of progression. The advantage of knowing the rate of disease progression is that, together with the remaining visual field and the estimated life expectancy of the patient, it provides a basis for evaluating the future development of vision and for adjusting therapy to avoid visual handicap.

The reduction of the visual field can be influenced by many factors. To ensure reliable results of the visual field examination, patients should be well-informed of the purpose and procedures of the test and the examiner should ensure that the patients can concentrate on performing the visual field examination. It is crucial to check the reliability of the results of visual field examination before interpreting them.

The available imaging techniques, such as OCT, HRT, and GDx, may usefully supplement the clinical examination of the optic disc and fundus. It is essential to become familiar with the instruments before starting to use them clinically; most importantly, one needs knowledge of the size and specifications of the normal database. If there are several OCTs from different manufacturers in the same clinic, it is important to be aware that the measurements from different OCTs are not always interchangeable [145].

Zhang et al. [146] found that in early stage glaucoma, OCT is more sensitive than visual field examination at detecting glaucoma progression. The sensitivity of the nerve fiber layer examination decreases in the late stage, while the ganglion cell complex retains its sensitivity, permitting the detection of progression in all stages of the glaucoma process [146]. Recent studies have shown that OCT findings in the macula [147] or central visual field [148] are related to vision-related quality of life. These methods may provide supplementary information about quality of life if the link between morphology and quality of life is confirmed by further studies.

As well as ophthalmic examinations similar to those for open-angle glaucoma, gonioscopy should be repeated during follow-ups for angle-closure glaucoma and for all eyes at risk of angle closure. It is recommended patients with angle-closure glaucoma be followed up approximately every 3–6 months and that patients with angle closure without optic nerve damage be followed up every 6–12 months (American Academy of Ophthalmology 2013).

Although there are many new emerging methods to evaluate IOP, Goldmann applanation tonometry is still the gold standard. If other methods are used, it is important that the same technique be used subsequently, as the measurement results of different instruments are not interchangeable [149–152]. It is reported that 16% of IOP peaks happen outside office hours in both treated glaucoma patients and healthy persons [58, 59]. It is therefore necessary to measure IOP at multiple time points, especially in the case of glaucomatous visual field progression despite low IOPs measured during office hours. Monocular testing to evaluate treatment effect may not be reliable, as the IOPs of both eyes of the same person may have different patterns of IOP variation [58, 59]. To check the variation in IOP, it may be necessary to take measurements several times a day and for several days, because the same eye may display different patterns of IOP variation on different days [58, 59].

Adjustment of Treatment

If there is reliable reduction of the visual field and it is caused by glaucoma, we should determine the possible factors causing the worsening. For example, are there problems with treatment compliance and, if so, why? Are there any other related factors, such as IOP peaking outside office hours [58, 59]? We may accept a certain rate of disease progression if the reduction of the visual field is unlikely to lead to visual handicap during the patient's lifetime.

If treatment adjustment is indicated, then we may consider various alternatives: Should we switch to or add a new medication, should we undertake laser treatment or perform surgery? A new baseline and new rate of progression should be estimated after each successful lowering of the IOP, as the previous rate of progression indicates the disease status only at the previous IOP level.

Similar to visual field progression, a loss of retinal nerve fibers visualized with imaging techniques may also indicate worsening of glaucoma and justify the adjustment of IOP-lowering treatment. However, it is not yet known what rate of retinal nerve fiber thinning is acceptable or what level of retinal nerve fiber loss corresponds to functional handicap. The relationship between IOP and rate of visual field progression is well established (1 mmHg ≥10% progression) [40, 112, 115, 116], whereas the relationship between IOP and rate of retinal nerve fiber layer thinning is not yet known. Consequently, fine adjustment of the target IOP based on retinal nerve fiber layer thinning is less well established.

When adjusting treatment, we should consider the general status of the patient and not focus solely on one parameter, for example, a single IOP reading. We may accept a minor to moderate worsening of visual field in one eye of an aged patient with poorer general health, especially if the other eye is relatively healthy. An acceptable rate of progression should be determined based on the general status of the patient and the basal visual field index or MD of the affected eye [153].

9.1.2.4 Vision-Related Quality of Life

Maintaining the vision-related quality of life of glaucoma patients is our ultimate aim in glaucoma care. Quality of life can be defined differently depending on the area of interest. WHO defines quality of life as "an individual's perception of their position in life in the context of the culture and value systems in which they live and in relation to their goals, expectations, standards and concerns. It is a broad ranging concept affected in a complex way by the person's physical health, psychological state, personal beliefs, social relationships and their relationship to salient features of their environment." [153]. The feeling of well-being can vary among individuals and change longitudinally within a person [154]. A visual field index of 50%, corresponding to an MD of less than approximately −18 dB, in the best eye is regarded as the threshold for severe reduction of the vision-related quality of life [46]. Glaucoma causes a worsening of quality of life, even at an early stage [24, 52, 155–160], impairing reading abilities [161–163], increasing the risk of falling [164], and causing difficulties in daily activities and driving [164, 165]. It has been shown that defects in the inferior visual field are a significant predictor of direct disability [52]. Even treatment, either medical or surgical, can reduce the quality of life [51, 52]. However, many glaucoma patients can still live relatively normal lives. In a survey organized by Glaukomforbundet, the Swedish glaucoma patients' association, all members of the association received a questionnaire on their quality of life and quality of care. The response rate was 73% and 1888 patients completed the questionnaire. The most important question concerned how the glaucoma patients experienced the influence of glaucoma on their daily lives. The answers revealed that approximately 70% of Glaukomförbundet members still drove, 90% had no problem watching TV, 78% experienced no difficulties reading, and most of them had no problems taking a walk outside the home. None of them perceived any difficulties regarding contact and communication with friends and with family members such as children and grandchildren [67]. Although there was selection bias, as members of Glaukomförbundet are usually active patients and approximately 30% of the members did not complete the questionnaire, these results still reflect some patients' view of the disease and at least some aspects of their lives.

Although a questionnaire can capture some aspects of the quality of life of glaucoma patients, personal contact and discussion is still essential to obtain a comprehensive overview of each patient. A patient-centered approach is essential and effective for this purpose [100, 109, 166]. A welfare officer or a specialist counselor is of great assistance for achieving such an overview in our hectic clinical activities.

One way to get information about quality of life is to ask patients how they spend their time in their daily life, for example, reading, professional activities, and recreational activities during the light and dark periods of the day. This can be done via a questionnaire sent to patients before clinic visits or by asking them to complete one in the waiting room. The results of such surveys, together with the clinical findings, could provide a basis for determining the level of assistance the patient needs and for tracking changes in the patient's quality of life. We need also consider the type of interaction between the patient and the care providers [49] during the process.

Because vision-related quality of life is influenced by geographic, ethnic, and cultural–demographic factors, there are no universally applicable outcome measures. It is essential that we discuss matters with our patients, to find out how much assistance they need in their daily lives and offer help according to the situation. For example, can patients take care of themselves inside and outside the home? Can they prepare meals and handle personal hygiene? Do the patients have any aids and do they use them properly? In addition, are the patients' homes adapted to accommodate the patient's disability?

9.1.2.5 Quality of Care

It is essential that the care be patient centered at both the individual and group levels, and that the care provider balance the provided services between these two levels based on medical considerations and available resources. Feedback from our patients on how they feel in the care system can constitute a basis for establishing this balance. Quality of care could be evaluated by the patients by means of a personal interview or questionnaire. To improve care, we should know, for example, how the patients feel when communicating with care providers, whether they are participating in care decisions, whether they feel that they are receiving enough information about glaucoma and its treatment, and their overall impressions of the care they receive. A questionnaire could be sent periodically to randomly selected patients, asking questions such as: Do you feel that you are being treated with respect and in a thoughtful way? Are you receiving information about your diagnosis or explanations of your illness? Do you feel that you are as involved as you would like in the decisions about your care and treatment? When interpreting the answers, we should keep in mind that patients behave differently when interacting with care providers [49]. These considerations are essential when discussing matters with patients, and feedback from the patients and information given to them are important in our effort to continually improve the care they receive.

9.1.2.6 Cooperation with Glaucoma Patients

Cooperation with glaucoma patients throughout the care process is mutually beneficial, and glaucoma care would be much better if patients could take a more active role in it. Many glaucoma patients are retired, still have relatively good general health, and are still active in the community; they are often aware of the consequences of glaucoma damage and the importance of glaucoma care. Many of them are interested in participating actively in the care process and are willing to do something to prevent further visual impairment and blindness. The most suitable patients are probably those manifesting the behavior type "independent and engaged" or "worried and engaged" [49], while patients of the behavior type "traditional and indifferent" or "vulnerable and worried" [49] may need more encouragement to get involved. Recent advances in medical technology such as home IOP measurement [58, 59, 167–170] make such cooperation clinically possible. Home measurement can collect IOP data outside office hours, provide IOP obtained in a "real life" situation, avoid the "white coat influence," measure the IOP for several days without hospitalization, and can probably improve adherence and persistence in topical treatment. Home IOP measurement saves time for the patients and their employers, saves resources for the care providers, and is economically beneficial to society. These measurements can even be applied in selected pediatric patients [171–173].

Furthermore, several types of computer-based home visual field tests are available on the Internet. Comparison between online perimetry (Peristat) and Humphrey perimetry has indicated good correlation at all stages of glaucoma damage [174]. Moreover, the results of visual field examination using a head-mounted perimeter are comparable to those obtained using a standard automated perimeter [175]. A recent study showed that home monitoring might detect rapid glaucomatous visual field progression earlier than clinic-based examination can [176]. The application of home-based measurements is even more valuable in remote areas where healthcare centers are scarce or unavailable. The quickly improving e-health system makes communication and data transfer convenient and safe, and patients can send their health data to their care providers without worrying about the security of their data.

9.1.2.7 Low-Vision Rehabilitation for Glaucoma Patients

Definition

According to a World Health Organization (WHO) report from 2017, 253 million people are affected by visual impairment worldwide; of them, 36 million are blind [177]. Visual impairment is defined as best corrected visual acuity (BCVA) between 0.05 (20/400) and 0.3 (20/60) in the better-seeing eye, whereas blindness is defined as a BCVA under 0.05 or a visual field of 10 degrees or less. Glaucoma is responsible for 2% of visual impairment and 8% of blindness in people, of whom 82% are over 50 years of age. Vision 2020: The Right to Sight is a global initiative of WHO and the International Agency for the Prevention of Blindness (IAPB) with the aim of eliminating avoidable blindness in the world. However, access to eye care services is unequal, depending on geographical (i.e., rural vs. urban) and economic limitations. Low income countries rely on nine ophthalmologists per one million inhabitants, whereas high-income countries offer an average of 79 ophthalmologists per one million (Resnikoff et al. 2012). However, living in a developed country is no guarantee of good access to eye care, as healthcare systems differ, sometimes offering limited coverage to low-income groups [178–180].

Impact of Low Vision

Visual impairment has huge consequences for the individual and the community [181, 182]. Young glaucoma patients need support throughout their lives to manage school and build a social life. Besides visual impairment, adult glaucoma patients may have economic difficulties due to limited working opportunities and medical expenditures. Older glaucoma patients need support to adapt to their limitations while remaining independent as long as possible. In developed countries, communities have more responsibility to provide support than in developing countries, where glaucoma patients rely more on their families. The amount of support is individual but communities have to implement strategies to meet glaucoma patient needs.

Low-Vision Rehabilitation

The UN Human Rights Convention stipulates that people with handicaps should have the same opportunities as others regarding access to information, communication, and transportation (UNGA, resolution 48/96, rule 4). Low vision due to glaucoma affects people's daily lives and requires structures to facilitate coping with the handicap. The aim of visual rehabilitation is to optimize patients' use of their remaining visual function to improve their quality of life. Visual rehabilitation consists of psychological, physical, and social support to sustain independent living. Low-vision rehabilitation centers provide individualized care in which professionals evaluate each patient's needs. Various categories of professionals can be involved in this rehabilitation: ophthalmologists assess the medical condition of the patients and classify their level of visual impairment; optometrists measure the visual potential of the patients to choose appropriate visual aids; technicians adapt devices and teach patients how to use them; and counselors give the psychological support needed to overcome vision loss and help in adapting to a new life situation.

Evaluation of Need

The most important factors for successful low-vision rehabilitation are a correct evaluation of patient needs and for patients to understand the rehabilitation plan. Depending on the resources available, various strategies can be adopted. To choose the most appropriate solutions for specific patients, a complete evaluation of distance and near visual acuity, contrast sensitivity, and visual field is required. It is also crucial to evaluate how much the visual impairment affects daily life. Each patient is affected differently depending on his or her age, social situation, and involvement in social activities. Vision-specific quality of life (QoL) questionnaires are helpful tools to discern how much help patients need in various areas, such as managing at home, work, or school and functioning socially. Questionnaires such as the Glaucoma Quality of Life-15 (GQL-15) and the National Eye Institute Visual Function Questionnaire (NEI VFQ-25) are useful instruments for assessing the level of visual impairment in daily life [183, 184]. As hearing well becomes crucial when vision ability decreases, patient auditory status should also be taken into account. In some cases, deaf–blindness support would be most appropriate.

Low-Vision Support

Glaucoma patients mostly complain about problems with reading [161], but glaucoma also affects mobility. Driving becomes challenging and walking becomes increasingly difficult, especially negotiating stairs, uneven ground, and obstacles [185]. A regular checkup of fitness for the driving license is essential to protect the patient and fellow road users from risk of car accidents.

Devices

Once the evaluation is completed, assistive devices and techniques can be implemented to enhance the quality of life. These usually require training to optimize their use. To facilitate reading, handheld magnifiers or typoscopes are available (Fig. 9.3). Books printed in Braille or talking books are other ways to have access to news and culture. CCTV or desktop magnifiers facilitate reading and writing (Figs. 9.4 and 9.5). In communications technology such as computers and cell phones, settings permit the adjustment of, for example, contrast, scale, and font size. Most cell phones nowadays offer voice-recognition alternatives to screen displays. Software is also available to translate to and from Braille. Assistive devices such as talking watches or compasses can also be helpful. To facilitate payments, coins and banknotes are of different sizes or incorporate tactile details to help in identification. When modern devices such as magnifiers and computers are unavailable, making simple adjustments can improve many everyday life activities, for example, the use of larger and bolder text that contrasts with the background might be useful (i.e., black on white or vice versa).

Environment

People who are visually impaired due to glaucoma have to adapt to their vision loss and learn how to carry on with personal care and household activities (Figs. 9.6 and 9.7). To facilitate independence, the domestic environment may require modification, for example, colorful stickers can be applied to light switches or contrast lines to the edges of stairs to make it easier to move around safely (Figs. 9.8, 9.9 and 9.10). Games such as

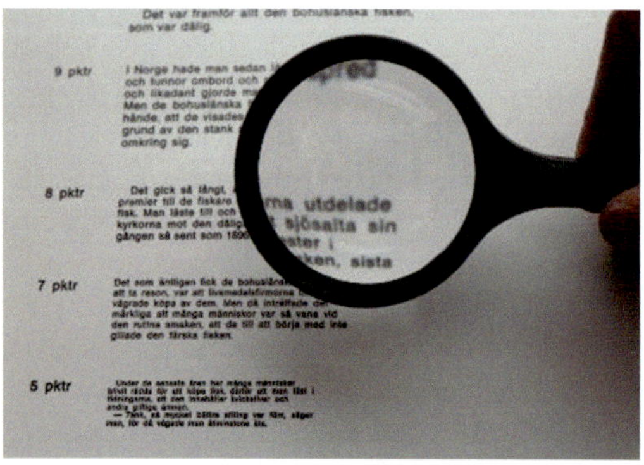

Fig. 9.3 Handheld magnifier

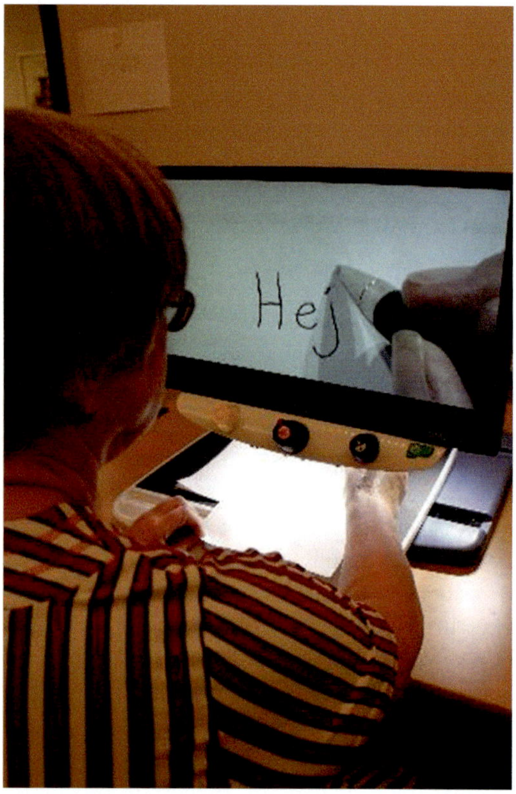

Fig. 9.4 CCTV

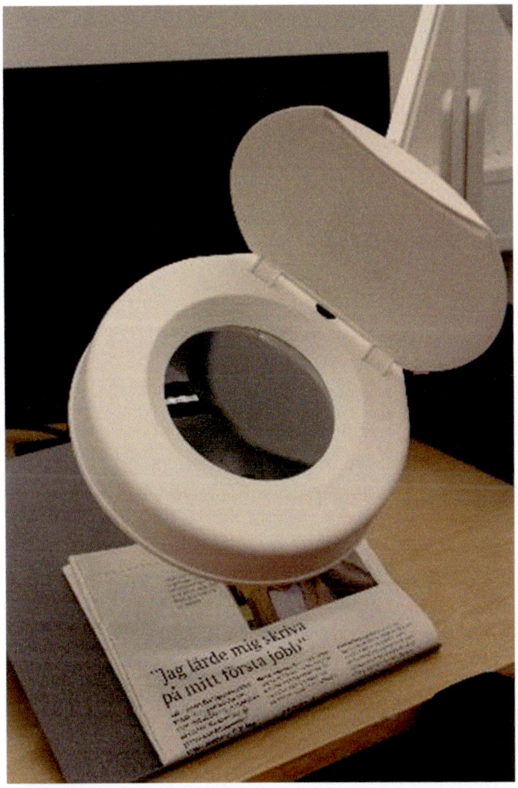

Fig. 9.5 Table-mounted magnifier

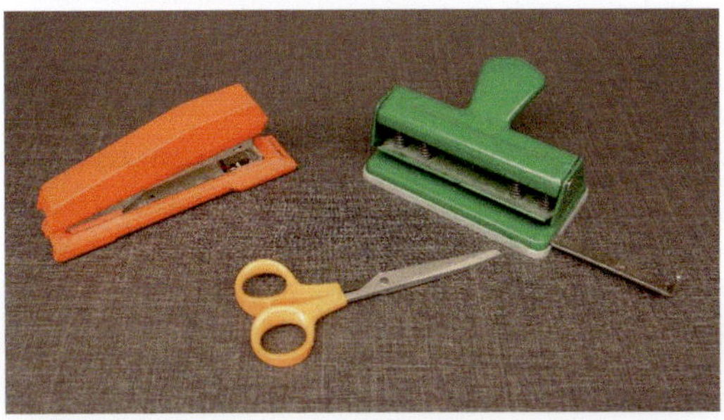

Fig. 9.6 High-contrast office equipment

chess or dice can be adapted to visual impairment by using tactile aids and Braille (Fig. 9.11). Extra attention should be paid to indoor lighting, especially reading lamps. Even meals can be served on plates that enhance contrasts, for example, rice served on a colorful plate or white porcelain placed on a colorful tablecloth (Fig. 9.12). When outdoors on a sunny day, a cap or hat with a large brim or well-fitting sunglasses can reduce glare (Fig. 9.13).

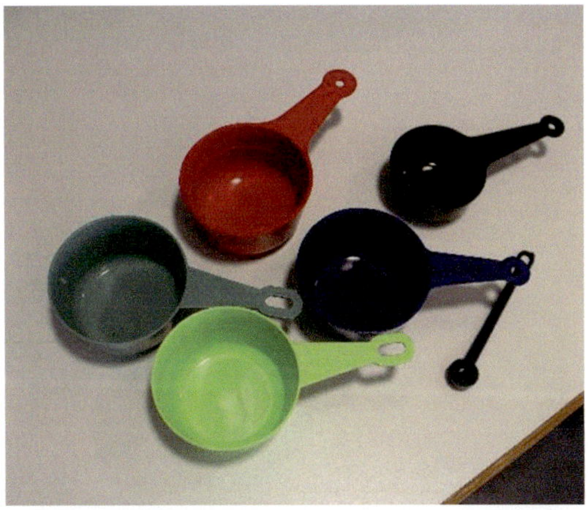

Fig. 9.7 High-contrast household implements

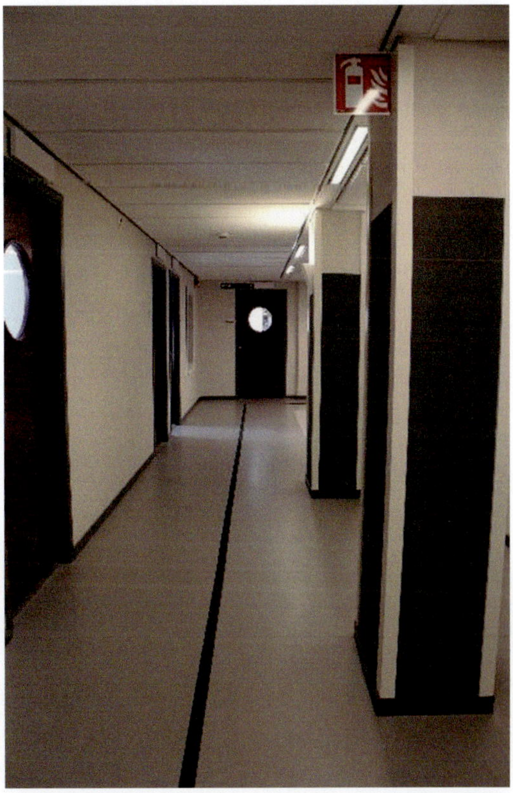

Fig. 9.8 High-contrast indoor design

Mobility

Low vision often affects mobility, leading some patients to restrict their geographic range of mobility [181]. Alongside sighted guides, white canes, and guide dogs can give some autonomy

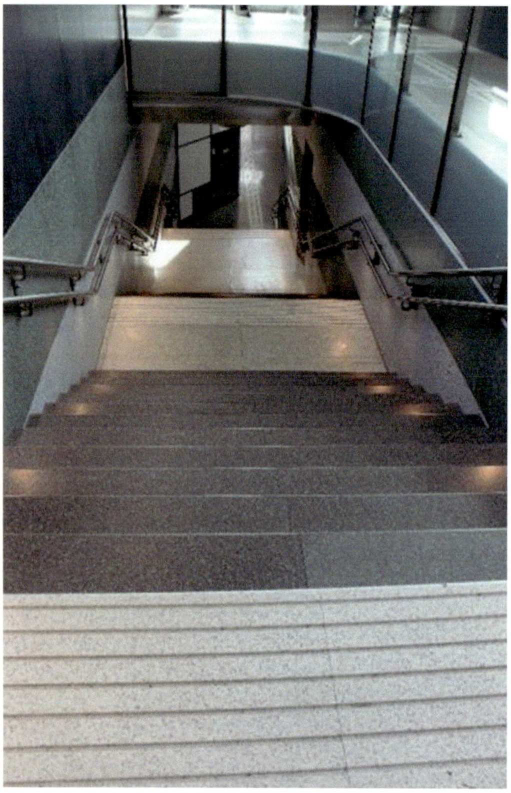

Fig. 9.9 Staircases with contrasting steps

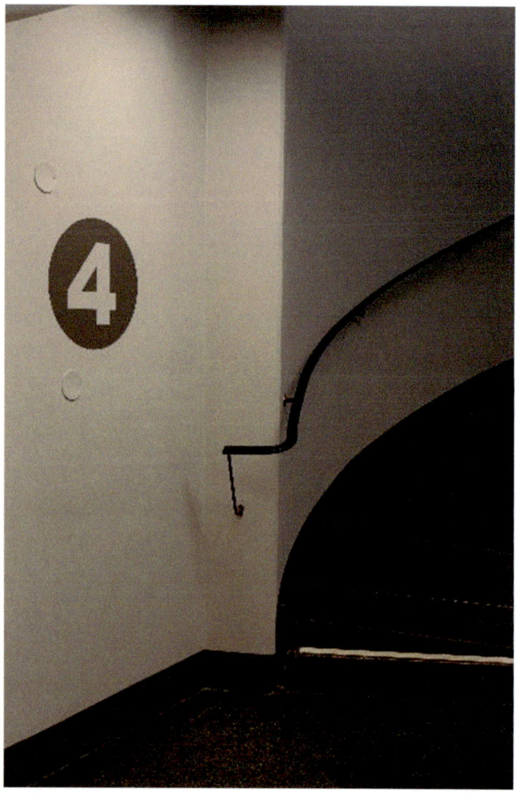

Fig. 9.10 High contrasting mark indicates the last step in the staircase

to visually impaired people. White canes are not only tools that help their users orient themselves in urban environments, they also signal visual impairment, leading to greater caution from others. These tools require practice and a trained ear to help their users get around on their own. New technologies such as cell phones and GPS can make it easier for the visually impaired to travel safely on their own.

Communities

To fulfill the UN Human Rights Convention, communities must adapt urban structures and infrastructure to facilitate the mobility of visually impaired people. It is advisable that patients with functional impairment be involved in designing such infrastructure (Figs. 9.14 and 9.15). Sounds are important to help the visually impaired orient themselves in the city. For example, pedestrian pushbuttons and audible traffic signals are helpful at crossroads, as are information buttons at bus stops that, when pressed, provide vocal information about what bus lines serve specific stops. Also helping visually impaired people navigate in an urban environment are pavements and curbs designed to incorporate tactile paving (Figs. 9.16 and 9.17). This helps people gauge where bus stops or zebra crossings are situated. In the city, where cyclists and pedestrians are numerous, it is advisable to have separate pedestrian lanes to ensure security for visually impaired people (Fig. 9.18). To satisfy most of their customers, industries can design products so that even visually impaired people find them easy to use, for example, by incorporating large text and contrasting colors. Nowadays, medicine packaging must be marked with Braille text, according to European Union regulations.

Psychological Support

Most glaucoma patients are over 70 years old and often suffer from other health problems. Physical

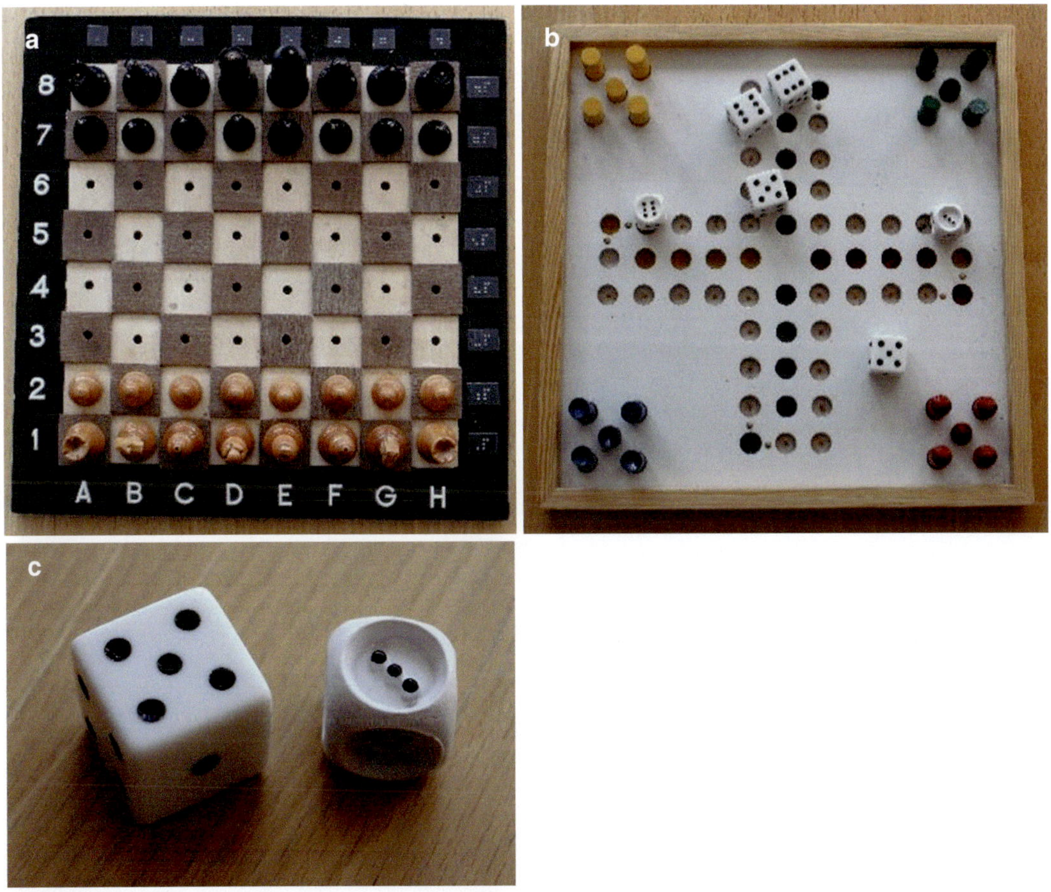

Fig. 9.11 (**a**–**c**) Board games and dice incorporating tactile aids or Braille

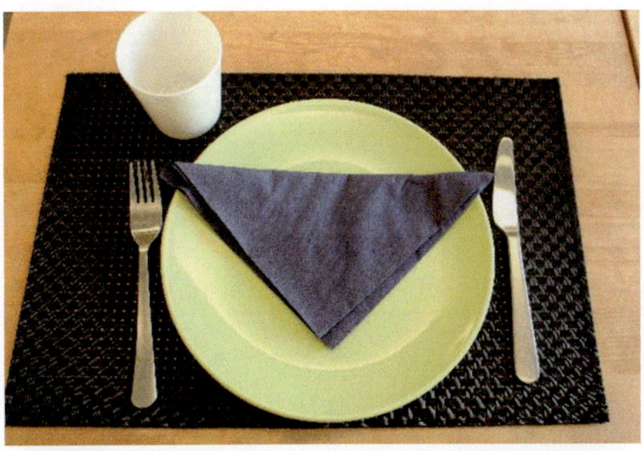

Fig. 9.12 High-contrast tableware

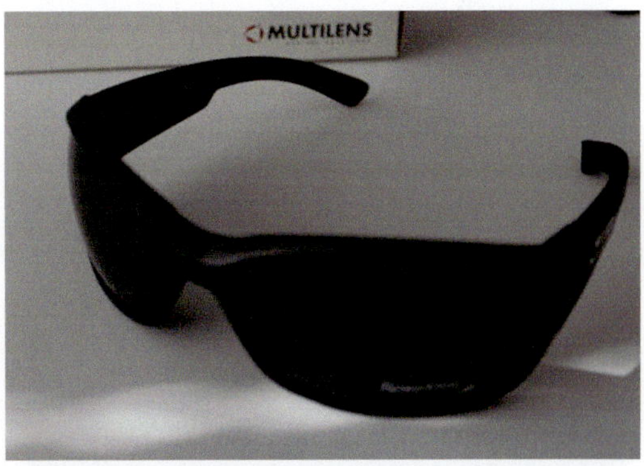

Fig. 9.13 Glare-reducing sunglasses

difficulties, such as rheumatism and hearing problems, might limit their ability to use visual aids, negatively influencing their quality of life. Psychological support is crucial in overcoming vision loss and avoiding depression. Low-vision rehabilitation should take into account all aspects of the glaucoma patient's life in endeavoring to facilitate an optimal quality of life. Low-vision support should not be implemented as a last

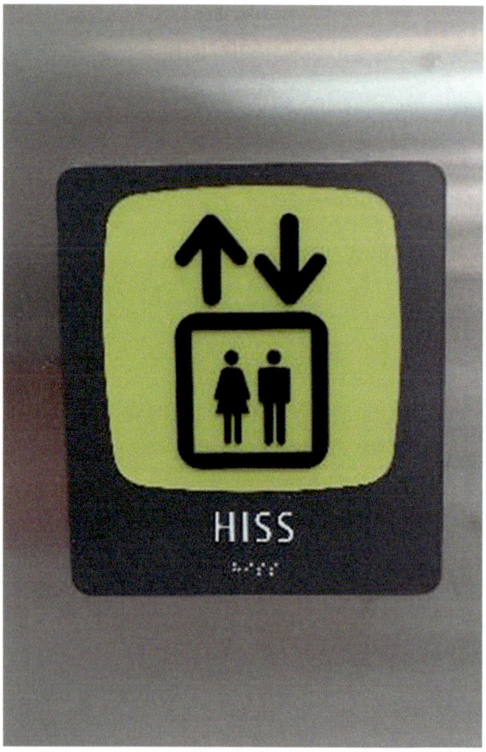

Fig. 9.14 High-contrast information with Braille text

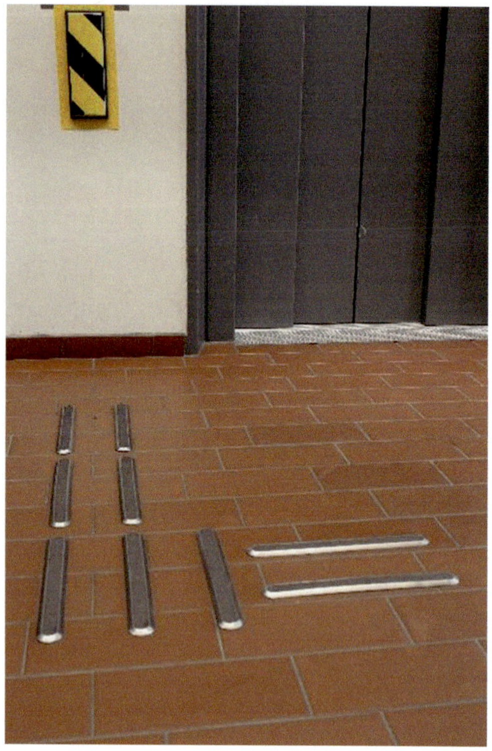

Fig. 9.16 Tactile paving

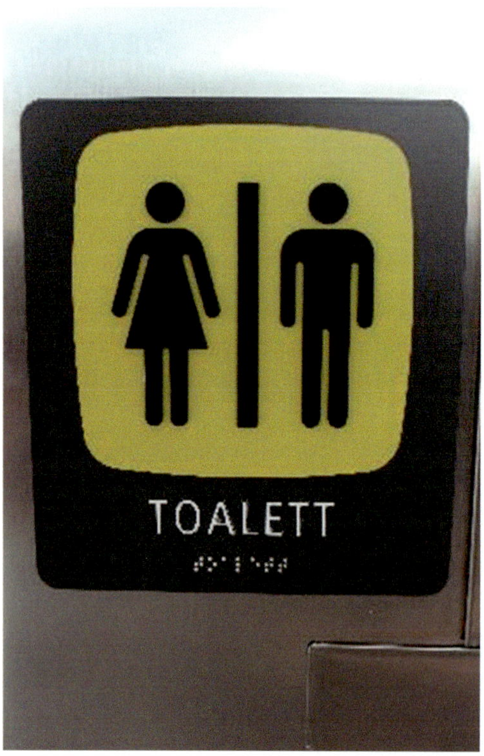

Fig. 9.15 High-contrast information with Braille text

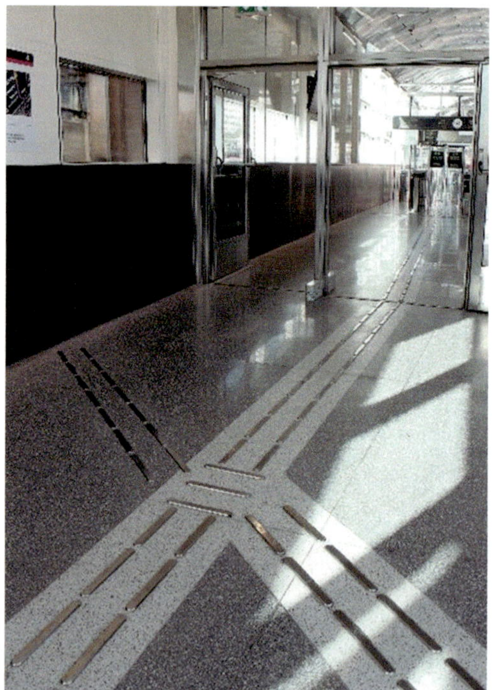

Fig. 9.17 Tactile paving

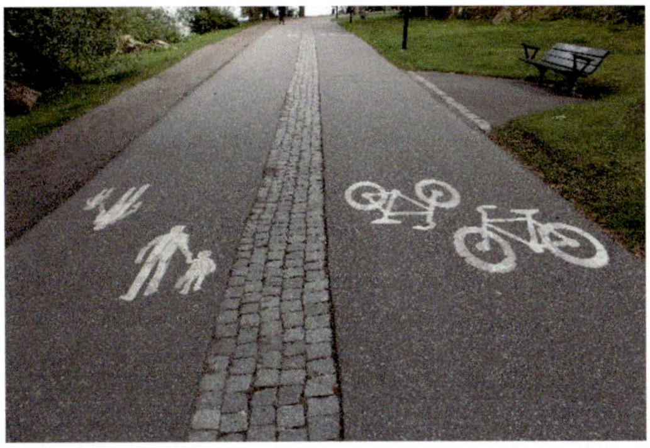

Fig. 9.18 Clearly marked pedestrian and bicycle lanes

resort when patients can no longer cope on their own. By contacting rehabilitation services at an early stage of their disease, glaucoma patients can become acquainted with devices such as magnifiers in a less urgent way.

We should encourage society to create an environment that suits everyone, including people with visual dysfunction [24].

9.1.3 Patient Data

The aim of data collection is to improve the care of each patient and of the patient group as a whole. Data collection should be based on a shared desire to improve patient care results and facilitate the work of care professionals and researchers. For "big data" collection, a hypothesis and working model should be established beforehand, in order to obtain clinically relevant causal relationships between factors. A meaningful analysis depends on standard criteria for defining glaucoma and on a clinically relevant, practical, and measurable outcome. A standard template of related parameters will facilitate the collection of data on relevant factors. Before starting a patient register, it is important to define the diagnostic criteria for glaucoma to avoid, for example, confusion between glaucoma and ocular hypertension. Patient safety and privacy should be prioritized during data collection. It is necessary to have a coordination group responsible for designing, coordinating, and monitoring the data collection and for analyzing the data collected. Various registers have been shown to be effective in improving care [186–189]. Big data analysis may provide us with insight into what treatment processes work and why. Involving patients in the data collection can form part of our cooperation with patients, possibly improving adherence to the treatment regimen.

Current documentation of glaucoma treatment success often centers on the IOP, because there is currently no universally accepted simple and effective method to document and compare vision-related quality of life between patients. A relevant, measurable, and easily accessible outcome measure is the visual field. Visual field status could be used to estimate the quality of life, while the rate of visual field reduction could be taken as an indicator of care quality.

As quality of life and quality of vision are the most essential parts of glaucoma care, development of a standardized questionnaire for estimating vision-related quality of life would be desirable. It is also essential to recall that there is educational, cultural, and socioeconomic variation among individuals, as well as possible longitudinal variation within the individual, when interpreting survey results. Big data analysis can help us identify trends and risk factors in a group. However, we should not be overconfident that we can measure everything in the healthcare system and believe that there is a simple solution to every problem. Big data analysis can only tell us about certain trends in a group; we must keep in mind that patient care should be individualized, as each patient is unique.

A standard definition of glaucoma and standardized patient-relevant outcome measures could permit the comparison of different treatment regimens, providing a basis for socioeconomic analysis with the aim of improving glaucoma care. Such an analysis could constitute a starting point for developing glaucoma care that is affordable to both patients and society [8, 63, 65, 190, 191].

Evaluating the results of different therapeutic regimens calls for a shared definition of successful glaucoma care, as various interest groups evaluate success differently based on their own points of view. Maintaining a high vision-related quality of life for glaucoma patients is our ultimate aim in glaucoma care.

References

1. Sima Q. (145-86 BCE). Records of Grand Historian.
2. Forsman E, Kivela T, Vesti E. Lifetime visual disability in open-angle glaucoma and ocular hypertension. J Glaucoma. 2007;16(3):313–9.
3. Peters D, Bengtsson B, Heijl A. Lifetime risk of blindness in open-angle glaucoma. Am J Ophthalmol. 2013;156(4):724–30.
4. Burr JM, Mowatt G, Hernandez R, Siddiqui MA, Cook J, Lourenco T, Ramsay C, Vale L, Fraser C, Azuara-Blanco A, Deeks J, Cairns J, Wormald R, McPherson S, Rabindranath K, Grant A. The clinical effectiveness and cost-effectiveness of screening for open angle glaucoma: a systematic review and economic evaluation. Health Technol Assess. 2007;11(41):iii–v.. ix–x, 1–190
5. Hernandez RA, Burr JM, Vale LD, OAG Screening Project Group. Economic evaluation of screening for open-angle glaucoma. Int J Technol Assess Health Care. 2008;24(2):203–11.
6. Quigley HA, Park CK, Tracey PA, Pollack IP. Community screening for eye disease by laypersons: the Hoffberger program. Am J Ophthalmol. 2002;133(3):386–92.
7. Tielsch JM, Katz J, Singh K, Quigley HA, Gottsch JD, Javitt J, Sommer A. A population-based evaluation of glaucoma screening: the Baltimore Eye Survey. Am J Epidemiol. 1991;134(10):1102–10.
8. Tuulonen A. Cost-effectiveness of screening for open angle glaucoma in developed countries. Indian J Ophthalmol. 2011;59(Suppl):S24–30.
9. Kyari F, Abdull MM, Bastawrous A, Gilbert CE, Faal H. Epidemiology of glaucoma in sub-saharan Africa: prevalence, incidence and risk factors. Middle East Afr J Ophthalmol. 2013;20(2):111–25.
10. Boland MV, Gupta P, Ko F, Zhao D, Guallar E, Friedman DS. Evaluation of frequency-doubling technology perimetry as a means of screening for glaucoma and other eye diseases using the National Health and Nutrition Examination Survey. JAMA Ophthalmol. 2016;134(1):57–62.
11. Chan MPY, Broadway DC, Khawaja AP, Yip JLY, Garway-Heath DF, Burr JM, Luben R, Hayat S, Dalzell N, Khaw KT, Foster PJ. Glaucoma and intraocular pressure in EPIC-Norfolk Eye Study: cross sectional study. BMJ. 2017;358:j3889.
12. Leske MC, Heijl A, Hyman L, Bengtsson B. Early Manifest Glaucoma Trial: design and baseline data. Ophthalmology. 1999;106(11):2144–53.
13. Mitchell P, Smith W, Chey T, Healey PR. Open-angle glaucoma and diabetes: the Blue Mountains eye study, Australia. Ophthalmology. 1997;104(4):712–8.
14. Tielsch JM, Sommer A, Katz J, Royall RM, Quigley HA, Javitt J. Racial variations in the prevalence of primary open-angle glaucoma. The Baltimore Eye Survey. JAMA. 1991;266(3):369–74.
15. Geimer SA. Glaucoma diagnostics. Acta Ophthalmol. 2013;91(1):1–32.
16. Fallon M, Valero O, Pazos M, Anton A. Diagnostic accuracy of imaging devices in glaucoma: a meta-analysis. Surv Ophthalmol. 2017;62(4):446–61.
17. Chong GT, Lee RK. Glaucoma versus red disease: imaging and glaucoma diagnosis. Curr Opin Ophthalmol. 2012;23(2):79–88.
18. Wahl J, Barleon L, Morfeld P, Lichtmess A, Haas-Brahler S, Pfeiffer N. The Evonik-Mainz Eye Care-Study (EMECS): development of an expert system for glaucoma risk detection in a working population. PLoS One. 2016;11(8):e0158824.
19. Muhammad H, Fuchs TJ, De Cuir N, De Moraes CG, Blumberg DM, Liebmann JM, Ritch R, Hood DC. Hybrid deep learning on single wide-field optical coherence tomography scans accurately classifies glaucoma suspects. J Glaucoma. 2017;26(12):1086–94.
20. Hagman J. Comparison of resource utilization in the treatment of open-angle glaucoma between two cities in Finland: is more better? Acta Ophthalmol. 2013;91(3):1–47.
21. Lorenz K, Wolfram C, Breitscheidel L, Shlaen M, Verboven Y, Pfeiffer N. Direct cost and predictive factors for treatment in patients with ocular hypertension or early, moderate and advanced primary open-angle glaucoma: the CoGIS study in Germany. Graefes Arch Clin Exp Ophthalmol. 2013;251(8):2019–28.
22. Traverso CE, Walt JG, Kelly SP, Hommer AH, Bron AM, Denis P, Nordmann JP, Renard JP, Bayer A, Grehn F, Pfeiffer N, Cedrone C, Gandolfi S, Orzalesi N, Nucci C, Rossetti L, Azuara-Blanco A, Bagnis A, Hitchings R, Salmon JF, Bricola G, Buchholz PM, Kotak SV, Katz LM, Siegartel LR, Doyle JJ. Direct costs of glaucoma and severity of the disease: a multinational long term study of resource utilisation in Europe. Br J Ophthalmol. 2005;89(10):1245–9.
23. Heijl A, Alm A, Bengtsson B, Bergstrom A, Calissendorff B, Lindblom B, Linden C, Swedish Ophthalmological Society. The glaucoma guidelines of the Swedish Ophthalmological Society. Acta Ophthalmol Suppl (Oxf). 2012;251:1–40.
24. Green J, Siddall H, Murdoch I. Learning to live with glaucoma: a qualitative study of diagnosis and the impact of sight loss. Soc Sci Med. 2002;55(2):257–67.
25. Hark L, Waisbourd M, Myers JS, Henderer J, Crews JE, Saaddine JB, Molineaux J, Johnson D, Sembhi H, Stratford S, Suleiman A, Pizzi L, Spaeth GL, Katz LJ. Improving access to eye care among persons at high-risk of glaucoma in philadelphia--design and methodology: the philadelphia glaucoma detection and treatment project. Ophthalmic Epidemiol. 2016;23(2):122–30.
26. Hourihan F, Mitchell P. Factors associated with use of glaucoma medications in a population of older people: The Blue Mountains Eye Study. Aust N Z J Ophthalmol. 1999;27(3–4):176–9.
27. Dandona L, Dandona R, Mandal P, Srinivas M, John RK, McCarty CA, Rao GN. Angle-closure glaucoma in an urban population in southern India. The Andhra Pradesh eye disease study. Ophthalmology. 2000;107(9):1710–6.

28. Dandona R, Dandona L, John RK, McCarty CA, Rao GN. Awareness of eye diseases in an urban population in southern India. Bull World Health Organ. 2001;79(2):96–102.
29. Vijaya L, George R, Arvind H, Baskaran M, Paul PG, Ramesh SV, Raju P, Kumaramanickavel G, McCarty C. Prevalence of angle-closure disease in a rural southern Indian population. Arch Ophthalmol. 2006;124(3):403–9.
30. Hennis A, Wu SY, Nemesure B, Honkanen R, Leske MC, Barbados Eye Studies Group. Awareness of incident open-angle glaucoma in a population study: the Barbados Eye Studies. Ophthalmology. 2007;114(10):1816–21.
31. WHO. Vision 2020 the right to sight, WHO. 2007. http://www.who.int/blindness/Vision2020_report.pdf?ua=1.
32. Katibeh M, Ziaei H, Panah E, Moein HR, Hosseini S, Kalantarion M, Eskandari A, Yaseri M. Knowledge and awareness of age related eye diseases: a population-based survey. J Ophthalmic Vis Res. 2014;9(2):223–31.
33. Lau JT, Lee V, Fan D, Lau M, Michon J. Knowledge about cataract, glaucoma, and age related macular degeneration in the Hong Kong Chinese population. Br J Ophthalmol. 2002;86(10):1080–4.
34. Thapa SS, Berg RV, Khanal S, Paudyal I, Pandey P, Maharjan N, Twyana SN, Paudyal G, Gurung R, Ruit S, Rens GH. Prevalence of visual impairment, cataract surgery and awareness of cataract and glaucoma in Bhaktapur district of Nepal: the Bhaktapur Glaucoma Study. BMC Ophthalmol. 2011;11:2.
35. Pfeiffer N, Krieglstein GK, Wellek S. Knowledge about glaucoma in the unselected population: a German survey. J Glaucoma. 2002;11(5):458–63.
36. Vad betyder ordet Glaukom?. Ögontrycket, Svenska Glaukomförbundet. 2010.
37. Dugast P, Thiboust P, Blumen-Ohana E, Nordmann JP. Is there a need for a therapeutic education with patients suffering with open-angle glaucoma? Preliminary inquiry regarding knowledge and patient adherence. J Fr Ophtalmol. 2016;39(6):527–34.
38. Kowing D, Messer D, Slagle S, Wasik A, V-POAG Study Group. Programs to optimize adherence in glaucoma. Optometry. 2010;81(7):339–50.
39. Leydhecker W, Akiyama K, Neumann HG. Intraocular pressure in normal human eyes. Klin Monbl Augenheilkd Augenarztl Fortbild. 1958;133(5):662–70.
40. Gordon MO, Beiser JA, Brandt JD, Heuer DK, Higginbotham EJ, Johnson CA, Keltner JL, Miller JP, Parrish RK 2nd, Wilson MR, Kass MA. The Ocular Hypertension Treatment Study: baseline factors that predict the onset of primary open-angle glaucoma. Arch Ophthalmol. 2002;120(6):714–20; discussion 829-730.
41. Kass MA, Heuer DK, Higginbotham EJ, Johnson CA, Keltner JL, Miller JP, Parrish RK 2nd, Wilson MR, Gordon MO. The ocular hypertension treatment study: a randomized trial determines that topical ocular hypotensive medication delays or prevents the onset of primary open-angle glaucoma. Arch Ophthalmol. 2002;120(6):701–13; discussion 829-730.
42. Prum BE Jr, Herndon LW Jr, Moroi SE, Mansberger SL, Stein JD, Lim MC, Rosenberg LF, Gedde SJ, Williams RD. Primary angle closure preferred practice pattern((R)) guidelines. Ophthalmology. 2016;123(1):P1–P40.
43. Tuulonen A, Airaksinen PJ, Erola E, Forsman E, Friberg K, Kaila M, Klemetti A, Makela M, Oskala P, Puska P, Suoranta L, Teir H, Uusitalo H, Vainio-Jylha E, Vuori ML. The Finnish evidence-based guideline for open-angle glaucoma. Acta Ophthalmol Scand. 2003;81(1):3–18.
44. Odberg T, Jakobsen JE, Hultgren SJ, Halseide R. The impact of glaucoma on the quality of life of patients in Norway. I. Results from a self-administered questionnaire. Acta Ophthalmol Scand. 2001;79(2): 116–20.
45. Mills RP, Budenz DL, Lee PP, Noecker RJ, Walt JG, Siegartel LR, Evans SJ, Doyle JJ. Categorizing the stage of glaucoma from pre-diagnosis to end-stage disease. Am J Ophthalmol. 2006;141(1):24–30.
46. Peters D, Heijl A, Brenner L, Bengtsson B. Visual impairment and vision-related quality of life in the Early Manifest Glaucoma Trial after 20 years of follow-up. Acta Ophthalmol. 2015;93(8):745–52.
47. Peters D, Bengtsson B, Heijl A. Factors associated with lifetime risk of open-angle glaucoma blindness. Acta Ophthalmol. 2014;92(5):421–5.
48. NEI. 2010 U.S. Age-Specific Prevalence Rates for Glaucoma by Age and Race/Ethnicity. https://nei.nih.gov/eyedata/glaucoma (2010).
49. Norin O, Enström J, de Gosson de Varennes S. Beteende och behov hos personer i kontakt med vården. Website of Sveriges Kommuner och Landstning: https://skl.se/download/18.5e588ed415aa6ecabde9f48f/1489484509965/Beteenden%20och%20behov%20hos%20personer%20i%20kontakt%20med%20v%C3%A5rden.pdf (2017).
50. European glaucoma society terminology and guidelines for glaucoma, 4th edition - Chapter 3: treatment principles and options Supported by the EGS Foundation: Part 1: Foreword; Introduction; Glossary; Chapter 3 treatment principles and options. Br J Ophthalmol. 2017;101(6):130–95.
51. Kalouda P, Keskini C, Anastasopoulos E, Topouzis F. Achievements and limits of current medical therapy of glaucoma. Dev Ophthalmol. 2017;59:1–14.
52. Matsuura M, Hirasawa K, Hirasawa H, Yanagisawa M, Murata H, Mayama C, Asaoka R. Developing an item bank to measure quality of life in individuals with glaucoma, and the results of the interview with patients: the effect of visual function, visual field progression rate, medical, and surgical treatments on quality of life. J Glaucoma. 2017;26(2):e64–73.
53. Williams AM, Muir KW, Rosdahl JA. Readability of patient education materials in ophthalmology: a single-institution study and systematic review. BMC Ophthalmol. 2016;16:133.

54. Fukuchi T, Yoshino T, Sawada H, Seki M, Togano T, Tanaka T, Ueda J, Abe H. The relationship between the mean deviation slope and follow-up intraocular pressure in open-angle glaucoma patients. J Glaucoma. 2013;22(9):689–97.
55. Heijl A, Leske MC, Bengtsson B, Hyman L, Bengtsson B, Hussein M, Early Manifest Glaucoma Trial Group. Reduction of intraocular pressure and glaucoma progression: results from the Early Manifest Glaucoma Trial. Arch Ophthalmol. 2002;120(10):1268–79.
56. Nouri-Mahdavi K, Hoffman D, Coleman AL, Liu G, Li G, Gaasterland D, Caprioli J, Advanced Glaucoma Intervention Study. Predictive factors for glaucomatous visual field progression in the Advanced Glaucoma Intervention Study. Ophthalmology. 2004;111(9):1627–35.
57. Clement CI, Bhartiya S, Shaarawy T. New perspectives on target intraocular pressure. Surv Ophthalmol. 2014;59(6):615–26.
58. Chen E, Querat L, Akerstedt C. Self-tonometry as a complement in the investigation of glaucoma patients. Acta Ophthalmol. 2016;94(8):788–92.
59. Querat L, Chen E. Monitoring daily intraocular pressure fluctuations with self-tonometry in healthy subjects. Acta Ophthalmol. 2017;95(5):525–9.
60. Jampel HD. Target pressure in glaucoma therapy. J Glaucoma. 1997;6(2):133–8.
61. Zeyen T. Target pressures in glaucoma. Bull Soc Belge Ophtalmol. 1999;274:61–5.
62. Stalmans I, Sunaric Megevand G, Cordeiro MF, Hommer A, Rossetti L, Goni F, Heijl A, Bron A. Preservative-free treatment in glaucoma: who, when, and why. Eur J Ophthalmol. 2013;23(4):518–25.
63. Tuulonen A, Kataja M, Syvanen U, Miettunen S, Uusitalo H. Right services to right patients at right time in right setting in Tays Eye Centre. Acta Ophthalmol. 2016;94(7):730–5.
64. Nordmann JP, Auzanneau N, Ricard S, Berdeaux G. Vision related quality of life and topical glaucoma treatment side effects. Health Qual Life Outcomes. 2003;1:75.
65. Tuulonen A. Is more always better? Acta Ophthalmol Scand. 2004;82(4):377–9.
66. Lee BW, Murakami Y, Duncan MT, Kao AA, Huang JY, Lin S, Singh K. Patient-related and system-related barriers to glaucoma follow-up in a county hospital population. Invest Ophthalmol Vis Sci. 2013;54(10):6542–8.
67. Gott bemötande av vården där Stockholmare känner sig mest trygga med sin ögonsjukvård. Ögontrycket, Svenska Glaukomförbundet. 2016.
68. Ekstrom C. Prevalence of open-angle glaucoma in central Sweden. The Tierp Glaucoma Survey. Acta Ophthalmol Scand. 1996;74(2):107–12.
69. Quigley HA. Number of people with glaucoma worldwide. Br J Ophthalmol. 1996;80(5):389–93.
70. Ramakrishnan R, Nirmalan PK, Krishnadas R, Thulasiraj RD, Tielsch JM, Katz J, Friedman DS, Robin AL. Glaucoma in a rural population of southern India: the Aravind comprehensive eye survey. Ophthalmology. 2003;110(8):1484–90.
71. Vijaya L, George R, Arvind H, Baskaran M, Raju P, Ramesh SV, Paul PG, Kumaramanickavel G, McCarty C. Prevalence and causes of blindness in the rural population of the Chennai Glaucoma Study. Br J Ophthalmol. 2006;90(4):407–10.
72. Abu Hussein NB, Eissa IM, Abdel-Kader AA. Analysis of factors affecting patients' compliance to topical antiglaucoma medications in Egypt as a developing country model. J Ophthalmol. 2015;2015:234157.
73. Rotchford AP, Murphy KM. Compliance with timolol treatment in glaucoma. Eye (Lond). 1998;12(Pt 2):234–6.
74. Schwartz GF. Compliance and persistency in glaucoma follow-up treatment. Curr Opin Ophthalmol. 2005;16(2):114–21.
75. Tsai JC. A comprehensive perspective on patient adherence to topical glaucoma therapy. Ophthalmology. 2009;116(11 Suppl):S30–6.
76. Vanelli M, Pedan A, Liu N, Hoar J, Messier D, Kiarsis K. The role of patient inexperience in medication discontinuation: a retrospective analysis of medication nonpersistence in seven chronic illnesses. Clin Ther. 2009;31(11):2628–52.
77. Hwang DK, Liu CJ, Pu CY, Chou YJ, Chou P. Persistence of topical glaucoma medication: a nationwide population-based cohort study in Taiwan. JAMA Ophthalmol. 2014;132(12):1446–52.
78. Lusthaus JA, Goldberg I. Investigational and experimental drugs for intraocular pressure reduction in ocular hypertension and glaucoma. Expert Opin Investig Drugs. 2016;25(10):1201–8.
79. Reardon G, Schwartz GF, Mozaffari E. Patient persistency with ocular prostaglandin therapy: a population-based, retrospective study. Clin Ther. 2003;25(4):1172–85.
80. Yousuf SJ, Jones LS. Adherence to topical glaucoma medication during hospitalization. J Glaucoma. 2011;20(9):573–6.
81. The effectiveness of intraocular pressure reduction in the treatment of normal-tension glaucoma. Collaborative Normal-Tension Glaucoma Study Group. Am J Ophthalmol. 1998;126(4):498–505.
82. Norell SE, Granstrom PA, Wassen R. A medication monitor and fluorescein technique designed to study medication behaviour. Acta Ophthalmol (Copenh). 1980;58(3):459–67.
83. Gurwitz JH, Glynn RJ, Monane M, Everitt DE, Gilden D, Smith N, Avorn J. Treatment for glaucoma: adherence by the elderly. Am J Public Health. 1993;83(5):711–6.
84. Kass MA, Meltzer DW, Gordon M, Cooper D, Goldberg J. Compliance with topical pilocarpine treatment. Am J Ophthalmol. 1986;101(5):515–23.
85. Nordstrom BL, Friedman DS, Mozaffari E, Quigley HA, Walker AM. Persistence and adherence with topical glaucoma therapy. Am J Ophthalmol. 2005;140(4):598–606.
86. Olthoff CM, Hoevenaars JG, van den Borne BW, Webers CA, Schouten JS. Prevalence and determinants of non-adherence to topical hypotensive treatment in Dutch glaucoma patients. Graefes Arch Clin Exp Ophthalmol. 2009;247(2):235–43.

87. Olthoff CM, Schouten JS, van de Borne BW, Webers CA. Noncompliance with ocular hypotensive treatment in patients with glaucoma or ocular hypertension an evidence-based review. Ophthalmology. 2005;112(6):953–61.
88. Schwartz GF, Reardon G, Mozaffari E. Persistency with latanoprost or timolol in primary open-angle glaucoma suspects. Am J Ophthalmol. 2004;137(1 Suppl):S13–6.
89. Deokule S, Sadiq S, Shah S. Chronic open angle glaucoma: patient awareness of the nature of the disease, topical medication, compliance and the prevalence of systemic symptoms. Ophthalmic Physiol Opt. 2004;24(1):9–15.
90. Mehari T, Giorgis AT, Shibeshi W. Level of adherence to ocular hypotensive agents and its determinant factors among glaucoma patients in Menelik II Referral Hospital, Ethiopia. BMC Ophthalmol. 2016;16:131.
91. Movahedinejad T, Adib-Hajbaghery M. Adherence to treatment in patients with open-angle glaucoma and its related factors. Electron Physician. 2016;8(9):2954–61.
92. Okeke CO, Quigley HA, Jampel HD, Ying GS, Plyler RJ, Jiang Y, Friedman DS. Interventions improve poor adherence with once daily glaucoma medications in electronically monitored patients. Ophthalmology. 2009;116(12):2286–93.
93. Hahn SR. Patient-centered communication to assess and enhance patient adherence to glaucoma medication. Ophthalmology. 2009;116(11 Suppl):S37–42.
94. Tsai JC, McClure CA, Ramos SE, Schlundt DG, Pichert JW. Compliance barriers in glaucoma: a systematic classification. J Glaucoma. 2003;12(5):393–8.
95. Chawla A, McGalliard JN, Batterbury M. Use of eyedrops in glaucoma: how can we help to reduce non-compliance? Acta Ophthalmol Scand. 2007;85(4):464.
96. Tsai JC. Medication adherence in glaucoma: approaches for optimizing patient compliance. Curr Opin Ophthalmol. 2006;17(2):190–5.
97. Tsai JH, Derby E, Holland EJ, Khatana AK. Incidence and prevalence of glaucoma in severe ocular surface disease. Cornea. 2006;25(5):530–2.
98. Sleath B, Robin AL, Covert D, Byrd JE, Tudor G, Svarstad B. Patient-reported behavior and problems in using glaucoma medications. Ophthalmology. 2006;113(3):431–6.
99. Ngan R, Lam DL, Mudumbai RC, Chen PP. Risk factors for noncompliance with follow-up among normal-tension glaucoma suspects. Am J Ophthalmol. 2007;144(2):310–1.
100. Friedman DS, Hahn SR, Gelb L, Tan J, Shah SN, Kim EE, Zimmerman TJ, Quigley HA. Doctor-patient communication, health-related beliefs, and adherence in glaucoma results from the Glaucoma Adherence and Persistency Study. Ophthalmology. 2008;115(8):1320–27, 1327 e1321–1323.
101. Budenz DL. A clinician's guide to the assessment and management of nonadherence in glaucoma. Ophthalmology. 2009;116(11 Suppl):S43–7.
102. Tatham AJ, Sarodia U, Gatrad F, Awan A. Eye drop instillation technique in patients with glaucoma. Eye (Lond). 2013;27(11):1293–8.
103. Schwartz GF, Hollander DA, Williams JM. Evaluation of eye drop administration technique in patients with glaucoma or ocular hypertension. Curr Med Res Opin. 2013;29(11):1515–22.
104. Dietlein TS, Jordan JF, Luke C, Schild A, Dinslage S, Krieglstein GK. Self-application of single-use eyedrop containers in an elderly population: comparisons with standard eyedrop bottle and with younger patients. Acta Ophthalmol. 2008;86(8):856–9.
105. Kholdebarin R, Campbell RJ, Jin YP, Buys YM. Multicenter study of compliance and drop administration in glaucoma. Can J Ophthalmol. 2008;43(4):454–61.
106. Mohindroo C, Ichhpujani P, Kumar S. How 'Drug Aware' are our glaucoma patients? J Curr Glaucoma Pract. 2015;9(2):33–7.
107. Linden C, Bengtsson B, Alm A, Calissendorff B, Eckerlund I, Heijl A. Glaucoma management in Sweden -- results from a nationwide survey. Acta Ophthalmol. 2013;91(1):20–4.
108. Friedman DS, Cramer J, Quigley H. A more proactive approach is needed in glaucoma care. Arch Ophthalmol. 2005;123(8):1134–5.
109. Friedman DS, Hahn SR, Quigley HA, Kotak S, Kim E, Onofrey M, Eagan C, Mardekian J. Doctor-patient communication in glaucoma care: analysis of videotaped encounters in community-based office practice. Ophthalmology. 2009;116(12):2277–85, e2271–2273.
110. Leske MC, Heijl A, Hyman L, Bengtsson B, Komaroff E. Factors for progression and glaucoma treatment: the Early Manifest Glaucoma Trial. Curr Opin Ophthalmol. 2004;15(2):102–6.
111. Stewart WC, Kolker AE, Sharpe ED, Day DG, Konstas AG, Hollo G, Astakhov YS, Teus MA, Stewart JA. Long-term progression at individual mean intraocular pressure levels in primary open-angle and exfoliative glaucoma. Eur J Ophthalmol. 2008;18(5):765–70.
112. Chauhan BC, Mikelberg FS, Balaszi AG, LeBlanc RP, Lesk MR, Trope GE, Canadian Glaucoma Study Group. Canadian Glaucoma Study: 2. risk factors for the progression of open-angle glaucoma. Arch Ophthalmol. 2008;126(8):1030–6.
113. Garway-Heath DF, Crabb DP, Bunce C, Lascaratos G, Amalfitano F, Anand N, Azuara-Blanco A, Bourne RR, Broadway DC, Cunliffe IA, Diamond JP, Fraser SG, Ho TA, Martin KR, McNaught AI, Negi A, Patel K, Russell RA, Shah A, Spry PG, Suzuki K, White ET, Wormald RP, Xing W, Zeyen TG. Latanoprost for open-angle glaucoma (UKGTS): a randomised, multicentre, placebo-controlled trial. Lancet. 2015;385(9975):1295–304.

114. Heijl A, Buchholz P, Norrgren G, Bengtsson B. Rates of visual field progression in clinical glaucoma care. Acta Ophthalmol. 2013;91(5):406–12.
115. Leske MC, Heijl A, Hussein M, Bengtsson B, Hyman L, Komaroff E, Early Manifest Glaucoma Trial Group. Factors for glaucoma progression and the effect of treatment: the early manifest glaucoma trial. Arch Ophthalmol. 2003;121(1):48–56.
116. Miglior S, Torri V, Zeyen T, Pfeiffer N, Vaz JC, Adamsons I, E. Group. Intercurrent factors associated with the development of open-angle glaucoma in the European glaucoma prevention study. Am J Ophthalmol. 2007;144(2):266–75.
117. Bengtsson B, Heijl A. A visual field index for calculation of glaucoma rate of progression. Am J Ophthalmol. 2008;145(2):343–53.
118. Rossetti L, Goni F, Denis P, Bengtsson B, Martinez A, Heijl A. Focusing on glaucoma progression and the clinical importance of progression rate measurement: a review. Eye (Lond). 2010;24(Suppl 1):S1–7.
119. Harju M. Intraocular pressure and progression in exfoliative eyes with ocular hypertension or glaucoma. Acta Ophthalmol Scand. 2000;78(6):699–702.
120. Heijl A, Bengtsson B, Hyman L, Leske MC, Early Manifest Glaucoma Trial Group. Natural history of open-angle glaucoma. Ophthalmology. 2009;116(12):2271–6.
121. Konstas AG, Hollo G, Astakhov YS, Teus MA, Akopov EL, Jenkins JN, Stewart WC. Factors associated with long-term progression or stability in exfoliation glaucoma. Arch Ophthalmol. 2004;122(1):29–33.
122. Leske MC, Heijl A, Hyman L, Bengtsson B, Dong L, Yang Z, EMGT Group. Predictors of long-term progression in the early manifest glaucoma trial. Ophthalmology. 2007;114(11):1965–72.
123. Broman AT, Quigley HA, West SK, Katz J, Munoz B, Bandeen-Roche K, Tielsch JM, Friedman DS, Crowston J, Taylor HR, Varma R, Leske MC, Bengtsson B, Heijl A, He M, Foster PJ. Estimating the rate of progressive visual field damage in those with open-angle glaucoma, from cross-sectional data. Invest Ophthalmol Vis Sci. 2008;49(1):66–76.
124. Leske MC, Wu SY, Hennis A, Honkanen R, Nemesure B, B. E. S. Group. Risk factors for incident open-angle glaucoma: the Barbados Eye Studies. Ophthalmology. 2008;115(1):85–93.
125. Prata TS, De Moraes CG, Teng CC, Tello C, Ritch R, Liebmann JM. Factors affecting rates of visual field progression in glaucoma patients with optic disc hemorrhage. Ophthalmology. 2010;117(1):24–9.
126. Bonomi L, Marchini G, Marraffa M, Bernardi P, Morbio R, Varotto A. Vascular risk factors for primary open angle glaucoma: the Egna-Neumarkt Study. Ophthalmology. 2000;107(7):1287–93.
127. Chung HS, Harris A, Evans DW, Kagemann L, Garzozi HJ, Martin B. Vascular aspects in the pathophysiology of glaucomatous optic neuropathy. Surv Ophthalmol. 1999;43(Suppl 1):S43–50.
128. Jurgens C, Grossjohann R, Tost F. Distribution of mean, systolic and diastolic ocular perfusion pressure in telemedical homemonitoring of glaucoma patients. Ophthalmic Res. 2012;48(4):208–11.
129. McGlynn MM, Ehrlich JR, Marlow ED, Chee RI, Silva FQ, Van Tassel SH, Radcliffe NM. Association of blood and ocular perfusion pressure with structural glaucomatous progression by flicker chronoscopy. Br J Ophthalmol. 2013;97(12):1569–73.
130. Okumura Y, Yuki K, Tsubota K. Low diastolic blood pressure is associated with the progression of normal-tension glaucoma. Ophthalmologica. 2012;228(1):36–41.
131. Ramdas WD, Wolfs RC, Hofman A, de Jong PT, Vingerling JR, Jansonius NM. Ocular perfusion pressure and the incidence of glaucoma: real effect or artifact? The Rotterdam Study. Invest Ophthalmol Vis Sci. 2011;52(9):6875–81.
132. Tielsch JM, Katz J, Sommer A, Quigley HA, Javitt JC. Hypertension, perfusion pressure, and primary open-angle glaucoma. A population-based assessment. Arch Ophthalmol. 1995;113(2):216–21.
133. Bengtsson B, Heijl A. Diurnal IOP fluctuation: not an independent risk factor for glaucomatous visual field loss in high-risk ocular hypertension. Graefes Arch Clin Exp Ophthalmol. 2005;243(6):513–8.
134. Bengtsson B, Leske MC, Hyman L, Heijl A, Early Manifest Glaucoma Trial Group. Fluctuation of intraocular pressure and glaucoma progression in the Early Manifest Glaucoma Trial. Ophthalmology. 2007;114(2):205–9.
135. Caprioli J. Intraocular pressure fluctuation: an independent risk factor for glaucoma? Arch Ophthalmol. 2007;125(8):1124–5.
136. Caprioli J, Coleman A. Pressure fluctuation. Ophthalmology. 2009;116(4):817.
137. Caprioli J, Coleman AL. Intraocular pressure fluctuation a risk factor for visual field progression at low intraocular pressures in the advanced glaucoma intervention study. Ophthalmology. 2008;115(7):1123–29, e1123.
138. De Moraes CG, Juthani VJ, Liebmann JM, Teng CC, Tello C, Susanna R Jr, Ritch R. Risk factors for visual field progression in treated glaucoma. Arch Ophthalmol. 2011;129(5):562–8.
139. Hong S, Seong GJ, Hong YJ. Long-term intraocular pressure fluctuation and progressive visual field deterioration in patients with glaucoma and low intraocular pressures after a triple procedure. Arch Ophthalmol. 2007;125(8):1010–3.
140. Nouri-Mahdavi K, Medeiros FA, Weinreb RN. Fluctuation of intraocular pressure as a predictor of visual field progression. Arch Ophthalmol. 2008;126(8):1168–69; author reply 1169–1170.
141. Borger PH, van Leeuwen R, Hulsman CA, Wolfs RC, van der Kuip DA, Hofman A, de Jong PT. Is there a direct association between age-related eye diseases and mortality? The Rotterdam Study. Ophthalmology. 2003;110(7):1292–6.

142. Klein BE, Klein R, Meuer SM, Goetz LA. Migraine headache and its association with open-angle glaucoma: the Beaver Dam Eye Study. Invest Ophthalmol Vis Sci. 1993;34(10):3024–7.
143. Lee AJ, Wang JJ, Kifley A, Mitchell P. Open-angle glaucoma and cardiovascular mortality: the Blue Mountains Eye Study. Ophthalmology. 2006;113(7):1069–76.
144. Wu SY, Nemesure B, Hennis A, Schachat AP, Hyman L, Leske MC, Barbados Eye Studies Group. Open-angle glaucoma and mortality: the Barbados Eye Studies. Arch Ophthalmol. 2008;126(3):365–70.
145. Knight OJ, Chang RT, Feuer WJ, Budenz DL. Comparison of retinal nerve fiber layer measurements using time domain and spectral domain optical coherent tomography. Ophthalmology. 2009;116(7):1271–7.
146. Zhang X, Dastiridou A, Francis BA, Tan O, Varma R, Greenfield DS, Schuman JS, Huang D, Advanced Imaging for Glaucoma Study Group. Comparison of glaucoma progression detection by optical coherence tomography and visual field. Am J Ophthalmol. 2017;184:63–74.
147. Prager AJ, Hood DC, Liebmann JM, De Moraes CG, Al-Aswad LA, Yu Q, Cioffi GA, Blumberg DM. Association of glaucoma-related, optical coherence tomography-measured macular damage with vision-related quality of life. JAMA Ophthalmol. 2017;135(7):783–8.
148. Blumberg DM, De Moraes CG, Prager AJ, Yu Q, Al-Aswad L, Cioffi GA, Liebmann JM, Hood DC. Association between undetected 10-2 visual field damage and vision-related quality of life in patients with glaucoma. JAMA Ophthalmol. 2017;135(7):742–7.
149. Hong J, Xu J, Wei A, Deng SX, Cui X, Yu X, Sun X. A new tonometer--the Corvis ST tonometer: clinical comparison with noncontact and Goldmann applanation tonometers. Invest Ophthalmol Vis Sci. 2013;54(1):659–65.
150. Kotecha A, White E, Schlottmann PG, Garway-Heath DF. Intraocular pressure measurement precision with the Goldmann applanation, dynamic contour, and ocular response analyzer tonometers. Ophthalmology. 2010;117(4):730–7.
151. Lee YG, Kim JH, Kim NR, Kim CY, Lee ES. Comparison between tonopachy and other tonometric and pachymetric devices. Optom Vis Sci. 2011;88(7):843–9.
152. Nakao Y, Kiuchi Y, Okimoto S. A comparison of the corrected intraocular pressure obtained by the corvis ST and Reichert 7CR tonometers in glaucoma patients. PLoS One. 2017;12(1):e0170206.
153. WHO. WHOQOL: measuring quality of life. World Health Organization. http://www.who.int/healthinfo/survey/whoqol-qualityoflife/en/.
154. van der Krieke L, Blaauw FJ, Emerencia AC, Schenk HM, Slaets JP, Bos EH, de Jonge P, Jeronimus BF. Temporal dynamics of health and well-being: a crowdsourcing approach to momentary assessments and automated generation of personalized feedback. Psychosom Med. 2017;79(2):213–23.
155. Fenwick EK, Ong PG, Man REK, Sabanayagam C, Cheng CY, Wong TY, Lamoureux EL. Vision impairment and major eye diseases reduce vision-specific emotional well-being in a Chinese population. Br J Ophthalmol. 2017;101(5):686–90.
156. McKean-Cowdin R, Wang Y, Wu J, Azen SP, Varma R, Los Angeles Latino Eye Study Group. Impact of visual field loss on health-related quality of life in glaucoma: the Los Angeles Latino Eye Study. Ophthalmology. 2008;115(6):941–48 e941.
157. Nelson P, Aspinall P, Papasouliotis O, Worton B, O'Brien C. Quality of life in glaucoma and its relationship with visual function. J Glaucoma. 2003;12(2):139–50.
158. Quaranta L, Riva I, Gerardi C, Oddone F, Floriano I, Konstas AG. Quality of life in glaucoma: a review of the literature. Adv Ther. 2016;33(6):959–81.
159. Wilson MR, Coleman AL, Yu F, Bing EG, Sasaki IF, Berlin K, Winters J, Lai A. Functional status and well-being in patients with glaucoma as measured by the Medical Outcomes Study Short Form-36 questionnaire. Ophthalmology. 1998;105(11):2112–6.
160. Viswanathan AC, McNaught AI, Poinoosawmy D, Fontana L, Crabb DP, Fitzke FW, Hitchings RA. Severity and stability of glaucoma: patient perception compared with objective measurement. Arch Ophthalmol. 1999;117(4):450–4.
161. Burton R, Crabb DP, Smith ND, Glen FC, Garway-Heath DF. Glaucoma and reading: exploring the effects of contrast lowering of text. Optom Vis Sci. 2012;89(9):1282–7.
162. Ramulu PY, West SK, Munoz B, Jampel HD, Friedman DS. Glaucoma and reading speed: the Salisbury Eye Evaluation project. Arch Ophthalmol. 2009;127(1):82–7.
163. Murata N, Miyamoto D, Togano T, Fukuchi T. Evaluating silent reading performance with an eye tracking system in patients with glaucoma. PLoS One. 2017;12(1):e0170230.
164. Haymes SA, Leblanc RP, Nicolela MT, Chiasson LA, Chauhan BC. Risk of falls and motor vehicle collisions in glaucoma. Invest Ophthalmol Vis Sci. 2007;48(3):1149–55.
165. Janz NK, Musch DC, Gillespie BW, Wren PA, Niziol LM, Collaborative Initial Glaucoma Treatment Study (CIGTS) Investigators. Evaluating clinical change and visual function concerns in drivers and nondrivers with glaucoma. Invest Ophthalmol Vis Sci. 2009;50(4):1718–25.
166. Stryker JE, Beck AD, Primo SA, Echt KV, Bundy L, Pretorius GC, Glanz K. An exploratory study of factors influencing glaucoma treatment adherence. J Glaucoma. 2010;19(1):66–72.
167. Asrani S, Chatterjee A, Wallace DK, Santiago-Turla C, Stinnett S. Evaluation of the ICare rebound

tonometer as a home intraocular pressure monitoring device. J Glaucoma. 2011;20(2):74–9.

168. Rosentreter A, Jablonski KS, Mellein AC, Gaki S, Hueber A, Dietlein TS. A new rebound tonometer for home monitoring of intraocular pressure. Graefes Arch Clin Exp Ophthalmol. 2011;249(11):1713–9.
169. Sood V, Ramanathan US. Self-monitoring of intraocular pressure outside of normal office hours using rebound tonometry: initial clinical experience in patients with normal tension glaucoma. J Glaucoma. 2016;25(10):807–11.
170. Termuhlen J, Mihailovic N, Alnawaiseh M, Dietlein TS, Rosentreter A. Accuracy of measurements with the iCare HOME rebound tonometer. J Glaucoma. 2016;25(6):533–8.
171. Flemmons MS, Hsiao YC, Dzau J, Asrani S, Jones S, Freedman SF. Home tonometry for management of pediatric glaucoma. Am J Ophthalmol. 2011;152(3):470–8. e472
172. Gandhi NG, Jones SK, Freedman SF. Icare ONE home tonometry in children with and without known glaucoma. J Glaucoma. 2016;25(2):e66–9.
173. Hsiao YC, Dzau JR, Flemmons MS, Asrani S, Jones S, Freedman SF. Home assessment of diurnal intraocular pressure in healthy children using the Icare rebound tonometer. J AAPOS. 2012;16(1):58–60.
174. Lowry EA, Hou J, Hennein L, Chang RT, Lin S, Keenan J, Wang SK, Ianchulev S, Pasquale LR, Han Y. Comparison of peristat online perimetry with the humphrey perimetry in a clinic-based setting. Transl Vis Sci Technol. 2016;5(4):4.
175. Matsumoto C, Yamao S, Nomoto H, Takada S, Okuyama S, Kimura S, Yamanaka K, Aihara M, Shimomura Y. Visual field testing with head-mounted perimeter 'imo'. PLoS One. 2016;11(8):e0161974.
176. Anderson AJ, Bedggood PA, George Kong YX, Martin KR, Vingrys AJ. Can home monitoring allow earlier detection of rapid visual field progression in glaucoma? Ophthalmology. 2017;124(12):1735–42.
177. WHO. Vision impairment and blindness. World Health Organization. 2017. http://www.who.int/mediacentre/factsheets/fs282/en/.
178. Baker RS, Bazargan M, Bazargan-Hejazi S, Calderon JL. Access to vision care in an urban low-income multiethnic population. Ophthalmic Epidemiol. 2005;12(1):1–12.
179. Holahan J, Cook A. Changes in economic conditions and health insurance coverage, 2000–2004. Health Aff (Millwood) 2005;Suppl Web Exclusives:W5-498–508.
180. Zhang X, Andersen R, Saaddine JB, Beckles GL, Duenas MR, Lee PP. Measuring access to eye care: a public health perspective. Ophthalmic Epidemiol. 2008;15(6):418–25.
181. Glen FC, Crabb DP. Living with glaucoma: a qualitative study of functional implications and patients' coping behaviours. BMC Ophthalmol. 2015;15:128.
182. Ramulu P. Glaucoma and disability: which tasks are affected, and at what stage of disease? Curr Opin Ophthalmol. 2009;20(2):92–8.
183. Goldberg I, Clement CI, Chiang TH, Walt JG, Lee LJ, Graham S, Healey PR. Assessing quality of life in patients with glaucoma using the Glaucoma Quality of Life-15 (GQL-15) questionnaire. J Glaucoma. 2009;18(1):6–12.
184. Nassiri N, Mehravaran S, Nouri-Mahdavi K, Coleman AL. National Eye Institute Visual Function Questionnaire: usefulness in glaucoma. Optom Vis Sci. 2013;90(8):745–53.
185. Popescu ML, Boisjoly H, Schmaltz H, Kergoat MJ, Rousseau J, Moghadaszadeh S, Djafari F, Freeman EE. Age-related eye disease and mobility limitations in older adults. Invest Ophthalmol Vis Sci. 2011;52(10):7168–74.
186. Algvere PV, Jahnberg P, Textorius O. The Swedish retinal detachment Register. I. A database for epidemiological and clinical studies. Graefes Arch Clin Exp Ophthalmol. 1999;237(2):137–44.
187. Artzen D, Lundstrom M, Behndig A, Stenevi U, Lydahl E, Montan P. Capsule complication during cataract surgery: case-control study of preoperative and intraoperative risk factors: Swedish Capsule Rupture Study Group report 2. J Cataract Refract Surg. 2009;35(10):1688–93.
188. Behndig A, Montan P, Stenevi U, Kugelberg M, Lundstrom M. One million cataract surgeries: Swedish National Cataract Register 1992–2009. J Cataract Refract Surg. 2011;37(8):1539–45.
189. Clark A, Ng JQ, Morlet N, Semmens JB. Big data and ophthalmic research. Surv Ophthalmol. 2016;61(4):443–65.
190. Tuulonen A, Azuara-Blanco A. Cost-effectiveness. Ophthalmology. 2009;116(1):166–7.
191. Tuulonen A. Challenges of glaucoma care – high volume, high quality, low cost. Acta Ophthalmol. 2013;91(1):3–5.

Concluding Comments/Authors' Preferences for the Guidelines

10

Xinghuai Sun and Yi Dai

Abstract

Glaucoma is a group of diseases that require long-term and even life-long treatment. Each ophthalmologist should master the art of glaucoma medical therapy based on scientific understanding of the etiology of glaucoma and the pharmacological mechanisms of anti-glaucoma medications.

Keywords

Visual function · Individualized treatment Quality of life · Target pressure

Currently, the goal of managing patients with glaucoma is to maintain useful visual function during the lifetime, that is, to protect the optic nerve and visual function from further damage, and to maintain a patient's health related quality of life. In many risk factors related with glaucoma, intraocular pressure (IOP) and IOP fluctuations are two factors which can be controlled and can effectively delay the progression of glaucoma [1, 2]. Managements to control the IOP include medication, laser, and surgery. Topical medical therapies are most likely to be accepted by doctors and patients, especially due to the emergence of hypotensive agents with greatly increased efficacy and compliance.

IOP-lowering medications for glaucoma can be applied as a stand-alone treatment. They also can be used in combination with laser or surgical treatment. Since the 1990s, many ocular hypotensive agents have become commercially available, enriching the field of medical treatment for glaucoma. During clinical application, some interesting phenomena related with medical therapy of

X. Sun (✉)
Department of Ophthalmology and Visual Science, Eye and ENT Hospital, Shanghai Medical College, Fudan University, Shanghai, China

NHC Key Laboratory of Myopia, Fudan University, Shanghai, China

Key Laboratory of Myopia, Chinese Academy of Medical Sciences, Shanghai, China

Shanghai Key Laboratory of Visual Impairment and Restoration, Fudan University, Shanghai, China

State Key Laboratory of Medical Neurobiology, Institutes of Brain Science and Collaborative Innovation Center for Brain Science, Fudan University, Shanghai, China
e-mail: xhsun@shmu.edu.cn

Y. Dai
Department of Ophthalmology and Visual Science, Eye and ENT Hospital, Shanghai Medical College, Fudan University, Shanghai, China

NHC Key Laboratory of Myopia (Fudan University), Key Laboratory of Myopia, Chinese Academy of Medical Sciences, Shanghai, China

Shanghai Key Laboratory of Visual Impairment and Restoration (Fudan University), Shanghai, China
e-mail: ydai@fudan.edu.cn

X. Sun, Y. Dai (eds.), *Medical Treatment of Glaucoma*,
https://doi.org/10.1007/978-981-13-2733-9_10

glaucoma emerge worthy of further investigation, such as retinal neuroprotection of brimonidine drops, and expansion of the Schlemm's canal lumen after topical application of prostaglandin analogues. Meanwhile, several problems related with irrational use of medicines need to be further regulated. With the marketing promotion of these ocular hypotensive agents, further understanding, even re-exploring, the mechanism of action and drug features is necessary. To effectively control the progression of glaucoma, more rational strategies of medical treatment are needed to develop for different types, different stages, and different patients in glaucoma.

Clinically, a single medication can achieve good result for some glaucoma patients, while in other cases three or more kinds of anti-glaucoma drugs are needed to get reluctant control of IOP. It is a real problem facing ophthalmologists every day that how to prescribe appropriate IOP-lowering medication for different glaucoma patients. Clinical optimization of glaucoma medication needs "science plus art." To this end, it should be based on considerations for both the patient and the ophthalmologist. To promote more rational use of IOP-lowering medications or combined managements, a comprehensive idea of the patient's condition and a thorough understanding of the hypotensive agents are the prerequisites. Specifically, one should first fully understand each patient's type of glaucoma, disease characteristics, and severity, the patient's overall medical states (age, gender, associated ocular or systemic diseases, other medication, etc.) and follow-up conditions, even occupation, economic status, lifestyle, and other factors. Moreover, doctors should also fully know/understand a variety of anti-glaucoma medications: pharmacological mechanism of IOP reduction, the characteristics of different categories of drugs, the characteristics of different agents in one category, as well as the concentration, dosage, duration, possible adverse reactions, market sources, and cost-effectiveness.

In addition, how to achieve the best clinical results with the least amount of medication? Aside from the individualized treatment options for different types and stages of glaucoma in different patients, it is necessary to pay attention to patient's compliance, tolerability, and sustainability of treatment. The value of "safe target IOP" formulated during the course of treatment is not static and should be adjusted according to the disease progression and the overall condition of the patients observed during regular follow-up. The goal of treatment is to maximally maintain the visual function of glaucoma patients.

Since the target IOP is affected by many factors, the recommended target IOP in glaucoma guidelines is not the same in different regions and countries [3–6] (Table 10.1).

With regard to the long-term even life-long disease and the variability of disease progression, the aim of glaucoma medical therapy is to stabilize the glaucomatous optic neuropathy. It is important to lower IOP significantly enough toward the target IOP. It is also important that

Table 10.1 Recommended rules for setting target IOP in different glaucoma guidelines

Guidelines	Target IOP
American Academy of Ophthalmology Preferred Practice Pattern (2015)	A reasonable initial treatment in a POAG patient is to reduce IOP at least 25% below baseline. Choosing a lower target IOP can be justified if there is more severe optic nerve damage, if the damage is progressing rapidly, or if other risk factors such as family history, age, or disc hemorrhages are present.
European Glaucoma Society (EGS) (2014)	In early glaucoma, an IOP of ≤21 mmHg with a reduction of at least 20%; in moderate glaucoma, an IOP of ≤18 mmHg with a reduction of at least 30%; factors to consider also include IOP level before treatment, stage of glaucoma, rate of progression, age and life expectancy, etc.
Asian Pacific Glaucoma Society (APGS) (2016)	Glaucoma with high risk progressive visual function loss: IOP reduction ≥40% or 1–2 SD below the population mean (9–12 mmHg); moderate risk: IOP reduction ≥30% or population mean, whichever is lower; glaucoma suspect at moderate risk: IOP reduction ≥20% or 1 SD above the population mean; glaucoma suspect at low risk: monitor, do not treat.
Chinese Glaucoma Society (CGS) (2014)	Setting the individualized target IOP possibly for each patient

not only a 24-h IOP fluctuation can be controlled stably, but a long-term IOP variation can be controlled in a safe range as well. That is a stable diurnal and long-term control of IOP [7].

One of the issues needs to be reflected on when following these guidelines is the characteristics of glaucoma and the availability of IOP-lowering medications in different countries and geographical regions [8]. EGS, PPP, and other guidelines represent advancedness and scientificness. However, for developing countries and backward areas, the applicability of these guidelines should be re-examined. It should also take into account the hygiene economics and patient satisfactions during the course of glaucoma medical therapy [9].

A reminder to clinician: an important aspect of primary angle-closure glaucoma treatment is to protect and open the anterior chamber angle with functional aqueous humor drainage. Medication to constrict pupil is crucial until iris bombe and pupillary block are released by laser or surgery. It is also necessary to use miotics in angle-closure glaucoma where there is a pronounced plateau iris configuration. During acute attacks, managements to control IOP should emphasize both angle protection (including miotics and anti-inflammatory corticosteroid therapies, both are important) and reopening the angle as soon as possible (including miotics and/or laser peripheral iridoplasty with iridotomy). It is the management principle of angle-closure glaucoma, which differs considerably from that used in open angle glaucoma [10].

Each ophthalmologist should master the art of glaucoma medical therapy based on scientific understanding of the etiology of glaucoma and the pharmacological mechanisms of anti-glaucoma medications.

All chapters in this book are contributed by individuals with expertise in the medical therapy and basic research of glaucoma. The book is intended to provide comprehensive introductions to various types of IOP-lowering medications in glaucoma, and a deep re-understanding of IOP-lowering medications in practice. It is to be hoped that this book will serve as a useful reference for ophthalmologists, optometrists, and health care providers in the medical treatment of glaucoma. At the same time, a number of potential new agents, new dosage forms, and new methods under research and development in the field of glaucoma medical therapy were also introduced and evaluated in this book. The ultimate goal of glaucoma medical treatment is to maintain the patient's visual function at present. It may become possible to improve the impaired visual function with new agents available in future. Through scientists and clinicians work together in various fields, we look forward to the arrival of such a bright and beautiful day!

Acknowledgment This book was supported by the top priority of Clinical Medicine Center of Shanghai (2017ZZ01020).

References

1. Heijl A, Leske MC, Bengtsson B, Hyman L, Bengtsson B, Hussein M. Reduction of intraocular pressure and glaucoma progression. Arch Ophthalmol. 2002;120:1268–79.
2. The AGIS Investigators. The advanced glaucoma intervention study (AGIS): the relationship between control of intraocular pressure and visual field deterioration. Am J Ophthalmol. 2000;130:429–40.
3. American Academy of Ophthalmology. Preferred practice pattern. 3rd ed. 2015.
4. European Glaucoma Society. Terminology and guidelines for glaucoma. 4th ed. 2014.
5. Asia-Pacific Glaucoma Society. Asia Pacific glaucoma guidelines. 3rd ed. 2016.
6. Chinese Glaucoma Society. Expert consensus on the diagnosis and treatment for primary glaucoma. Chin J Ophthalmol. 2014;50(5):382–3.
7. Asrani S, Zeimer R, Wilensky J, Gieser D, Vitale S, Lindenmuth K. Large diurnal fluctuations in intraocular pressure are an independent risk factor in patients with glaucoma. J Glaucoma. 2000;9(2):134–42.
8. Hedman K, Larsson L-I. The effect of Latanoprost compared with Timolol in African-American, Asian, Caucasian, and Mexican open-angle glaucoma or ocular hypertensive patients. Surv Ophthalmol. 2002;47(Suppl 1):S77–89.
9. Sun X, Lin M, Duan X, Zhang C, Ming J. Patient satisfaction with fixed-combination bimatoprost/timolol ophthalmic solution: a survey study in patients with glaucoma in China. Patient Prefer Adherence. 2017;28(11):845–52.
10. Sun X, Dai Y, Chen Y, Yu D-Y, Cringle SJ, Chen J, Kong X, Wang X, Jiang C. Primary angle closure glaucoma: What we know and what we don't know. Prog Retin Eye Res. 2017;57:26–45.

GPSR Compliance

The European Union's (EU) General Product Safety Regulation (GPSR) is a set of rules that requires consumer products to be safe and our obligations to ensure this.

If you have any concerns about our products, you can contact us on ProductSafety@springernature.com

In case Publisher is established outside the EU, the EU authorized representative is:

Springer Nature Customer Service Center GmbH
Europaplatz 3
69115 Heidelberg, Germany

Batch number: 10165433

Printed by Printforce, the Netherlands